Health Informatics

(formerly Computers in Health Care)

Kathryn J. Hannah   Marion J. Ball
Series Editors

Health Informatics Series
(formerly Computers in Health Care)

Series Editors
Kathryn J. Hannah   Marion J. Ball

James G. Anderson   Carolyn E. Aydin

Editors

Evaluating the Organizational Impact of Healthcare Information Systems

Second Edition

With 48 Illustrations

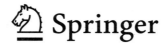 Springer

James G. Anderson, PhD
Professor of Medical Sociology
Professor of Health Communication
Fellow, American College of
    Medical Informatics
Co-Director of the Rural Center
    for AIDS/STD Prevention
Department of Sociology and Anthropology
Purdue University
West Lafayette, IN 47907
USA

Carolyn E. Aydin, PhD
Research Scientist
Nursing Research and Development
Cedars-Sinai Medical Center and Burns
    and Allen Research Institute
Los Angeles, CA 90048
USA

Series Editors:

Kathryn J. Hannah, PhD, RN
Adjunct Professor, Department
    of Community Health Sciences
Faculty of Medicine
The University of Calgary
Calgary, Alberta T2N 4N1
Canada

Marion J. Ball, EdD
Vice President, Clinical Informatics
    Strategies
Healthlink, Inc.
Baltimore, MD 21210
USA
and
Adjunct Professor
The Johns Hopkins University
    School of Nursing
Baltimore, MD 21205
USA

Library of Congress Control Number: 2005923548

ISBN 10: 0-387-24558-8   Printed on acid-free paper.
ISBN 13: 978-0387-24558-4

Printed in the United States of America.   (BS/MVY)

9 8 7 6 5 4 3 2 1   SPIN 10972649

springeronline.com

Series Preface

This series is directed to healthcare professionals who are leading the transformation of health care by using information and knowledge to advance the quality of patient care. Launched in 1988 as *Computers in Health Care*, the series offers a broad range of titles: some are addressed to specific professions such as nursing, medicine, and health administration; others to special areas of practice such as trauma and radiology. Still other books in the series focus on interdisciplinary issues, such as the computer-based patient record, electronic health records, and networked healthcare systems.

Renamed *Health Informatics* in 1998 to reflect the rapid evolution in the discipline now known as health informatics, the series continues to add titles that contribute to the evolution of the field. In the series, eminent experts, serving as editors or authors, offer their accounts of innovation in health informatics. Increasingly, these accounts go beyond hardware and software to address the role of information in influencing the transformation of healthcare delivery systems around the world. The series also increasingly focuses on "peopleware" and the organizational, behavioral, and societal changes that accompany the diffusion of information technology in health service environments.

These changes will shape health services in the new millennium. By making full and creative use of the technology to tame data and to transform information, health informatics will foster the development of the knowledge age in health care. As coeditors, we pledge to support our professional colleagues and the series readers as they share the advances in the emerging and exciting field of health informatics.

Kathryn J. Hannah, PhD, RN
Marion J. Ball, EdD

Preface

Information systems pervade complex organizations. In healthcare organizations such as hospitals, the U.S. Congressional Office of Technology Assessment has estimated that computerized systems, when fully implemented, account for 4% to 8% of an institution's total operating budget. As healthcare costs continue to spiral upward, healthcare institutions are under increasing pressure from purchasers and payers of services to create a cost effective system by controlling operating costs while maintaining quality of care and service. The Institute of Medicine also estimates that as many as 98,000 deaths occur each year because of medical errors. Information systems are being marketed to healthcare organizations to provide management information, control costs, facilitate total quality management and continuous quality improvement programs, and improve patient safety. Cost control and improvements in safety and quality are the two major premises on which decisions to purchase information systems are based.

There is mounting evidence, however, that the implementation of many information systems has resulted in unforeseen costs, unfulfilled promises, and disillusionment. There is also the growing realization that information systems affect the structure and functioning of organizations, the quality of work life of employees within them, and ultimately the cost and quality of the goods and services they provide. Professionals who develop, implement, and evaluate clinical computer systems, however, frequently address only the technical aspects of these systems, while the success of implementation and utilization depends upon integration of the computer system into a complex organizational setting. Without an evaluation strategy that goes beyond the technical aspects of the system, an institution has no means of knowing how well it is actually functioning within the organization and no firm basis for developing specific interventions to enhance system success. Including these issues in systems evaluations will increase the likelihood of implementing a system that is cost effective for the organization as a whole.

The purpose of this book is to provide computer system developers, administrators, healthcare policy analysts, chief information officers, investigators, and others with a guide for evaluating the impacts of computerized information systems on (1) the structure and functioning of healthcare organizations, (2) the quality of work life of individual healthcare professionals and others working within the organization, and (3) the cost-effective delivery of health care. Evaluating information system impacts requires not only an understanding of computer technology, but also an understanding of the social and behavioral processes that affect and are affected by the introduction of this technology into organizational settings. Investigators in the social sciences have developed theoretical foundations and analytical approaches to help understand the impact and use of information systems, but few guidelines exist to help developers, administrators, and evaluators design evaluation strategies and select appropriate methods to study system outcomes.

This book is designed as a practical guide for determining appropriate questions to ask and the most effective methods available to answer those questions. The book begins with the premise that any evaluation must be preceded by a clear statement of study objectives. Next, investigators should recognize their own perspective and assumptions concerning how information systems affect and are affected by the organizational setting in which they are implemented. Only at this point are investigators ready to review and select appropriate methodologies to answer their research questions.

The selection of appropriate methodologies is critical to the successful outcome of any investigation. Given the complex interrelationships between computer systems and their organizational environments, there is no one best method for evaluation. Rather, the selection of methods will be determined by the evaluation objectives. This book advocates a pluralistic approach, providing the reader with detailed information on a number of methods that can be used to evaluate healthcare information systems. More than one evaluation strategy may be brought to bear on the same problem domain, with each method providing a different, complementary view of the issues under study. The book is designed to assist an investigator in selecting among different methods to build the specific approach that will be most fruitful for investigating a given situation or problem. The chapters also provide a practical overview of established research guidelines for sampling, data collection procedures and instruments, and analytic techniques.

The material presented in this book draws on more than two decades of empirical studies in healthcare computing conducted by the contributors and others. Individual chapters review specific methods for organizational evaluation such as direct observations, use of archival data, interviewing strategies, survey research, cognitive approaches, work sampling, simulation, and social network analysis. Part I begins with an overview of theoretical perspectives and evaluation questions, followed by eight chapters covering different methods for evaluating the impacts of information systems using examples specific to healthcare organizations. Each of the eight chapters provides the reader with a detailed overview of a specific method, followed by annotated references at the end of the chapter for further reading. The example studies in Part II illustrate different evaluation methods and provide the reader with an understanding of the nature and scope of evaluation research and its importance in studying the impact of information systems, including providing information for practical decision-making and interventions.

The book also draws from a variety of social science disciplines to integrate the study of information systems with social science theory and methods. We argue that investigators in the social sciences have developed theoretical frameworks and analytical approaches that can help understand how the introduction of computer systems in healthcare settings affect the quality of the work environment, tasks and skills of health professionals, social interactions among professionals in the organization, and the effective delivery of medical care. We hope to make the developers and users of medical information systems more aware of (1) the extent to which the success of these systems depends upon complex social processes, and (2) the contributions the social sciences can make in helping to understand these processes.

The study of information systems, however, also requires social scientists themselves to develop new theories, data collection techniques, and analytic methods. This book should provide investigators and students with a starting point for new theoretical and policy oriented research into the impact of information systems on healthcare organizations. We also hope to initiate a dialogue between adherents of different research approaches, helping to clarify the range of methods and their appropriateness, strengths and weaknesses, and the understanding that can be acquired by combining different methods in a single research endeavor.

Finally, there is growing awareness at colleges and universities of the importance of studying and evaluating the use and impact of information systems as evidenced by the growth of curricula and faculty positions in the information sciences; medical, dental, and nursing informatics; and healthcare administration. Moreover, some schools are developing joint teaching and research programs that draw from diverse disciplines such as medicine, computer science, information systems, library sciences, organizational behavior, operations, management, and social sciences. This book is meant to provide a useful guide to the research and evaluation of systems for this wide variety of disciplines as well as to system developers, administrators, and practitioners.

We wish to thank Marilyn M. Anderson for her assistance in coordinating and assembling the various contributions to this book.

James G. Anderson, PhD
Carolyn E. Aydin, PhD

Acknowledgments

The editors gratefully acknowledge that the following material has been reprinted with kind permission.

Chapter 7 reprinted from:
Sittig, DF. Work-Sampling: a statistical approach to evaluation of the effect of computers on work patterns in healthcare. *Methods Inf Med* 1993;32:167–74.

Chapters 8 and 9 reprinted from:
Computers in Biology and Medicine 32(3):151–164, 179–193. Anderson JG. © 2002 Elsevier Ltd.

Chapter 10 reprinted from:
Aydin, Carolyn E., Anderson, James G., Rosen, Peter N., Felitti, Vincent J., Weng, Hui-Ching. "Computers in the Consulting Room: a case study of clinician and patient perspectives." *Health Care Management Science* 1 (1998) 61–74. Balzer Science Publishers BV.

Chapter 11 reprinted from:
Massaro, Thomas A. Introducing Physician Order entry at a Major Academic Medical Center 1 and 2. *Academic Medicine.* Vol. 68, No. 1, January 1993, pp. 20–30.

Chapter 12 reprinted from:
Journal of the American Medical Informatics Association, V9(5):479–490, Anderson JG et al: "Evaluating the capability of information technology to prevent adverse drug events: A computer simulation approach." © 2002 American Medical Informatics Association.

Chapter 13 reprinted from:
Aydin, C.E., & Forsythe, D.E. (1997). Implementing Computers in Ambulatory Care: Implications of Physician Practice Patterns for System Design. Proceedings of the 1997 AMIA Fall Symposium, Nashville, TN, pp. 677–681. (*Journal of the American Medical Informatics Association*, Symposium Supplement. © 1997 American Medical Informatics Association.)

Chapter 14 reprinted from:
Korst, Lisa M, Eusebio-Angeja, Alea C., Chamorro, Terry, Aydin, Carolyn E., Gregory, Kimberly D. "Nursing Documentation Time during Implementation of an Electronic Medical Record." *Jrnl of Nsg Admin* 2003;33(1):24–30.

Chapter 15 reprinted from:
Andrews, Robert D., Gardner, Reed M., Metcalf, Sandy M., Simmons, Deon. "Computer Charting: An Evaluation of a Respiratory Care Computer System." *Respiratory Care*, August 1985, Vol. 30, No. 8, pp. 695–708.

Contents

xi

Contributors

JAMES G. ANDERSON, PhD
Professor of Medical Sociology, Professor of Health Communication, Fellow, American College of Medical Informatics, Co-Director of the Rural Center for AIDS/STD Prevention, Department of Sociology and Anthropology, Purdue University, West Lafayette, IN 47907, USA

MARILYN M. ANDERSON, BA
Anderson Consulting, West Lafayette, IN 47906, USA

ROBERT D. ANDREWS, MA, MT (ASCP)
Information Technology Specialist, Department of Veterans Affairs, Salt Lake City, UT 84113, USA

CAROLYN E. AYDIN, PhD
Research Scientist, Nursing Research and Development, Cedars-Sinai Medical Center and Burns and Allen Research Institute, Los Angeles, CA 90048, USA

ERIN BRADNER, PhD
AutoDesk, San Rafael, CA 94903, USA

TERRY CHAMORRO, RN, MN
Consultant, Clinical Information Systems, Cedars-Sinai Health System, Los Angeles, CA 90048, USA

ALEA C. EUSEBIO-ANGEJA, MD
Kaiser Permanente Medical Center, South San Francisco, CA 94880, USA

GUNTHER EYSENBACH, MD
Senior Scientist, Centre for Global eHealth Innovation, Division of Medical Decision Making and Health Care Research, Toronto General Research Institute of the UHN, Toronto, ON M5S 1A1, Canada; Associate Professor, Department of Health Policy, Management and Evaluation, University of Toronto, Toronto, ON M5S 1A1, Canada

VINCENT J. FELITTI, MD
Co-Principal Investigator, Adverse Childhood Experiences Study; Clinical Professor of Medicine, Department of Medicine, University of California, San Diego, San Diego, CA 92093, USA

DIANA E. FORSYTHE, PhD (DECEASED)
Formerly Associate Adjunct Professor, Department of Medical Anthropology, University of California, San Francisco, San Francisco, CA 94143, USA

REED M. GARDNER, PhD
Professor and Chairman, Department of Medical Informatics, University of Utah, Salt Lake City, UT 84112, USA

KIMBERLY D. GREGORY, MD, MPH
Director of Maternal Fetal Medicine and Women's Health Services Research, Cedars-Sinai Medical Center, Los Angeles, CA 90048; Associate Professor-in-Residence, Department of Obstetrics and Gynecology, David Geffen School of Medicine, University of California, Los Angeles, Los Angeles, CA 90095, USA

THADDEUS J. HUNT, JD
Law Office of Thaddeus Hunt, Chicago, IL 60603, USA

STEPHEN J. JAY, MD
Professor and Chair, Department of Public Health, School of Medicine, Indiana University, Indianapolis, IN 46202, USA

BONNIE KAPLAN, PhD
Lecturer, Yale Center for Medical Informatics, Yale University School of Medicine, New Haven, CT 06520; President, Kaplan Associates, Hamden, CT 06517, USA

LISA M. KORST, MD, PhD
Associate Professor, Department of Pediatrics, Division of Research on Children, Youth, and Families, Childrens Hospital Los Angeles, Los Angeles, CA 90027, USA

ANDRE W. KUSHNIRUK, PhD
Associate Professor and Director, School of Health Information Science,
University of Victoria, BC V8W 2Y2, Canada

THOMAS A. MASSARO, MD, PhD
Director of Performance Improvement, University of Virginia Medical
Center, Charlottesville, VA 22908; Associate Dean for Graduate Medical
Education and Professor, Department of Pediatrics, School of Medicine,
University of Virginia, Charlottesville, VA 22908, USA

JOSEPH A. MAXWELL, PhD
Associate Professor, Graduate School of Education, George Mason
University, Fairfax, VA 22030, USA

SANDY M. METCALF, RRT, BS
Quality Consultant for Surgical Services, Urban Central Region,
Intermountain Health Care, Salt Lake City, UT 84111, USA

VIMLA L. PATEL, PhD
Professor, Department of Biomedical Informatics, Columbia University,
New York, NY 10032; Professor, Department of Psychiatry, New York State
Psychiatric Institute, New York, NY 10032; Adjunct Professor of Psychology
and Education, Columbia Teachers College, New York, NY 10027, USA

MADHU REDDY, PhD
Assistant Professor, Department of Information Science and Technology,
School of Management and Information Systems, University of Missouri,
Rolla, MO 65409, USA

PETER N. ROSEN, MD
Director, Laboratory for Visual Performance Assessment, University of
California, San Diego, San Diego, CA 92093, USA

DEON SIMMONS, RRT
Assistant Director, Department of Respiratory Care, LDS Hospital, Salt
Lake City, UT 84143, USA

DEAN F. SITTIG, PhD
Director of Applied Research in Medical Informatics, Northwest
Permanente, Portland, OR 97232, USA

HUI-CHING WENG, PhD
Assistant Professor, Department of Health Management, I-Shou
University, Taiwan 840

Part I
Evaluating Healthcare Information Systems: A Multimethod Approach

Part Introduction

Despite the fact that they are technologically sound, more than half of medical information systems fail due to user and staff resistance. Although implementation success depends heavily on the integration of the computer system into a complex organizational setting, few guidelines exist for designing effective evaluation strategies and selecting appropriate methods to examine outcomes of system use.

Predicting organizational changes resulting from information systems requires an understanding of dynamic social and political processes that occur within organizations as well as the characteristics of individuals, work groups, and the information system. Chapter 1 outlines how theories about the impacts of information systems on organizations and the people in them can guide research and evaluation. Models of change based on different assumptions can aid in understanding the implementation of information systems and guide the selection of methodological tools for assessing their organizational impacts. Three general models are discussed. The first views the computer system as an *external force* that brings about predictable change in the behavior of individuals and organizational units. A second perspective views the design of information systems as being *determined by the information needs* of managers and clinicians. It is assumed that the organization has control over the technical aspects of the system and the consequences of its implementation. A third theoretical perspective holds that *complex social interactions* within the organization determine the use and impact of medical computer systems. The chapter concludes with 12 suggested areas for evaluation of healthcare information systems and an overview of appropriate research methodologies.

Chapters 2 through 9 discuss the major methods that can be used to evaluate an information system. Given the scope and complexity of these projects, there is no "one best approach" to evaluation. The selection of a methodology must be determined by the overall objectives of the evaluation. At the same time, the selection of a methodology for a particular project is critical to the success of the project. In order to select an appropriate methodology, the investigator needs to be aware of the various methods that are available as well as their advantages and limitations. Each chapter provides an overview of a specific approach to evaluation. Examples provide the reader with a resource for understanding the nature and scope of the specific approach. Extensive references at the end of each chapter provide useful sources for the reader to learn more about each method.

Chapter 2 provides an overview of qualitative research methods. These methods attempt to understand the process by which organizational change occurs after the introduction of an information system from the point of view of the participants and their social and institutional context. Major advantages of qualitative methods include (1) understanding how users perceive and evaluate the system; (2) understanding the influence of the social and cultural context on system use; (3) investigating causal processes; (4) providing information that can be used to improve a system under development; and (5) providing information to decision makers. These issues are illustrated by a study of a clinical laboratory information system.

Chapter 3 outlines ways to evaluate how well healthcare information systems support collaboration of healthcare team members. Most evaluations of information technology focus only on the individual user. At the same time, each team member brings different backgrounds, perspectives, and skills to the team. These skills and perspectives have implications for the adoption and use of healthcare information systems. In order to fully understand the impact of technology, it is necessary to use a variety of techniques and methods in evaluation. These techniques are illustrated by a study of the use of an information system by members of a surgical intensive care unit.

Chapter 4 provides a guide to survey methods that can be used to evaluate the impacts of computer systems on the functioning of healthcare organizations and the work life of individuals within them. Survey research involves gathering information from a sample of a population using standardized instruments. The author points out that, where possible, standard measures with established validity and reliability should be used. The chapter describes a number of survey instruments drawn from the literature on information systems, organizations and organizational behavior, and work attitudes and values. These instruments have been developed and used in healthcare organizations and other organizational settings and have documented reliabilities and validities. Many of the instruments are included in the Appendix or references are provided to enable the reader to obtain a copy of the instrument.

Chapter 5 discusses ways in which the Internet can be used in the research and evaluation process. The Internet can be used as a source for qualitative research and to use the Web to conduct surveys. Three different research methodologies for qualitative research on the Web are described. Passive analysis studies information patterns on websites and/or interactions in newsgroups, mailing lists, and chat rooms without the researchers being actively involved themselves. Active analysis is where the researcher directly participates in the communication process. For example, when introducing a healthcare information system, developers may integrate discussion boards in the system where users can ask for assistance, discuss the system, and make suggestions for improvement. Also, surveys can be conducted using the Internet by means of interviews or questionnaires designed for self-completion.

Chapter 6 provides an overview of cognitive approaches to evaluation. These approaches focus on understanding the processes involved in decision making and reasoning by healthcare workers as they interact with information systems in carrying out a range of tasks. Methodologies are described for using evaluation throughout the system design and development life cycle. The chapter also illustrates how research in cognitive science can be used to drive the development of new conceptual frameworks for evaluation of healthcare information systems. Specific examples of the application of cognitive approaches for the laboratory analysis of user interactions with complex information systems such as electronic medical records and Web-based information resources are described.

Chapter 7 describes techniques that have been developed to evaluate the impact of healthcare information systems on the work patterns of healthcare workers. These techniques include: time-motion analysis, subjective evaluations, review of departmental statistics, personal activity records, and work sampling. A step-by-step description of work sampling is provided.

Chapter 8 describes social network approaches to evaluating healthcare information systems. Social network analysis comprises a set of methods that can be used to analyze the relationships among people, departments, and organizations. These patterns of relationships affect both individual and organizational attitudes and behavior such as the adoption, diffusion, and use of new medical informatics applications. An introduction is provided to the concepts and methods of social network analysis and several applications are described.

Chapter 9 describes the use of computer simulation models to evaluate healthcare information systems. In instances where these applications cannot be evaluated by traditional methods, computer simulation provides a flexible approach to evaluation. The process involved in developing and validating a simulation model is described and several examples of simulation studies are discussed.

1
Overview: Theoretical Perspectives and Methodologies for the Evaluation of Healthcare Information Systems

JAMES G. ANDERSON and CAROLYN E. AYDIN

Introduction

Evaluating the impact of computer-based medical information systems requires not only an understanding of computer technology but also an understanding of complex social and behavioral processes. Different theories about the impacts of information systems on organizations guide research and evaluation. This chapter discusses three different theoretical perspectives. The first perspective views the computer information system as an *external force* that affects individuals and the organization. The second perspective assumes that *managers and clinicians can control* the design, implementation, and impact of information systems. A third perspective holds that *complex social interactions* within the organization determine the use and impact of information systems. The discussion of these perspectives is followed by suggested evaluation questions and an overview of appropriate research methods.

In addition to this theoretical framework and the perspectives detailed below, the reader may wish to review Lorenzi et al.'s [1] comprehensive review of the behavioral and business disciplines that offer data and information potentially valuable to evaluating the introduction of new information technologies in healthcare. Related references include Lorenzi and Riley [2] on change management, Snyder-Halpern's [3] organizational readiness approach, Southon, Sauer, and Dampney's [4] articles on a failed information systems initiative in large complex distributed organizations, Lauer et al.'s [5] use of an equity implementation model, Kaplan's [6] 4Cs of evaluation, Berg's [7] myths that hamper implementation, Aarts and Peel's [8,9] articles using a descriptive model of the stages of change, Doolan et al.'s [10] case series on computers in clinical care, and Ash et al.'s [11] qualitative study on physician order entry. Since the first edition of this book was published in 1994, increased recognition of the organizational issues involved in technology implementation has also resulted in the cre-

5

ation of active working groups in both the International Medical Informatics Association (IMIA) in 1993 and the American Medical Informatics Association (AMIA) in 1996 [12].

The Need for Evaluation

Since 1994, the pace of computerization in healthcare has accelerated [13–17], while reports of system failures have continued [4,18–20]. Healthcare organizations are considering many new information technology applications in the hope of increasing efficiency, reducing costs, and improving patient care and safety [21]. These products include a growing number of medical computer applications in which healthcare providers interact directly with the computer. These applications are referred to generally as medical or clinical information systems or electronic medical records (EMRs). Medical information systems involve computer-stored databases containing patient information to support medical order entry, results reporting, decision support systems, clinical reminders, and other healthcare applications [22,23]. In some healthcare organizations, a comprehensive system coordinates patient care activities by linking computer terminals in patient care areas to all departments through a central or integrated information system. Other organizations use smaller separate systems that link patient care areas to only one department such as the laboratory, radiology, or the pharmacy. These systems provide communication networks between departments as well as storage and retrieval of medical information. Other computerized databases or expert systems may serve a single department or group of practitioners.

Concerns about patient safety have also accelerated the implementation of computerized physician order entry (CPOE). In California, for example, Senate Bill 1875 requires as a condition of licensure that all hospitals adopt a formal plan to reduce medication-related errors. With the exception of small rural hospitals, this plan "shall include technology implementation, such as, but not limited to, computerized physician order entry . . ." [24]. The Institute of Medicine's 2003 report entitled "Patient Safety: Achieving a New Standard for Care" [25] states that only a fraction of hospitals have implemented a comprehensive electronic health record, but views the necessary technology information infrastructure as a critical component of safe care.

A recent survey of 626 hospitals in the United States found that computerized physician order entry was not available to physicians in 84% of the hospitals [26]. Moreover, these systems often fail because developers frequently emphasize the technological and economic aspects of the systems and neglect social and political considerations such as the organizational environment, social interactions, political issues, and hidden costs such as interruptions of established organizational routines [27–32]. Dowling [33] found in a survey of 40 randomly selected hospitals that 45%

of the information systems failed due to user resistance and staff interference despite the fact that they were technologically sound. Lyytinen [34] and Lyytinen and Hirschheim [35] also report a 50% failure rate for information systems. The authors suggest that failure may be due to technical problems; problems with the format and content of the data; user problems related to skills, competence, and motivations; and organizational problems.

There are few published studies about the reasons for failure and their relative importance. In the March/April 2004 issue of the *Journal of the American Medical Informatics Association* focusing on "perspectives on CPOE and patient care information systems," Berger and Kichak [36], Ash et al. [37], and McDonald et al. [38] address different aspects of computerized physician order entry and its possible unintended consequences. Winkelman and Leonard [39] move further by providing an evaluation framework for considering adaptation of electronic patient records systems for use by patients. In addition, organizations such as the California Healthcare Foundation, VHA, and Alberta Heritage Foundation for Medical Research have conducted recent studies on topics such as the diffusion of innovation in healthcare, use of computer-based patient records, computerized physician order entry, and health technology assessment [13,40–43].

At the same time that organizations move to implement CPOE and other systems, the emphasis on cost effectiveness requires organizations to justify expenditures through detailed evaluations of the impacts of new information systems. Although implementation success depends heavily on the integration of the computer system into a complex organizational setting, professionals who develop, implement, and evaluate healthcare computer systems have few guidelines for designing effective evaluation strategies and selecting appropriate methods to examine the outcomes of system use in healthcare organizations. To ensure that newly adopted systems accomplish their intended purpose, vendors and purchasers alike need to develop detailed plans prior to system implementation for ongoing implementation and postinstallation evaluation to examine the use and long-term impacts of these systems.

Evaluating the impact of computer-based medical information systems requires not only an understanding of computer technology, but also an understanding of the social and behavioral processes that affect and are affected by the introduction of the technology into the practice setting. As technological developments result in the widespread use of computers in healthcare, the social and behavioral sciences can provide an important perspective to guide the establishment of research agendas and the conduct of policy-relevant investigations. According to the conceptual framework developed by Ives, Hamilton, and Davis [44] and Kraemer and Dutton [45], for example, research and evaluation of information systems may involve any or all of the following categories: (1) the external environment of the organization; (2) the internal environment of the organization; (3) the information system users; (4) the systems development environment and staff; (5)

the management and operational environment of the system; (6) the nature of the system including the information processed; (7) patterns of utilization; (8) organizational impacts; (9) and social impacts. These impacts may be direct or indirect, intended or unintended. The following sections outline how different theories about the impacts of information systems influence research and evaluation by suggesting different research questions and demanding different methodological tools for assessing their impacts on organizations and the people in them. Despite 10 years of research since the first edition of this book, the following sections continue to provide a useful framework and examples for the planning and implementation of an effective evaluation of computerization in healthcare organizations.

Assumptions About Change

Theories about change embody conceptions of the nature and direction of causal influences. Information systems research may be based on a number of different theories or models of change with different or competing assumptions. These models of change influence which research questions will and will not be asked and guide the selection of research methodologies [46].

Three common "storylines" with contrasting assumptions characterize the consequences associated with computer systems: optimist, pessimist, and pluralist [28,47]. The optimist position predicts increased productivity, improved skill requirements, more interdependent jobs, and enhanced communication (i.e., workers share information with workers in other departments by means of common access to a system). The pessimist position, on the other hand, predicts that information technology will rob workers of their expertise and decrease their interactions through job routinization and fragmentation (i.e., workers access information only remotely through computer terminals), and generate conflicts about control over information and other resources [28,47,48]. The present book adopts the third or pluralist position that, while computer systems can have both isolating and integrating capabilities, actual impacts depend on what the organization and its members do with the technology and how the implementation is managed.

According to this position, the introduction of computer systems in healthcare organizations may be accompanied by changes on several different levels. These include changes for: (1) individuals and their jobs, (2) departments as a whole and how each department's work is performed, (3) the structure and functioning of the entire organization, and (4) the quality of both the service patients receive and the medical care that is delivered. Some of these changes may be immediate and evident in the performance of the daily work of healthcare. Other changes may occur slowly and be more difficult to detect. The changes that occur, however, are not simply caused by the computer system. Rather, these changes are viewed as a result of complex interactions between the capabilities of the system itself, administrative decisions on how to use the system in a particular organization, and actions of individual employees as they adapt to the system in their everyday work [28,49–51].

The pluralist perspective also maintains that research about the effects of computers on managerial decision making, authority and control; the work environment, productivity, and job enhancement; the frequency, nature, and quality of interpersonal relationships among organizational members; and relations between organizations and their environment can enhance our insights into the complex effects of introducing computers into organizational settings [52,53]. To date, however, research findings suggest that these effects are complicated, diverse, and contingent on the specific organizational context. In some instances the availability of the new technology even generates new organizational needs to which it is applied [27]. Understanding the changes that may occur, however, can help analysts predict impacts of individual systems, including both desired and unanticipated effects on the organization in which it is being implemented.

Evaluation Research and Models of Change

Evaluation research differs from scientific inquiry. While both use the same logic of inquiry and research procedures, scientific studies focus primarily on meeting specific research standards. Although scientific rigor is important in evaluation studies as well, evaluation research must also recognize the interests of organizational stakeholders and be conducted in a way that is most useful to decision makers. While evaluation studies may strive to meet the criteria for scientific rigor, the primary purpose of evaluation research is to provide information to organization stakeholders and decision makers [54].

Although evaluation studies may not specify an explicit paradigm or theoretical framework, underlying and often unconscious assumptions about models of change may influence both the questions selected for study and the accompanying research strategies [55]. Different assumptions will lead researchers to ask different questions and focus on different outcomes to the computer implementation process. Thus it is important that evaluation researchers also recognize the influence of their own and the organization stakeholders' underlying assumptions about change in selecting specific questions for investigation.

The following sections detail three different models of change prevalent in information systems research, including: (1) the computer system as an external force, (2) system design determined by user information needs, and (3) complex social interactions as determinants of system use. Examples are also included to illustrate the different theoretical perspectives. Many of these examples, as well as those cited in subsequent chapters, both meet the rigorous requirements of scientific investigation and provide evaluation information to stakeholders in the organization under study as well [56].

The Computer System as an External Force

Theories about how information systems affect organizations imply quite different conceptions of what causes change to occur [28,50,55,57–59]. The simplest approach views the computer system as an exogenous or external force that brings about change in the behavior of individuals and organizational units. Information systems are developed and implemented to support management goals. Participants who are expected to use the new technology are viewed as passive or as resistant or dysfunctional if they fail to use the system. Evaluation in this instance usually focuses on technical performance (e.g., cost, speed, accuracy, etc.). Studies are frequently undertaken in the laboratory using controlled clinical trials and there may be little or no investigation of how systems fit into the daily work of the organization into which they will be introduced [60].

In general, studies based on this theoretical perspective treat organizational and technological characteristics as invariant rather than as changing over time. They also fail to include characteristics of the organizational environment and social interaction that may have important effects on outcomes [31]. A variant of this theoretical approach, however, does include the examination of the impact of the computer on specific characteristics of the organization. Leifer and McDonough [61], for example, found that departments that used a computer system were more centralized, less complex, and less uncertain about their environment to begin with than departments that didn't use the system, even when task routineness was controlled.

System Design Determined by User Information Needs

A second theoretical perspective views the design of information systems as determined by the information needs of managers and clinicians [55,57]. In this view, the information system is considered to be endogenous to the organization with organization members having control over the technical aspects of the system and the consequence of its implementation. According to this theory, change occurs in a rational fashion as needs are identified and problems solved. Much of the literature from this perspective is optimistic about the amount of influence that designers and implementers have over system capabilities and characteristics [62,63].

Complex Social Interactions Determine System Use

A third theoretical perspective holds that complex social interations within the organization determine the use and impact of medical computer systems [29,55,57,64,65]. This theoretical perspective is more complex than the two perspectives outlined above. According to this view, the way technology is ultimately implemented and utilized in a particular organizational setting depends on conflicting objectives, preferences, and work demands. From this viewpoint, predicting organizational change resulting from information systems requires a understanding of the dynamic social and political processes that occur within organizations as well as the characteristics of individuals and the information system. The prediction of outcomes requires knowledge of the processes that occur during system planning, implementation, and use rather than simply the levels of independent variables hypothesized to predict change [57,66].

Barley [67], for example, focused on social interactions in his study of the introduction of computerized tomography scanners in two community hospitals. Results showed that the new technology challenged traditional role relations and patterns of interaction among radiologists and radiological technologists in both settings. Only one of the departments, however, became more decentralized as a result. Moreover, professionals who adopt an innovation may adapt it to their own specific needs and organizational contexts, in a sense "reinventing" the innovation [55,64,68,69].

In another example, Lundsgaarde, Fischer, and Steele [70] studied the reactions of physicians, nurses, and ancillary personnel to the implementation of the PROMIS medical information system. Physicians resisted using the system due to fears that it would disrupt traditional staff relations. Nurses and other staff readily accepted the system, however, because it allowed them to utilize their professional expertise more fully. Aydin [71] also addressed social interactions in her study of the effects of a computerized medical information system on the pharmacy and nursing departments in two hospitals. The results indicated changes in tasks and greater interdependence between the two departments.

Awareness of these different models of change can help system evaluators recognize their own implicit assumptions and consider additional areas of study and the research strategies that accompany them. The next section outlines 12 general research questions suggested by these and other theoretical perspectives. The questions are followed by a discussion of the research methodologies appropriate to each of the different perspectives.

Evaluation Questions and Research Methods

In evaluating the impacts of a new computer system, an essential step is to determine what questions to ask. This section suggests a number of potential questions for evaluation studies. The selection of appropriate questions will be determined by both implicit assumptions about change and the explicit purpose of the evaluation for the organization itself.

The suggested questions cover a variety of theoretical frameworks, including those detailed above. Research on the relationship between acceptance of a computer system and individual variables such as personality style or resistance to change, for example, treats the computer as an exogenous force and adds a psychological framework in which the investigator assumes that individual differences will influence actions in the work place [72]. In contrast, investigators who look for differences between professions or departments in acceptance of medical systems focus on social interactions and the political nature of information systems, making the assumption that professional or departmental issues will be important in determining individual reactions to new computer systems [49,73,74]. The use of network methods (see Chapter 8) in investigating computer impacts, on the other hand, implies a diffusion model in which acceptance of the innovation is transmitted through channels of communication, over time, among members of a social system.

The 12 questions detailed below, while not exhaustive, provide a beginning framework for addressing system impacts. Additional questions and approaches are suggested in later chapters in the book. Recognizing the purpose of a specific system evaluation will also help determine the focus of the investigation. If, for example, the organization is committed to maintaining the system, evaluators will most likely focus on issues such as how to encourage more individuals to use the system, ensure adequate training, enhance satisfaction with improved system support, encourage the formation of user groups, and so on. If, on the other hand, discontinuing the system is an option, the focus may be on determining how well the system is functioning, the level of system use, and its cost-efficacy. The evaluator who is knowledgeable about different models of change may also be able to suggest additional questions that may provide important information for the decisions to be made for the organization.

The suggested areas for evaluation are organized around the following 12 questions. These questions and the detailed issues they encompass are meant to encourage system evaluators to go beyond obvious questions of user attitudes and system acceptance and attempt to address some of the more difficult issues that will, in the long run, prove important in the implementation of successful, cost effective systems. Table 1.1 links each question with the models of change detailed above and includes suggested evaluation methods. The final section in the chapter provides an overview of the evaluation methods, which are described in detail in subsequent chapters of the book.

Evaluation Questions

1. Does the system work technically as designed?

The first step is usually to determine whether the system actually works. For an order entry system, for example, does the computer actually transmit the needed information about physician orders between nursing stations and the appropriate ancillary department? Does a physician expert system provide the physician with the necessary information to arrive at a

TABLE 1.1. Evaluation questions, models of change, and suggested research methods.

Evaluation question	Models of change	Suggested methods	Further description
1. Does the system work as designed?	External force User needs Interactions	Qualitative (interviews, observation, documents) Survey Cognitive approaches Work sampling	Chapters 2, 3 Chapter 4 Chapter 6 Chapter 7
2. Is the system used as anticipated?	External force User needs Interactions	Qualitative (interviews, observation, documents) Survey Internet survey Cognitive approaches Work sampling	Chapters 2, 3 Chapter 4 Chapter 5 Chapter 6 Chapter 7
3. Does the system produce the desired results?	External forces User needs Interactions	Qualitative (interviews observation, documents) Survey Work sampling	Chapters 2, 3 Chapter 4 Chapter 7
4. Does the system work better than the procedures it replaced?	External force User needs	Qualitative (interviews observation, documents) Survey Cognitive approaches Work sampling Simulation	Chapters 2, 3 Chapter 4 Chapter 6 Chapter 7 Chapter 9
5. Is the system cost effective?	External force User needs	Work sampling Simulation	Chapter 7 Chapter 9
6. How well have individuals been trained to use the system?	External force User needs	Qualitative (interviews, observation, documents) Survey Cognitive approaches	Chapters 2, 3 Chapter 4 Chapter 6
7. What are the anticipated long-term impacts on how departments interact?	Interactions	Qualitative (interviews, observation) Survey Network analysis	Chapters 2, 3 Chapter 4 Chapter 8
8. What are the long-term effects on the delivery of medical care?	User needs Interactions	Qualitative (interviews, observation, documents) Survey Work sampling	Chapters 2, 3 Chapter 4 Chapter 7
9. Will the system have an impact on control in the organization?	Interactions	Qualitative (interviews, documents) Survey Network analysis	Chapters 2, 3 Chapter 4 Chapter 8
10. To what extent do impacts depend on practice setting?	Interactions	Qualitative (interviews, observation, documents) Survey	Chapters 2, 3 Chapter 4
11. What are the impacts on the healthcare system at large?	Interactions	Qualitative (interviews, observations, documents) Survey Internet survey	Chapters 2, 3 Chapter 4 Chapter 5
12. How will the system affect patient safety	Interactions	Qualitative (interviews, observations, documents) Survey Cognitive approaches	Chapters 2, 3 Chapter 4 Chapter 6

diagnosis and make treatment decisions? Do the appropriate professionals actually use the system?

A system that seems to work perfectly in tests or simulations may encounter a number of difficulties when actually implemented in a hospital or medical practice. For the purposes of the present volume, we will assume that the technical aspects of the system are operating correctly and focus on evaluating system impacts that stem from determining who actually uses the system, how they use it, and the impacts of its use on individuals, groups, and the delivery of medical care.

2. Is the system being used as anticipated?

Who uses the system, how much, and for what purposes? If system use is optional, is the system used by enough individuals to warrant continuation? Who uses it and who doesn't? What factors influence individual decisions to use the system (e.g., personality styles, professional issues, age, departmental norms for how work should be done, communication networks)? What is its impact on individual jobs (e.g., work overload, job satisfaction, new skills development, new job classifications, etc.)?

Even systems that work are often not used as anticipated. Thus it is important to determine whether the system (1) meets the needs of projected users, (2) is convenient and easy to use, and (3) fits work patterns of the professionals for whom it is intended. These issues are particularly important for computer systems designed for healthcare professionals. In other industries such as banking, insurance, or travel, for example, workers may be required to use a computer system continuously in order to perform their work. Healthcare systems, on the other hand, are frequently an adjunct to enhance or speed medical work performed on and for patients. Using the computer may require changes in daily work patterns that healthcare professionals may be unwilling or unable to make if the system is inconvenient or difficult to use. Other systems may potentially meet user needs, but be too confusing or complicated to encourage use, particularly if individuals only need to use the system on a sporadic basis. For example, a physician with admitting privileges at several different hospitals may be unwilling or unable to learn and remember different computer protocols for each hospital. Furthermore, even when computer use is required, errors are likely when the system is not tailored to the needs of the user. All of these are issues for consideration when evaluating system impacts.

3. Does the system produce the desired results?

Desired by whom? Administrators? Physicians? Other professionals or departments? What competing interests are involved? [75]. Decisions to adopt centralized systems are often made by hospital administrators with varying amounts of consultation with the departments and individuals who will use the system. Ideally, however, system implementation will be preceded by agreement on expected system outcomes for the organization as a whole. Individual departments may actually agree to the adoption of a system that does not meet their own specific needs, but provides benefits for the institution. Sometimes these agreements involve other negotiated benefits for the department in question.

Aydin [71], for example, found that the pharmacy department in a major medical center agreed to use what it considered to be a "nursing" order entry system. In return for agreeing to the system, the pharmacy negotiated a return to the expanded consultant role that they had been forced to give up under previous budget cuts. In contrast, however, the PROMIS system was discontinued despite its use by radiologists, pharmacists, and nurses because it lacked acceptance by the medical staff, the primary decision-making power in the organization [55,70].

4. Does the system work better than the procedures it replaced?

Computer system implementation requires expenditures for hardware, software, and user training, as well as possible increases in staff for data entry tasks, especially where more information is being gathered and stored than in the past. Thus system evaluators must address system benefits as well as operating efficiency. Has computerization resulted in cost savings in staff time spent in data collection and analysis? If not, are the additional data and analysis made possible by computerization worth the time and money spent (e.g., to meet regulatory requirements, control other costs, increase patient or physician satisfaction, or deliver better healthcare to patients)?

5. Is the system cost effective?

For whom? Individual practitioners? Departments? Patients? The organization as a whole? Medical information systems have the potential to reduce costs by improving information flows between departments as well as by providing information that may not have been readily available before the implementation of the system. On the other hand, costs may increase for employee training and higher salaries when new computer skills are added to job descriptions. Increased personnel expenses in nursing for clerks to enter orders in the computer, for example, may be balanced by cost savings in the pharmacy where the order entry system automatically bills patients for pharmacy charges. On the other hand, direct order entry by physicians may save clerical costs. Order entry may also result in the "capture" of charges that were frequently "lost" with manual systems.

6. How well have individuals been trained to use the system?

How many errors occur? Are data entry errors widespread, or limited to a few users? Do individuals communicate with colleagues about new ways to use the computer system? Is system support readily available when problems arise? Are improvements needed in the training provided, user-friendliness of the system, time available for users to practice and become familiar with the system, communication with users, and support in solving system problems?

7. What are the anticipated long-term impacts on how departments linked by computer interact with each other?

Is communication and coordination between departments more or less efficient using the computer system? If departments worked well together before the computer system, has computer implementation created any new problems? Has the computer system resolved ongoing problems such as slow transmission of orders, and so on? Are lab results reported faster with the computer system? Does one department feel they are bearing more than their share of the new job responsibilities related to the computer system (e.g., nurses or clerical staff doing order entry for pharmacy or radiology)? Is another department concerned with errors in order entry (e.g., errors in radiology orders made by clerical staff on nursing units)? Do these issues affect system effectiveness?

8. What are the anticipated long-term effects on the delivery of medical care?

Will lab/radiology results reporting be faster? If so, will the increases in efficiency be evident in decreased lengths of stay? Will computer-based monitoring of physician orders eliminate duplicate and/or unnecessary tests? If so, what will be the impact on the cost or quality of care? On physician satisfaction? If an order entry system, for example, requires nurses, clerks or physicians to enter the reason for requesting a specific radiology test along with the order, will radiologists be able to document that having this information enables them to better meet physicians' diagnostic needs?

9. Will system implementation have an impact on control in the organization?

Will the new system enable administrators to monitor or control physician practice behavior, decrease departmental independence in professional decision making, and so on? If so, what is the impact on physician attitudes, cost of medical care, and so on? Is there a shift in the balance of power between clinical personnel and managers, between departments, between the institution and attending physicians? Is there an impact on the competitive position of the institution? Who determines what information is to be included in new systems and how it is to be collected and used? [76].

10. To what extent do medical information systems have impacts that depend on the practice setting in which they are implemented?

Under what circumstances and in what organizational settings do certain effects occur? How common are these effects? What are the impacts of organization, size, culture, values, and so forth on system outcomes? What evaluation questions are appropriate in different settings?

11. What are the impacts on the healthcare system at large?

A report by the Institute of Medicine identified computer-based patient records (CPRs) as a key infrastructural requirement to support a reformed healthcare system [14]. It has been estimated that these systems when implemented nationwide could save $80 billion per year. However, at present there are few studies that have investigated the financial, organizational, and behavioral changes that will need to be made at the national, state, and institutional levels in order to overcome barriers to this information technology. Questions to be asked include: Will the system better enable patients to manage their own healthcare? Will the system help to control costs? Will the system improve care?

12. How will the medical information system affect patient safety?

A number of reports estimate that as many as 98,000 to 195,000 people in the United States die in hospitals due to potentially preventable errors [71–74,77–80]. Many of these errors could be prevented by implementing information technology that is currently available. Questions that should be raised include: Will the electronic health record system be integrated with other systems such as laboratory, pharmacy, radiology? Will the system provide decision support to physicians when they enter orders? Can the system detect potential adverse events and issue alerts and reminders to providers to avoid harm to patients? What unanticipated impacts on patient safety might occur as a result of the medical information system?

The following section provides a brief overview of some of the research methods appropriate to these evaluation questions and the models of change they represent (see Table 1.1).

Research Methods

Numerous research methods are available to support investigation of the research questions and the underlying models of change described above. This section provides a brief overview of some of these methods with examples of their contributions to research on information systems in healthcare organizations. The discussion includes qualitative methods, multiple research strategies to evaluate information systems in collaborative healthcare environments, survey research methods, cognitive approaches to evaluation, work sampling, social network analysis, computer simulation, and research strategies that combine quantitative and qualitative methodologies. Each of these methods is described in detail in subsequent chapters of the book.

Qualitative research, described in detail in Chapter 2, is conducted in natural settings and is characterized by the use of data in the form of words rather than numbers, primarily from observations, interviews, and documents. These methods attempt to understand change from the point of view of the participants and their social and institutional context. Qualitative methods are particularly useful in determining *how* and *why* specific outcomes occur [81]. In instances where the investigator is attempting to build a theory of how a medical information system affects the organization and its members, for example, these methods provide important insights into the reasons for change. While particularly useful when the major purpose of the investigator is theory building, however, qualitative methods are equally important in theory testing [82]. Case studies, which may combine quantitative and qualitative methods, are used both for theory construction [81,83–84], and for testing theories or hypotheses about causes and effects [85,86]. In theory testing, specific theoretical propositions need to be developed in advance to guide data-collection and hypothesis testing [87].

Qualitative methods are also particularly useful in collecting and analyzing data pertinent to the design of medical information systems. Fafchamps [88], for example, describes an ethnographic work flow analysis of physician behavior in the clinics of two healthcare institutions. Information about physician needs, practice behavior, and the clinical setting was collected by (1) asking physicians to describe what they were doing and conducting a guided tour of the clinics, (2) structured observations of meetings and interpersonal interactions, (3) focused interviews, and (4) analyzing formal and informal notes and reports. These data were analyzed and used to help design a physician workstation.

Multiple research techniques need to be used to evaluate the impact of information systems on different members of the healthcare team (see Chapter 3). For example, a study of an electronic patient record system in a surgical intensive care unit examined the patient care team of residents, fellow, attending physicians, pharmacists, and nurses [89]. Each team member brought different backgrounds, perspectives and skills to the team. These different skills and perspectives had implications for the adoption and use of the patient record system on their unit.

Survey research methodologies are also widely used to study the impact of information systems (see Chapter 4). In survey research, responses to predefined questions or items are collected from a sample of individuals, departments, or organizations to produce quantitative descriptions of population characteristics or of relationships between variables. Zmud and Boynton [90] provide summary data and statistical analysis on 119 scales that have been used to study information systems.

In considering attitudes toward computers, for example, a comparative survey of physicians, pharmacists, lawyers, and CPAs by Zoltan-Ford and Chapanis [91] found that physicians and lawyers expressed dissatisfaction with what they perceived to be the depersonalizing nature of computers and with the complexity of computer languages. Surveys by Teach and Shortliffe [92] and Singer et al. [93] concluded that physicians generally accept applications that enhance their patient management capabilities, but tend to oppose applications that automate clinical activities traditionally performed by physicians themselves. Anderson et al.'s [94] survey of medical students, residents, and practicing physicians found that, while physicians recognize the potential of computers to improve patient care, they express concerns about the possibility of increased control over their practices, threats to privacy, and legal and technical problems.

Surveys can also be used to collect descriptive data needed to establish policies or to solve problems. Survey data may indicate the existence of problems, as well as their seriousness and pervasiveness. In this instance the methodology is problem-driven [45]. Kaiser and King [95], for example, used survey research in their study of the emerging role of information analysts. Kraemer and Dutton [45] provide a useful propositional inventory based on a meta-analysis of the findings from a large number of surveys. In general, studies based on surveys fail to examine the relationships between information systems and their external environments, the dynamics of how change takes place, and societal impacts of the information system.

The *Internet* also provides a new research tool (see Chapter 5). First the Internet is a rich source of qualitative research that can be used to identify research issues, generate hypotheses, or for needs assessment. Second, electronic interviews can be conducted via e-mail or in chat rooms. Also, surveys can be administered by e-mail or posted in newsgroups or discussion forums or on the Web.

Cognitive approaches to evaluation focus on understanding the processes involved in decision making and reasoning of healthcare workers as they interact with information systems in carrying out a range of tasks (see Chapter 6). Methods that have been developed in the areas of usability engineering and cognitive task analysis have important implications for the assessment of cognition involved in complex medical tasks and the impact of information systems.

Work sampling provides evaluation tools that can be used to assess the effects of clinical computer systems on the work patterns of healthcare workers (see Chapter 7). These techniques permit the investigator to address questions such as (1) How and by whom is the system used? (2) How much time is spent using the system? (3) What effect does the system have on other work-related activities? (4) How long should it take to use the system? (5) How can work patterns be improved so as to use utilize each member of the healthcare team's knowledge and training to the fullest extent?

Another approach to the study of social interactions, frequently termed *social network analysis* or structural analysis, focuses on interactions that occur between individuals and/or departments as a medical information system is adopted and its use diffuses throughout the organization (see Chapter 8). The network or structural approach hypothesizes that individuals' responses to the information system are affected and constrained by their positions and roles in the social system of which they are a part. Individual adoption and use is seen as dependent on group interaction [55,64,96,97]. This perspective differs fundamentally from those that assume that individuals and organizational units are somewhat independent of one another in the ways in which they respond to and use an information system. Instead, this approach attempts to identify the communication structure or the underlying social structure, generally unknown to organizational participants, by collecting and analyzing relational data. Network analysis methods are based on graph theory, clustering methods, and multidimensional scaling, and are described in detail in Chapter 8.

Anderson and Jay [68], for example, used network analysis in their study of the time-of-adoption of a computer-based hospital information system. Medical doctors adopted the innovation (i.e., began entering their orders) in clusters, with all of the doctors in a clique adopting at about the same time. "Network location was found to have a significant effect on the adoption and utilization of the HIS (the computer-based-innovation) independently of background and practice characteristics of physicians" [68,98,99]. In other words, the network variable increased unexplained variance in innovativeness in addition to that explained by such individual characteristics of the doctors such as age and medical specialty. Furthermore, utilization patterns were similar among physicians belonging to each group.

Computer simulation models can also be used to study medical information systems (see Chapter 9). This approach provides researchers with a relatively inexpensive means to study operational effectiveness and predict the effects of changing the operational environment without actually interfering with the ongoing work of the organization. In one study, Anderson, Jay, Schweer, and Anderson [100] developed a mathematical model to characterize the process by which physicians change their use of a medical information system. A structural equation model was constructed using data collected from members of a hospital medical staff. The model indicated that consultation with other physicians on the hospital service led to greater exposure to and a more favorable attitude toward potential computer applications. Physicians who were more knowledgeable about computers were more likely to tailor the system to their individual practices. All of these factors resulted in increased use of the system by physicians. The results of the study led to a number of policy recommendations regarding strategies for introducing computer technology to physicians.

In a second study, a computer simulation model of the order entry process for a hospital information system was developed and used to perform computer simulation experiments to estimate the effects of two methods of order entry on several outcome measures [101–103]. The results indicated that the development and use of personal order sets for order entry could result in a significant reduction in staffpower, salaries, fringe benefits, and errors for the hospital.

Combining Methods

Studies that attempt to examine complex social interactions as determinants of system use generally require a combination of qualitative and quantitative methods. Qualitative data, for example, can be used to gain critical insights into motivations and interactions within the organization. Detailed observations in the actual organizational setting can also be used to interpret the findings and explain how and why information systems bring about changes. Subsequently, qualitative data, surveys, and experimental methods can all be used for empirical testing of hypotheses. This combination of qualitative and quantitative methods produces insights that neither method alone can provide. Furthermore, the findings are considered to be more robust and generalizable [104].

In one example, both qualitative and quantitative methods were used to study the impact of a clinical laboratory computer system [104–106]. Quantitative results showed differences between technicians in their reactions to the computer system. Shedding further light on these differences, qualitative data indicated that laboratory employees differed in their orientation to the nature of their work. One group of technicians focused on work load increases, the other emphasized improved results reporting and service. The users' response to the computer system depended on their perception of the extent to which the system supported or interfered with the performance of their job as they defined it.

Conclusion

Each of the methods described above is explained in detail, with sample evaluation instruments where appropriate, in Chapters 2 through 9. The chapters also include examples of studies that make different theoretical assumptions, address different evaluation questions, and employ different research methodologies. Each study also has important practical policy implications for the organization under study.

Additional Readings

The Social Impact of Computers

Anderson and Jay [65] and Anderson [22,23] review evaluation studies of the use and impact of healthcare information systems. Dunlop and Kling [107] provide an important collection of readings outlining the different positions in the debates about social issues surrounding computerization.

Evaluation and Models of Change

Kling [28], Kling and Scacchi [29], Lyytinen [31], and Markus and Robey [57] provide detailed theoretical research frameworks for information systems and research dealing with information systems problems.

Rice's [108] chapter is a detailed review of the different paradigms and theoretical frameworks adopted by information system researchers.

Research Methods

The three volumes from the Harvard Business School Research Colloquium on research methodologies that can be used to study information systems cover qualitative research methods [109], experimental research methods [110], and survey research methods [111].

Nissen, Klein, and Hirschheim's [112] edited volume provides comprehensive documentation of current research methods and approaches in information systems today.

Rossi and Freeman [54] is an excellent textbook on evaluation research. Patton [113] provides an excellent introduction to qualitative approaches to evaluation. Yin [81] is an excellent monograph on case study research.

Scott [97] provides a good readable introduction to network analysis.

A special issue of *Computers in Biology and Medicine* [114] provides a good review of evaluation methods in health informatics.

Friedman and Wyatt's text on evaluation methods in medical informatics [115] provides a detailed course on the evaluation of informatics in healthcare organizations and is an excellent complement to the present volume.

Future Directions in Evaluation

Kaplan and Shaw [116] provide an up-to-date review of evaluation literature on the people, organizational, and social issues related to the implementation of information technology in health care, including recommendations for future research.

References

[1] N.M. Lorenzi, R.T. Riley, A.J.C. Blythe, G. Southon, and B.J. Dixon. Antecedents of the people and organizational aspects of medical informatics: Review of the literature, Journal of the American Medical Informatics Association 4 (1997) 79–93.

[2] N.M. Lorenzi and R.T. Riley. Managing change: An overview, Journal of the American Medical Informatics Association 7 (2000) 116–124.

[3] R. Snyder-Halpern. Indicators of organizational readiness for a clinical information technology/systems innovation: A Delphi study, International Journal of Medical Informatics 63 (2001) 179–204.

[4] F.C.G. Southon, C. Sauer, and C.N.G. Dampney. Information technology in complex health services: Organizational impediments for successful technology transfer and diffusion, Journal of the American Medical Informatics Association 4 (1997) 112–124.

[5] T.W. Lauer, K. Joshi, and T. Browdy. Use of the equity implementation model to review clinical system implementation efforts: A case report, Journal of the American Medical Informatics Association 7 (2000) 91–102.

[6] B. Kaplan. Addressing organizational issues in the evaluation of medical systems, Journal of the American Medical Informatics Association 4 (1997) 94–101.

[7] M. Berg. Implementing information systems in healthcare organizations: Myths and challenges, International Journal of Medical Informatics 64 (2001) 143–156.

[8] J. Aarts and V. Peel. Using a descriptive model of change when implementing large scale clinical information systems to identify priorities for further research, International Journal of Medical Informatics 56 (1999) 43–50.

[9] J. Aarts, V. Peel, and G. Wright. Organizational issues in health informatics: A model approach, International Journal of Medical Informatics 52 (1998) 235–242.

[10] D.F. Doolan, D.W. Bates, and B.C. James. The use of computers for clinical care: A case series of advanced U.S. sites, Journal of the American Medical Informatics Association 10 (2003) 94–107.

[11] J.S. Ash, P.N. Gorman, M. Lavelle, T.H. Payne, T.A. Massaro, G.L. Frantz, and J.A. Lyman. A cross-site qualitative study of physician order entry, Journal of the American Informatics Association 10 (2003) 188–200.

[12] R.M. Braude. Editorial comments: People and organizational issues in health informatics, Journal of the American Informatics Association 4 (1997) 150–151.

[13] D.J. Brailer and E.L. Terasawa. *Use and Adoption of Computer-Based Patient Records* (California HealthCare Foundation, Oakland, CA, 2003).

[14] R.S. Dick, E.B. Steen, and D.E. Detmer, editors, *The Computer-Based Patient Record* (National Academy Press, Washington, DC, 1997).

[15] President's Information Technology Advisory Committee, HealthCare Delivery and Information Technology (HIT) subcommittee: Draft recommendations, www.nitrd.gov.pitac.

[16] W.A. Yasnoff, B.L. Humphreys, and J.M. Overhage, et al., A consensus action agenda for achieving the national health information infrastrucutre, Journal of the American Medical Informatics Association 11 (2004) 332–338.

[17] M.J. Barrett, B.J. Holmes, and S.E. McAulay. *Electronic Medical Records: A Buyer's Guide for Small Physician Practices* (Californa HealthCare Foundation, Oakland, CA, 2003).

[18] G. Southon, C. Sauer, and K. Dampney. Lessons from a failed information systems initiative: Issues for complex organizations, International Journal of Medical Informatics 55 (1999) 33–46

[19] B.L. Goddard. Termination of a contract to implement an enterprise electronic medical record system, Journal of the American Informatics Association 7 (2000) 564–568.

[20] E.G. Poon, D. Blumenthal, T. Jaggi, M.M. Honour, D.W. Bates, and R. Kaushal. Overcoming barriers to adopting and implementing computerized physician order entry in U.S. hospitals, Health Affairs 23(4) (2004) 184–190.

[21] R.H. Miller, I. Sim, and J. Newman. *Electronic Medical Records: Lessons from Small Physician Practices* (California HealthCare Foundation, Oakland, CA, 2003).

[22] J.G. Anderson. Computer-based ambulatory information systems: Recent developments, Journal of Ambulatory Care Management 23(2) (2000) 53–63.

[23] J.G. Anderson. Clinical information systems, in: A. Kent, editor, *Encyclopedia of Library and Information Science*, Vol. 69, Supplement 32 (Marcel Dekker, New York, 2000), pp. 33–53.

[24] SB1875, California Senate Bill 1975, 2000.

[25] Institute of Medicine, *Patient Safety: Achieving a New Standard for Care* (National Academy Press, Washington, DC, 2004).

[26] J.S. Ash, P.N. Gorman, V. Seshadri, and W.R. Hersh. Computerized physician order entry in U.S. hospitals: Results of a 2002 survey, Journal of the American Informatics Association 11 (2004) 95–99.

[27] J.L. King and K. Kraemer. *Cost as a Social Impact of Telecommunications and Other Information Technologies* (Public Policy Research Organization, Irvine, CA, 1980).

[28] R. Kling. Social analyses of computing: Theoretical perspectives in recent empirical research, Computing Surveys 12 (1980) 61–110.

[29] R. Kling and W. Scacchi. The web of computing: Computer technology as social organization, in: M.C. Yovits, editor, *Advances in Computers*, 21, pp. 2–90 (Academic Press, New York, 1982), pp. 2–90.

[30] K. Kumar and N. Bjorn-Andersen. A cross-cultural comparison of information systems designer values, Communications of the ACM 33 (1990) 528–538.

[31] K. Lyytinen. Different perspective on information systems: Problems and solutions, ACM Computing Surveys 19 (1987) 5–46.

[32] J. Mouritsen and N. Bjorn-Andersen. Understanding third wave information systems, in: C. Dunlop and R. Kling, editors, *Computerization and Controversy: Value Conflicts and Social Choices* (Academic Press, San Diego, CA, 1991), pp. 308–320.

[33] A.F. Dowling. Do hospital staff interfere with computer system implementation? Healthcare Management Review 5 (1980) 23–32.

[34] K. Lyytinen. Expectation failure concept and systems analysts' view of information systems failure: Results of an exploratory study, Information & Management 14 (1988) 45–56.

[35] K. Lyytinen and R. Hirschheim. Information systems failure: A survey and classification of empirical literature, Oxford Surveys in Information Technology 4 (1987) 257–309.

[36] R.G. Berger and J.P. Kichak. Computerized physician order entry: Helpful or harmful? Journal of the American Informatics Association 11 (2004) 100–103.

[37] J.S. Ash, M. Berg, and E. Cohera. Some unintended consequences of information technology in healthcare: The nature of patient care information system-related errors, Journal of the American Informatics Association 11 (2004) 104–112.

[38] C.J. McDonald, J.M. Overhage, B.W. Mamlin, P.D. Dexter, and W.M. Tierney. Physicians, information technology, and healthcare systems: A journey, not a destination, Journal American Medical Informatics Association 11 (2004) 121–124.

[39] W.J. Winkelman and K.J. Leonard. Overcoming structural constraints to patient utilization of electronic medical records: A critical review and proposal for an evaluation framework, Journal of the American Informatics Association 11 (2004) 151–161.

[40] M. Cain and R. Mittman. *Diffusion of Innovation in Healthcare* (California Healthcare Foundation, Oakland, CA, 2002).

[41] B. Spurlock, M. Nelson, J. Paterno, and T. Sandeep. *Legislating Medication Safety: The California Experience* (California HealthCare Foundation, Oakland, CA, 2003).

[42] VHA, *New Tools, New Roles: The Fusion of Technology and Work Force* (VHA, Irving, TX, 2003).

[43] D. Hailey. *Elements of Effectiveness for Health Technology Assessment Programs* (Alberta Heritage Foundation for Medical Research, Edmonton, Alberta, Canada, 2003).

[44] B. Ives, S. Hamilton, and G.B. Davis. A framework for research in computer-based management information systems, Management Science 26 (1980) 910–934.

[45] K.L. Kraemer and W.H. Dutton. Survey research in the study of management information systems, in: K.L. Kraemer, editor, *The Information Systems Research Challenge: Survey Research Methods*, Vol. 3 (Harvard Business School, Boston, MA, 1991), pp. 3–57.

[46] T.S. Kuhn. *The Structure of Scientific Revolutions.* (University of Chicago Press, Chicago, 1962).

[47] R. Hirschheim. *Office Automation: A Social and Organizational Perspective* (John Wiley & Sons, New York, 1985).

[48] H. Braverman. *Labor and Monopoly Capital: The Degradation of Work in the Twentieth Century* (Monthly Review Press, New York, 1974).

[49] C.E. Aydin and R.E. Rice. Bringing social worlds together: Computers as catalysts for non-interactions in healthcare organizations, Journal of Health and Social Behavior 33 (1992) 168–185.

[50] M.L. Markus. Power, politics, and MIS implementation, Communications of the ACM 26 (1983) 430–444.

[51] M.L. Markus. *Systems in Organizations: Bugs and Features* (Pitman, Boston, MA, 1984).

[52] P. Attewel and J.B. Rule. Computing and organizations: What we know and what we don't know, Communications of the ACM 27 (1984) 1184–1192.

[53] K.L. Kraemer and J.N. Danziger. The impacts of computer technology on the worklife of information workers, Social Science Computer Review 8 (1990) 592–613.

[54] P.H. Rossi, M.W. Lipsey, and H.E. Freeman. *Evaluation: A Systematic Approach*, 7th ed. (Sage Publications, Thousand Oaks, CA, 2004).

[55] B. Kaplan. Models of change and information systems research, in: H.E. Nissen, H.K. Klein, and R. Hirschheim, editors, *Information Systems Research: Contemporary Approaches and Emergent Traditions* (North Holland, Amsterdam, 1991), pp. 593–611.

[56] J.G. Anderson, C.E. Aydin, and B. Kaplan. An analytical framework for measuring the effectiveness/impacts of computer-based patient record systems, in: J.F. Nunamaker, Jr., and R.H. Sprague, Jr., editors, *Proceedings of the 28th Hawaii International Conference on System Sciences, Vol. IV: Information Systems—Collaboration Systems and Technology Organizational Systems and Technology*, Los Alamitos, CA: IEEE Computer Society Press (1995), pp. 767–776.

[57] M.L. Markus and D. Robey. Information technology and organizational change: Causal structure in theory and research, Management Science 34 (1988) 583–598.

[58] J. Pfeffer. *Organizations and Organization Theory* (Pitman, Marshfield, MA, 1982).

[59] J.D. Slack. *Communication Technologies and Society: Conceptions of Causality and the Politics of Technological Intervention* (Ablex, Norwood, NJ, 1984).

[60] D.E. Forsyth and B.G. Buchanan. Broadening our approach to evaluating medical information systems, in: *Proceedings 15th Annual Symposium on Computer Applications in Medical Care*, Washington, DC (1992), pp. 8–12.

[61] R. Leifer and E.F. McDonough III. Computerization as a predominant technology effecting work unit structure, in: *Proceedings 6th Annual Conference on Information Systems* (1985), pp. 238–248.

[62] N. Bjorn-Andersen, K. Eason, and D. Robey. *Managing Computer Impact: An International Study of Management and Organization* (Ablex, Norwood, NJ, 1986).

[63] M.H. Olson. New information technology and organizational culture, MIS Quarterly 6 (1982) 71–92.

[64] E.M. Rogers. *Diffusion of Innovation*, 3rd ed. (The Free Press, New York, 1983).

[65] J.G. Anderson and S.J. Jay, editors, *Use and Impact of Computers in Clinical Medicine* (Springer-Verlag, New York, 1987).

[66] L.B. Mohr. *Explaining Organizational Behavior* (Jossey-Bass, San Francisco, 1982).

[67] S.R. Barley. Technology as an occasion for structuring: Evidence from observations of CT scanners and the social order of radiology departments, Administrative Science Quarterly 31 (1986) 78–108.

[68] J.G. Anderson and S.J. Jay. Computers and clinical judgment: The role of physician networks, Social Science and Medicine 10 (1985) 969–979.

[69] B.M. Johnson and R.E. Rice. Reinvention in the innovation process: The case of word processing, in: R.E. Rick and Associates, editors, *The New Media* (Sage, Beverly Hills, CA, 1984), pp. 157–183.

[70] H.P. Lundsgaarde, P.J. Fischer, and D.J. Steele. *Human Problems in Computerized Medicine* (University of Kansas Publications in Anthropology, No. 13, Lawrence, KS, 1981).

[71] C.E. Aydin. Occupational adaptation to computerized medical information systems, Journal of Health and Social Behavior 30 (1989) 163–179.

[72] M.A. Counte, K.H. Kjerulff, J.C. Salloway, and B. Campbell. Implementing computerization in hospitals: A case study of the behavioral and attitudinal impacts of a medical information system, Journal of Organizational Behavior Management 6 (1984) 109–122.

[73] C.E. Aydin and R.E. Rice. Social world, individual differences, and implementation: Predicting attitudes toward a medical information system, Information and Management 20 (1991) 119–136.

[74] R.E. Rice and C. Aydin. Attitudes toward new organizational technology: Network proximity as a mechanism for social information processing, Administrative Science Quarterly 36 (1991) 219–244.

[75] B. Griffin. Effects of work redesign on employee perceptions, attitudes, and behaviors: A long-term investigation, Academy of Management Journal 34 (1991) 425–435.

[76] B. Kaplan. National Health Service reforms: Opportunities for medical informatics research, in: K.C. Lun, et al., editors, *Proceedings of the 7th World Congress on Medical Informatics*, Amsterdam, Elsevier Science Publications (1992).

[77] P. Aspden, J.M. Corrigan, J. Wolcott, and S.M. Erickson. *Patient Safety: Achieving a New Standard for Care* (National Academy Press, Washington, DC, 2004).

[78] Institute of Medicine, *Crossing the Quality Chasm: A New Health System for the 21st Century* (National Academy Press, Washington, DC, 2001).

[79] L. Kohn, J.M. Corrigan, and M.S. Donaldson, editors, *To Err Is Human: Building a Safer Health System* (National Academy Press, Washington, DC, 2000).

[80] Health Grades, Inc., *Patient Safety in American Hospitals* (Health Grades, Inc., Denver, CO, 2004).

[81] R.K. Yin. *Case Study Research* (Sage, Beverly Hills, CA, 1984).

[82] J. VanMannen, J.M. Dabbs, and R.R. Faulkner. *Varieties of Qualitative Research* (Sage Publications, Newbury Park, CA, 1982).

[83] I. Benbasat, D.I. Goldstein, and M. Mead. The case research strategy in studies of information systems, MIS Quarterly 11 (1987) 369–386.

[84] A. George and T. McKeown. Case studies and theories of organizational decision making, in: R.F. Coulam and R.A. Smith, editors, *Advances in Information Processing in Organizations*, Vol. 6 (JAI Press, Greenwich, CT, 1985), pp. 21–58.

[85] M.L. Markus. Case selection in a disconfirmatory case study, in: J.I. Cash and P.R. Lawrence, editors, *The Information Systems Research Challenge: Qualitative Research Methods*, Vol. 1 (Harvard Business School, Boston, MA, 1989), pp. 20–26.

[86] L.B. Mohr. The reliability of the case study as a source of information, in: R.F. Coulam and R.A. Smith, editors, *Advances in Information Processing in Organizations*, Vol. 6 (JAI Press, Greenwich, CT, 1985), pp. 65–93.

[87] R.K. Yin. Research design issues in using the case study method to study management information systems, in: J.I. Cash and P.R. Lawrence, editors, *The Information Systems Research Challenge: Qualitative Research Methods*, Vol. 1 (Harvard Business School, Boston, MA, 1989), pp. 1–6.

[88] D. Fafchamps. Ethnographic workflow analysis: Specification for design, in: J.H. Bullinger, editor, *Proceedings of the 4th International Conference on Human-Computer Interaction, Amsterdam*, Elsevier Science Publishers (1991).

[89] M. Reddy, W. Pratt, and P. Dourish, et al., Asking questions: Information needs in a surgical intensive care unit, in: *Proceedings of the American Medical Informatics Association Fall Symposium*, San Antonio, TX (2002), pp. 651–655.

[90] R.W. Zmud and A.C. Boynton. Survey measures and instruments in MIS: Inventory and appraisal, in: K.L. Kraemer, editor, *The Information Systems Research Challenge: Survey Research Methods* Vol. 3, (Harvard Business School, Boston, MA, 1991), pp. 149–180.

[91] E. Zoltan-Ford and A. Chapanis. What do professional persons think about computers? Behaviour and Information Technology 1 (1982) 55–68.

[92] R.L. Teach and E.H. Shortliffe. An analysis of physician attitudes regarding computer-based clinical consultation systems. Computers and Biomedical Research 14 (1981) 542–558.

[93] J. Singer, H.S. Sacks, F. Lucente, and T.C. Chalmers. Physician attitudes toward applications of computer database systems, Journal of the American Medical Association 249 (1983) 1610–1614.

[94] J.G. Anderson, S.J. Jay, H.M. Schweer, and M.M. Anderson. Why doctors don't use computers: Some empirical findings, Journal of the Royal Society of Medicine 79 (1986b) 142–144.

[95] K.M. Kaiser and W.R. King. The manager-analyst interface in systems development, MIS Quarterly 6 (1982) 49–59.

[96] E.M. Rogers. Progress, problems and prospects for network research: Investigating relationships in the age of electronic communication technologies, Social Networks 9 (1987) 285–310.

[97] J. Scott. *Social Network Analysis. A Handbook.* (Sage Publications, Newbury Park, CA, 1991).

[98] J.G. Anderson, S.J. Jay, J. Perry, and M.M. Anderson. Diffusion of computer applications among physicians: A quasi-experimental study, Clinical Sociology Review 8 (1990) 116–127.

[99] J.G. Anderson, S.J. Jay, H.M. Schweer, M.M. Anderson, and D. Kassing. Physician communication networks and the adoption and utilization of computer applications in medicine, in: J.G. Anderson and S.J. Jay, editors, *Use and Impact of Computers in Clinical Medicine* (Springer-Verlag, New York, 1987), pp. 185–198.

[100] J.G. Anderson, S.J. Jay, H.M. Schweer and M.M. Anderson. Physician utilization of computers in medical practice: Policy implications based on a structural model, Social Science and Medicine 23 (1986a) 259–267.

[101] J.G. Anderson, S.J. Jay, L. Cathcart, S.J. Clevenger, D.R. Kassing, J. Perry, and M.M. Anderson. A computer simulation of physician use of a hospital information system, in: W.E. Hammond, editor, *Proceedings AAMSI Congress 1988*, San Francisco, CA (1988a), pp. 114–118.

[102] J.G. Anderson, S.J. Jay, S.J. Clevenger, D.R. Kassing, J. Perry, and M.M. Anderson. Physician utilization of a hospital information system: A computer simulation model, in: *Proceedings 12th Annual Symposium on Computer Applications in Medical Care*, Washington, DC (1988b), pp. 858–861.

[103] J.G. Anderson, S.J. Jay, M.M. Anderson, and T.J. Hunt. Evaluating the capability of information technology to prevent adverse drug events: A computer simulation approach, Journal American Medical Informatics Association 9 (2002) 479–490.

[104] B. Kaplan and D. Duchon. Combining qualitative and quantitative methods in information systems research: A case study. MIS Quarterly 12 (1988) 571–586.

[105] B. Kaplan. Initial impact of a clinical laboratory computer system: Themes common to expectations and actualities, Journal of Medical Systems 11 (1987) 137–147.

[106] B. Kaplan and D. Duchon. A job orientation model of impact on work seven months post-implementation, in: B. Barber, D. Cao, D. Qin, and G. Wagner, editors, *MEDINFO 89* (North Holland, Amsterdam, 1989), pp. 1051–1055.

[107] C. Dunlop and R. Kling. *Computerization and Controversy: Value Conflicts and Social Choices* (Academic Press, Boston, 1991).

[108] R.E. Rice. Contexts of research on organizational computer-mediated communication: A recursive review, in: H. Lea, editor, *Contexts of Computer-Mediated Communication* (Harvester-Wheatsheaf, United Kingdom, 1992).

[109] J.I. Cash and P.R. Lawrence. *The Information Systems Research Challenge: Qualitative Research Methods*: Harvard Business School Research Colloquium, Vol. 1 (Harvard Business School, Boston, MA, 1989).

[110] I. Benbasat. *The Information Systems Research Challenge: Experimental Research Methods*: Harvard Business School Research Colloquium, Vol. 2 (Harvard Business School, Boston, MA, 1989).

[111] K.L. Kraemer. *The Information Systems Research Challenge: Survey Research Methods*: Harvard Business School Research Colloquium, Vol. 3 (Harvard Business School, Boston, MA, 1991).

[112] H.E. Nissen, H.K. Klein, and R. Hirschheim, editors, *Information Systems Research: Contemporary Approaches and Emergent Traditions* (North Holland, Amsterdam, 1991).

[113] M.Q. Patton. Qualitative Research and Evaluation Methods, 2nd ed. (Sage Publications, Newbury Park, CA, 1990).

[114] J.H. Moehr. Special issue: Evaluation in health informatics, Computers in Biology and Medicine 32(3) (2002) 11–236.

[115] C.P. Friedman and J.C. Wyatt. *Evaluation Methods in Medical Informatics* (Springer, New York, 1997).

[116] B. Kaplan and N.T. Shaw. Future directions in evaluation research: People, organizational, and social issues, Methods of Information in Medicine 43 (2004) 215–231.

2
Qualitative Research Methods for Evaluating Computer Information Systems

Bonnie Kaplan and Joseph A. Maxwell

Introduction

Qualitative research methods are being used increasingly in evaluation studies, including evaluations of computer systems and information technology. This chapter provides an overview of the nature and appropriate uses of qualitative methods and of key considerations in conducting qualitative research.

The goal of qualitative research is understanding issues or particular situations by investigating the perspectives and behavior of the people in these situations and the context within which they act. To accomplish this, qualitative research is conducted in natural settings and uses data in the form of words rather than numbers. Qualitative data are gathered primarily from observations, interviews, and documents, and are analyzed by a variety of systematic techniques. This approach is useful in understanding causal processes, and in facilitating action based on the research results.

Qualitative methods are primarily inductive. Hypotheses are developed during the study so as to take into account what is being learned about the setting and the people in it. Qualitative methods may be combined with quantitative methods in conducting a study. Validity threats are addressed primarily during data collection and analysis.

The chapter discusses these points and uses an evaluation of a clinical laboratory information system to illustrate them.

Computer information systems can significantly improve patient care, hospital management and administration, research, and health and medical education. However, many systems do not achieve these goals. Dowling estimated that 45% of computer-based medical information systems failed due to user resistance, even though these systems were sound technologically. Thus, the stakes in developing, implementing, and evaluating such systems are high [1].

Different evaluation objectives require different methodological approaches. Many evaluations of medical computer information systems focus on impacts such as costs and benefits, timeliness, completeness, error rates, retrievability, usage rates, user satisfaction, and clinician behavior changes [2,3]. Quantitative methods are excellent for studying these kinds of evaluation questions, in which selected features of the information technology, the organization, the user, and the information needs generally are treated as independent, objective, and discrete entities, and as unchanging over the course of the study [4].

When a researcher or evaluator wishes to study issues that are not easily partitioned into discrete entities, or to examine the dynamics of a process rather than its static characteristics, qualitative methods are more useful than solely quantitative ones. The strengths of qualitative research methods lie in their usefulness for understanding the meaning and context of the phenomena studied, and the particular events and processes that make up these phenomena over time, in real-life, natural settings [5]. When evaluating computer information systems, these contextual issues include social, cultural, organizational, and political concerns surrounding an information technology; the processes of information systems development, installation, and use (or lack of use); and how all these are conceptualized and perceived by the participants in the setting where the study is being conducted [6]. Thus, qualitative methods are particularly helpful for any of the following:

- To determine what might be important to measure, why measured results are as they are, or if the subject of study cannot be measured easily
- To understand not only what happened, or what people are responding to, but why; to understand how people think or feel about something and why they think that way, what their perspectives and situations are and how those influence what is happening; to understand and explore what a technology (such as an newborn nursery telemonitoring system) or practice (such as using a computer to access health information) means to people
- To investigate the influence of social, organizational, and cultural context on the area of study, and vice versa
- To examine causal processes, and not simply what causal relationships exist
- To study processes as they develop and emerge, rather than in outcomes or impacts; for example, to investigate the development process for the application under study in parallel with that process so that you can improve the application development as it progresses.

Qualitative research methods have undergone significant development in recent years [7–10] and are being increasingly used in evaluation research both within and outside health care [6,10–13]. There also is a growing literature on combining qualitative and quantitative methods [14–22]. The purpose of this chapter is to explain what qualitative approaches can contribute to medical computer systems evaluations. We begin by describing the nature and goals of qualitative research and evaluation, and illustrate these with an example of the use of qualitative methods in computer information systems evaluation. We then discuss some key considerations in qualitative evaluation research and present the most important methods used in this approach.

The Nature of Qualitative Research

"Qualitative research" refers to a range of approaches that differ significantly among themselves, but that share some defining characteristics and purposes. These approaches are known by a variety of terms, some broad and some quite specific. The more general terms, which are more or less equivalent to "qualitative research," are "field research" and "naturalistic research." More specific terms, denoting particular types of qualitative research, are "interpretive research," "ethnographic research," "phenomenological research," "hermeneutic research," "humanistic research," and some kinds of case studies or action research [23]. We use "qualitative research" to refer to all of these.

Qualitative research typically involves systematic and detailed study of individuals in natural settings, instead of in settings contrived by the researcher, often using open-ended interviews intended to elicit detailed, in-depth accounts of the interviewee's experiences and perspectives on specific issues, situations, or events. Qualitative methods employ data in the form of words: transcripts of open-ended interviews, written observational descriptions of activities and conversations, and documents and other artifacts of people's actions. Such data are analyzed in ways that retain their inherent textual nature. This is because the goals of qualitative research typically involve understanding a phenomenon from the points of view of the participants, and in its particular social and institutional context. These goals largely are lost when textual data are quantified and aggregated [5].

Reasons for Qualitative Research

There five main reasons for using qualitative methods in evaluating computer information systems:

1. Understanding how a system's users perceive and evaluate that system and what meanings the system has for them

Users' perspectives generally are not known in advance. It is difficult to ascertain or understand these through purely quantitative approaches. By allowing researchers to investigate users' perspectives in depth, qualitative methods can contribute to the explanation of users' behavior with respect to the system, and thus to the system's successes and failures and even of what is considered a "success" or "failure" [6].

2. Understanding the influence of social and organizational context on systems use

Computer information systems do not exist in a vacuum; their implementation, use, and success or failure occur in a social and organizational context that shapes what happens when that system is introduced. Some researchers consider this so important as to treat "context" as intrinsically part of the object of study rather than as external to the information system. Because of "context," in important respects, a system is not the same system when it is introduced into different settings [24,25]. As is true for users' perspectives, the researcher usually does not know in advance what all the important contextual influences are. Qualitative methods are useful for discovering and understanding these influences, and also for developing testable hypotheses and theories.

3. Investigating causal processes

Although experimental interventions can demonstrate *that* causal relationships exist, they are less useful in showing *how* causal processes work [26–28]. Qualitative methods often allow the researcher to get inside the black box of experimental and survey designs and to discover the actual processes involved in producing the results of such studies. Qualitative research is particularly useful for developing explanations of the actual events and processes that led to specific outcomes [7], or when causality is multidirectional and there is no clear effect or impact of one factor on some specific outcome [6]. In this way, qualitative methods can yield theories and explanations of how and why processes, events, and outcomes occur [29].

4. Providing formative evaluation that is aimed at improving a program under development, rather than assessing an existing one

Although quantitative and experimental designs often are valuable in assessing outcomes, they are less helpful in giving those responsible for systems design and implementation timely feedback on their actions. Qualitative evaluation can help both in system design as well as in studies of system use [6]. Using qualitative methods can help in identifying potential problems as they are forming, thereby providing opportunities to improve the system as it develops. These evaluations also allow for varying and changing project definitions and how the system and organization are mutually transformative, thereby enabling learning by monitoring the many experiments that naturally occur spontaneously as part of the processes of implementation and use [6].

5. Increasing the utilization of evaluation results

Administrators, policy makers, systems designers, and practitioners often find purely quantitative studies of little use because these studies do not seem related to their own understanding of the situation and the problems they are encountering. Qualitative methods, by providing evaluation findings that connect more directly with these individuals' perspectives, can increase the credibility and usefulness of evaluations for such decision makers [10].

An Example: Evaluating a Clinical Laboratory Computer Information System

These attributes of qualitative research are illustrated by a study of a clinical laboratory computer information system used by different laboratories within one department of an academic medical center [16,30–32]. This system was evaluated by combining both quantitative and qualitative methods. A survey questionnaire was designed to assess the impact of the computer system on work in the laboratories. Qualitative data gathered from interviews, observations, and open-ended questionnaire questions were used to determine what changes were attributed to the computer system. Statistical analysis of the survey data initially revealed no differences among laboratory technologists' responses. Qualitative data analysis of their answers to open-ended questions indicated that laboratory technologists within each laboratory differed in their reactions to the system, as did laboratories as a whole. Some focused on work increases, whereas others emphasized improved laboratory results reporting and service.

Although the quantitative survey data provided no apparent reason for these differences, the qualitative data did, leading to further investigation. This investigation revealed that different technologists had different views of their jobs, and these different views affected their attitudes toward the computer system. For some technologists, the system enhanced their jobs, while for others, it interfered with their jobs, even though they ostensibly had the same jobs and were using the same system. Neither the researchers nor the laboratory personnel expected this finding, though the finding rang true. Further analysis of the quantitative data supported this explanation for the differences among laboratories and among technologists. In the original quantitative analysis, few differences were discernible among technologists or among laboratories from the quantitative data because standard quantitative measures of job characteristics assumed a uniformity of job situations and perceptions. However, this uniformity did not exist, as revealed in qualitative data that identified technologists' own views of their jobs and of the system.

This example illustrates several features of qualitative research. First, it was not possible to design, in advance, a quantitative study that would have tested the right hypotheses, because appropriate hypotheses could not be known in advance. A qualitative approach enabled the researchers to see how individuals construed the information technology, their jobs, and the interaction between the laboratory computer information system and their jobs. Thus, the researchers were able to generate productive hypotheses and theory.

Second, the qualitative data enabled the researchers to make sense of their quantitative findings. The qualitative data helped to explain why the quantitative results were as they were. This is one example of the point made above—that qualitative research often can uncover the causal processes that explain quantitative results.

Third, the qualitative data were able to serve these purposes because they helped the researchers understand the system from the points of view of those involved with it. These points of view are crucial to studying issues such as computer systems acceptance or rejection, or the changes that occur when a new system is introduced.

Fourth, a variety of human, contextual, and cultural factors affect system acceptance in actual use. Qualitative data enabled the researchers to understand the contexts in which the system was developed, installed, and used, and thus to understand differences among laboratories.

Finally, the results had face validity. They were believable to the laboratory director in the hospital where the study was done, to laboratory personnel in other hospitals, and even outside of hospitals where workers showed characteristics similar to the laboratory technologists'. Because the results were credible and the description of the laboratory technologists were recognizable, they were useful for others. This is the primary means by which qualitative studies can be generalized or results made transferable: not by statistical inference to some defined population, but through the development of a theory that has applicability beyond the setting studied [33], as was done in this study [16].

In the remainder of this chapter, we discuss some important considerations in designing and conducting evaluations that use qualitative methods.

Getting Started

The most important initial question for an evaluator is whether qualitative methods are appropriate for conducting the study. For this, it is important to consider what qualitative methods can add to an evaluation: what kinds of questions they are capable of answering, and what value they have.

Research Questions and Evaluation Goals

Qualitative methods typically are used to understand the perception of an information system by its users, the context within which the system is implemented or developed, and the processes by which changes occur or outcomes are generated. They usually focus on the description, interpretation, and explanation of events, situations, processes, and outcomes, rather than the correlation of variables, and tend to be used for understanding a particular case or for comparison of a small number of cases, rather than for generalization to a specified population. They are useful for systematically collecting so-called "anecdotal" evidence and turning the experiences they describe into data that can be rigorously collected and analyzed.

Thus, the questions posed in a qualitative study are initially framed as "what," "how," and "why" queries, rather than as whether a particular hypothesis is true or false. The fundamental question is "What is going on here?" This question is progressively narrowed, focused, and made more detailed as the evaluation proceeds. Qualitative studies may begin with specific concerns or even suppositions about what is going on, but major strengths of qualitative methods are avoiding tunnel vision, seeing the unexpected, disconfirming one's assumptions, and discovering new ways of making sense of what is going on. Qualitative evaluators typically begin with questions such as:

- What is happening here?
- Why is it happening?
- How has it come to happen in this particular way?
- What do the people involved think is happening?
- How are these people responding to what is happening?
- Why are these people responding that way?

To answer these questions, qualitative evaluators attempt to understand the way others construe, conceptualize, and make sense of what is happening in a particular situation. In doing this, they must become familiar with the everyday behaviors, habits, work routines, and attitudes of the people involved as these people go about their daily business. It also is important for evaluators to become familiar with the language or specialized jargon used by people involved with the study. Knowledge of behaviors, habits, routines, attitudes, and language provides a way of identifying key concepts and values. This knowledge enables the evaluator not only to better understand what is going on, but also to present findings in terms meaningful to the participants. Policy makers, department administrators, systems designers, and others will be able to recognize the situations being reported and, therefore, know better how to address them. In addition, individuals outside the organization where the evaluation is conducted will have sufficient context to develop a good understanding of it.

Further, qualitative methods can be used throughout the entire systems development and implementation process. They treat a computer information system project as a process, rather than as an object or event. By doing this, the evaluator can play an active role in the project, offering evaluations as the project progresses (formative evaluations) instead of having to wait until the project is completed (summative evaluations). In this way, evaluators can serve as a bridge between the interests of systems developers and systems users [6].

Recognizing diversity of perceptions also is important; "various individuals ... may perceive it [an innovation] in light of many possible sets of values" [34]. For example, in Lundsgaarde and colleague's [35,36] evaluation of PROMIS, individuals who thought their professional status was enhanced by the system were more positive than those who felt their status was lowered. Other values also can play a role; Hirschheim and Klein [37] illustrate this for systems developers, Kaplan [38–40] for the physician and developer values in systems development and use, while Sicotte and colleagues discuss a system failure in terms that contrast differences in values and goals among nurses and system developers [41,42]. A major strength of qualitative approaches is their sensitivity to this diversity and to unique events and outcomes.

Role of Theory

Theory is useful for guiding a study. Familiarity with the subject of study or with a wide range of theories and situations, for example, can help the researcher make sense of occurrences in the particular study being conducted. It can help the evaluator to not overlook important issues and help provide a set of constructs to be investigated. In this way, theory can shape research questions and focus. Theory also will guide a researcher's interpretation and focus. Theories of knowledge and epistemologies underlying research approaches influence how the project is conceived, how the research is carried out, and how it is reported. For example, Kaplan describes how three different theoretical perspectives would lead to different interpretations of Lundsgaarde, Fischer, and Steele's findings in their evaluation of PROMIS [43].

Theory may play different roles in qualitative research. Two different approaches may be taken, or combined. In the first, the evaluator works within an explicit theoretical frame. For example, postmodern and constructivist theories are becoming increasingly popular in studies of information systems [6,44]. In the second approach, the evaluator attempts to avoid prior commitment to theoretical constructs or to hypotheses formulated before gathering any data. Nevertheless, in each approach, qualitative researchers develop categories and hypotheses from the data. The two approaches may be combined. For example, an evaluator may start with research questions and constructs based on theory, but instead of being limited to or constrained by prior theory, also attempts to develop theory, hypotheses, and categories through using a strategy known as "grounded theory" [45,46].

Regardless of which approach is used, an evaluator cannot avoid a prior theoretical orientation that affects research and evaluation questions, as well as affecting the methods chosen for investigating those questions. The difference between the two approaches is not whether the evaluator has some prior theoretical bent—that is unavoidable—but whether the evaluator deliberately works within it or tries to work outside it.

Gaining Entry

An evaluation begins with the process of the researcher gaining access to the setting and being granted permission to conduct the evaluation. How this is done shapes the researcher's relationship with the participants in the study, and, consequently, affects the nature of the entire study [12,18]. Some of these effects bear on validity issues, as discussed below. In addition to practical and scientific issues, negotiating a research or evaluation study raises ethical ones [6,10,47]. To help address some of the ethical concerns, we believe that, to the extent possible, all participants in the setting being evaluated should be brought into the negotiation process. Furthermore, doing interviews or observations may intrude into people's private lives, work spaces, and homes, and probe their feelings and thoughts. Personal issues may easily arise, so the researcher needs sensitivity to respect people's privacy and sensibilities. Often confidentiality is promised, which may require significant steps to protect people's identities.

Qualitative Research Design

Qualitative research primarily is inductive in its procedures. Qualitative researchers assume that they do not know enough about the perspectives and situations of participants in the setting studied to be able to formulate meaningful hypotheses in advance, and instead develop and test hypotheses during the process of data collection and analysis. For the same reasons, qualitative evaluations tend to be in-depth case studies of particular systems.

Qualitative research design involves considerable flexibility [5,7], for two reasons. First, many aspects of the project change over time, including the processes being studied, evaluation goals, definitions of "success," and who the stakeholders may be [6]. As they change, the study itself also may need changing. Second, qualitative inquiry is inductive and often iterative in that the evaluator may go through repeated cycles of data collection and analysis to generate hypotheses inductively from the data. These hypotheses, in turn, need to be tested by further data collection and analysis. The researcher starts with a broad research question, such as "What effects will information systems engendered by reforms in the UK's National Health Service have on relative power and status among clinical and administrative staff in a teaching hospital?" [48]. The researcher narrows the study by continually posing increasingly specific questions and attempting to answer them through data already collected and through new data collected for that purpose. These questions cannot all be anticipated in advance. As the evaluator starts to see patterns, or discovers behavior that seems difficult to understand, new questions arise. The process is one of generating hypotheses and explanations from the data, testing them, and modifying them accordingly. New hypotheses may require new data, and, consequently, potential changes in the research design.

Data Collection

The most important principle of qualitative data collection is that everything is potential data. The evaluator does not rigidly restrict the scope of data collection in advance, nor use formal rules to decide that some data are inadmissible or irrelevant. However, this approach creates two potential problems: validity and data overload.

Validity issues are addressed below. The problem of data overload is in some ways more intractable. The evaluator must continually make decisions about what data are relevant and may change these decisions over the course of the project. The evaluator must work to focus the data collection process, but not to focus it so narrowly as to miss or ignore data that would contribute important insights or evidence.

Qualitative evaluators use three main sources for data: (1) observation, (2) open-ended interviews and survey questions, and (3) documents and texts. Qualitative studies generally collect data by using several of these methods to give a wider range of coverage [49]. Data collection almost always involves the researcher's direct engagement in the setting studied, what often is called "fieldwork." Thus, the researcher is the instrument for collecting and analyzing data; the researcher's impressions, observations, thoughts, and ideas also are data sources. The researcher incorporates these when recording qualitative data in detailed, often verbatim form as field notes or interview transcripts. Such detail is essential for the types of analysis that are used in qualitative research. We discuss each of these data sources in turn, drawing again on Kaplan and Duchon's study and several other studies for examples.

Observation

Observation in qualitative studies typically involves the observer's active involvement in the setting studied; it is usually called "participant observation" to distinguish it from passive or non-interactive observation. Participant observation allows the observer to ask questions for clarification of what is taking place and to engage in informal discussion with system users, as well as to record ongoing activities and descriptions of the setting. It produces detailed descriptive accounts of what was going on (including verbal interaction), as well as eliciting the system users' own explanations, evaluations, and perspectives in the immediate context of use, rather than retrospectively. Such observation often is crucial to the assessment of a system. For example, Kaplan and Duchon went to the laboratories to observe what technologists actually did, rather than simply depend on verbal reports or job descriptions; Forsythe [50,51], in her studies of physicians' information needs, attended hospital rounds and recorded each request for information.

Observation also can be conducted when evaluating the potential uses of a proposed computer information system. Kaplan, for example, observed how the flowsheets in the patient record were used in an intensive care unit when it was suggested that flowsheets be replaced by a computer terminal that would display laboratory data in graphic form. She observed that only the pharmacist consulted the flowsheets. When a physician came to see the patient, or a new nurse came on duty, he or she assessed the patient's condition by talking to the nurse who had been caring for that patient, rather than by consulting the patient's record. These observations raised a number of issues that would need addressing if a computer display of flowsheet information were to be implemented successfully. In another study preparatory to developing a system to make clinical images part of an online patient record, physician use of images was studied [52].

Open-Ended Interviews and Survey Questions

Open-ended interviewing requires a skillful and systematic approach to questioning participants. This can range from informal and conversational interviews to ones with a specific agenda. There are two distinctive feature of open-ended interviewing. First, the goal is to elicit the respondent's views and experiences in his or her own terms, rather than to collect data that are simply a choice among preestablished response categories. Second, the interviewer is not bound to a rigid interview format or set of questions, but should elaborate on what is being asked if a question is not understood, follow up on unanticipated and potentially valuable information with additional questions, and probe for further explanation.

For example, Kaplan and Duchon interviewed laboratory directors and chief supervisory personnel to determine what they expected the potential effects of the computer system would be on patient care, laboratory operations, and hospital operations. They asked such questions as "What effects do you expect the computer system to have?" so as not to constrain what the interviewees would answer. They also asked "What do you think this study should focus on?" so as to explore issues they had not anticipated.

A close analogue to open-ended interviewing, for large groups of respondents, is using open-ended survey questions. Kaplan and Duchon included in their survey such open-ended questions as "What important changes do you think the computer system has caused?" The final question on the survey was a request for any additional comments. Such questions are important to include in interviews and questionnaires to insure that unanticipated issues are explored.

Another way to investigate the views of groups of respondents is through focus groups. This involves interviewing several people together, and adds an opportunity for those present to react and respond to each others' remarks [53,54].

Documents and Texts

Documents, texts, pictures or photographs, and artifacts also can be valuable sources of qualitative data. For example, Nyce and Graves [55] analyzed published texts, case memoirs, and novels written by physicians in their study of the implications of knowledge construction in developing visualization systems in neurology. In Kaplan's studies of the acceptance and diffusion of medical information systems [38–40,56], she did close readings of original source documents: published research papers; populariza-tions in medical magazines, newsletters, and books; conference reports; memoirs of individuals who developed the systems; and books commis-sioned by federal agencies.

Data Analysis

The basic goal of qualitative data analysis is understanding: the search for coherence and order. The purpose of data analysis is to develop an under-standing or interpretation that answers the basic question of what is going on here. This is done through an iterative process that starts by developing an initial understanding of the setting and perspectives of the people being studied. That understanding then is tested and modified through cycles of additional data collection and analysis until an adequately coherent inter-pretation is reached [7,10].

Thus, in qualitative research, data analysis is an ongoing activity that should start as soon as the project begins and continue through the entire course of the research [5]. The processes of data collection, data analysis, interpretation, and even research design are intertwined and depend on each other.

As with data collection, data analysis methods usually cannot be precisely specified in advance. As noted previously, qualitative data collection and analysis have an inductive, cyclic character. As Agar describes it:

You learn something ("collect some data"), then you try to make sense out of it ("analysis"), then you go back and see if the interpretation makes sense in light of new experience ("collect more data"), then you refine your interpretation ("more analysis"), and so on. The process is dialectic, not linear [57].

All forms of qualitative data analysis presuppose the existence of detailed textual data, such as observational field notes, interview transcripts, or docu-ments. There also is a tendency to treat as "textual" other nonnumeric forms of data, such as diagrams or photographs. A necessary first step in data analy-sis, prior to all of the subsequent techniques, consists of reading the data. This reading is done to gain familiarity with what is going on and what people are saying or doing, and to develop initial ideas about the meaning of these state-ments and events and their relationships to other statements and events. Even at later stages in data analysis, it often is valuable to go back and reread the original data in order to see if the developing hypotheses make sense. All of the analysis techniques described below depend on this prior reading; they require the ongoing judgment and interpretation of the researcher.

There are four basic techniques of qualitative data analysis: (1) coding, (2) analytical memos, (3) displays, and (4) contextual and narrative analy-sis. They are used, separately and in combination, to help identify themes; develop categories; and explore similarities and differences in the data, and relationships among them. None of these methods is an algorithm that can be applied mechanically to the data to produce "results." We briefly discuss each of the four techniques.

Coding

The purpose of coding, in qualitative research, is different from that in experimental or survey research or content analysis. Instead of applying a preestablished set of categories to the data according to explicit, unambiguous rules, with the primary goal being to generate frequency counts of the items in each category, it instead involves selecting particular segments of data and sorting these into categories that facilitate insight, comparison, and the development of theory [46]. While some coding categories may be drawn from the evaluation questions, existing theory, or prior knowledge of the setting and system, others are developed inductively by the evaluator during the analysis, and still others are taken from the language and conceptual structure of the people studied. The key feature of most qualitative coding is that it is grounded in the data [45] (i.e., it is developed in interaction with, and is tailored to the understanding of, the particular data being analyzed).

Analytical Memos

An analytical memo is anything that a researcher writes in relationship to the research, other than direct field notes or transcription. It can range from a brief marginal comment on a transcript, or a theoretical idea incorporated into field notes, to a full-fledged analytical essay. All of these are ways of getting ideas down on paper, and of using writing as a way to facilitate reflection and analytical insight. Memos are a way to convert the researcher's perceptions and thoughts into a visible form that allows reflection and further manipulation [7,46]. Writing memos is an important analysis technique, as well as being valuable for many other purposes in the research [5], and should begin early in the study, perhaps even before starting the study [58].

Displays

Displays, such as matrices, flowcharts, and concept maps, are similar to memos in that they make ideas, data, and analysis visible and permanent. They also serve two other key functions: data reduction, and the presentation of data or analysis in a form that allows it to be grasped as a whole. These analytical tools have been given their most detailed elaboration by Miles and Huberman [7], but are employed less self-consciously by many other researchers. Such displays can be primarily conceptual, as a way of developing theory, or they can be primarily data oriented. Data-oriented displays, such as matrices, can be used as an elaboration of coding; the coding categories are presented in a single display in conjunction with a reduced subset of the data in each category. Other types of displays, such as concept maps, flowcharts, causal networks, and organizational diagrams, display connections among categories.

Contextual and Narrative Analysis

Contextual and narrative analysis has developed mainly as an alternative to coding (e.g., [59]). Instead of segmenting the data into discrete elements and resorting these into categories, these approaches to analysis seek to understand the relationships between elements in a particular text, situation, or sequence of events. Methods such as discourse analysis [60], narrative analysis [59,61], conversation analysis [62]; profiles [63], or ethnographic microanalysis [64] identify the relationships among the different elements in that particular interview or situation, and their meanings for the persons involved, rather than aggregating data across contexts. Coffey and Atkinson [65] review a number of these strategies.

Software

Qualitative methods produce large amounts of data that may not be readily amenable to manipulation, analysis, or data reduction by hand. Computer software is available that can facilitate the process of qualitative analysis [66,67]. Such programs perform some of the mechanical tasks of storing and coding data, retrieving and aggregating previously coded data, and making connections among coding categories, but do not "analyze" the data in the sense that statistical software does. All of the conceptual and analytical work of making sense of the data still needs to be done by the evaluator. There are different types of programs, some developed specifically for data analysis, and others (including word processors, textbase managers, and network builders) that can be used for some of the tasks of analysis. For relatively small-scale projects, some qualitative researchers advocate not using *any* software besides a good word processor. A very sophisticated and powerful program may be difficult to use if it has unneeded features, so it is advisable to carefully consider what the program needs to do before committing to its use. Weitzman and Miles [66] and Weitzman [67] provide a useful list of questions to consider in choosing software.

Validity

Validity in qualitative research addresses the necessarily "subjective" nature of data collection and analysis. Because the researcher is the instrument for collecting and analyzing data, the study is subjective in the sense of being different for different researchers. Different researchers may approach the same research question by collecting different data or by interpreting the same data differently.

Qualitative researchers acknowledge their role as research instruments by making it an explicit part of data collection, analysis, and reporting. As in collecting and analyzing any data, what the evaluator brings to the task—his or her biases, interests, perceptions, observations, knowledge, and critical faculties—all play a role in the study.

Qualitative researchers include in their studies specific ways to understand and control the effects of their background and role. They recognize that the relationships they develop with those studied have a major effect on the data that can be gathered and the interpretations that can be developed [8,12]. The researcher's relationships and rapport with study participants significantly influence what people will reveal in interviews and the extent to which they alter their behavior in response to an observer's presence. Similarly, researchers recognize that their personal experiences and theoretical bents influence their choice of evaluation questions, data, and interpretation. Qualitative researchers consider it their responsibility to carefully articulate previous beliefs and constantly question every observation and every interpretation so as to help avoid being blinded or misdirected by what they bring to the study [68]. They also report their backgrounds to study participants and the audience for the evaluation, including the research community, so that others may consider the potential influence on study results.

The product of any qualitative analysis is an interpretation, rather than a purely "objective" account. It often is valuable for several researchers to analyze the same data and compare results, but discrepancies between different researchers' interpretations do not automatically invalidate the results. Because of the flexibility and individual judgment inherent in qualitative methods, reliability generally is weaker than in quantitative designs, but validity often is stronger; qualitative researchers' close attention to meaning, context, and process make them less likely to ask the wrong questions or overlook or exclude important data [69]. Thus, the loss of reliability is counterbalanced by the greater validity that results from the researcher's flexibility, insight, and ability to use his or her tacit knowledge.

To further insure validity, qualitative researchers typically assess specific validity threats during data collection and analysis by testing these threats against existing data or against data collected specifically for this purpose [5,7,69–72]. Particular strategies include: (1) collecting rich data, (2) paying attention to puzzles, (3) triangulation, and (4) feedback or member checking, and (5) searching for discrepant evidence and negative cases. We discuss each of these in turn.

Rich Data

Rich data are data that are detailed and varied enough that they provide a full and revealing picture of what is going on, and of the processes involved [73]. Collecting rich data makes it difficult for the researcher to see only what supports his or her prejudices and expectations and thus provides a *test* of one's developing theories, as well as provides a basis for generating, developing, and supporting such theories.

Puzzles

One underlying assumption of qualitative methods is that things make sense [74]. They make sense to the people involved in the setting, who understand the situation in ways the research must discover or determine. Moreover, the evaluator must make sense of things. If the evaluator has not understood how sense is to be made of a situation, the evaluator has not yet achieved an adequate interpretation, perhaps because not enough data have been collected, or because the problem is being approached from the wrong perspective or theoretical framework. In particular, the evaluator must pay careful attention to resolving surprises, puzzles, and confusions as important in developing a valid interpretation [75].

Triangulation

Qualitative researchers typically collect data from a range of individuals and settings. Multiple sources and methods increase the robustness of results. Using more than one source of data and more than one method of data collection allows findings to be strengthened by cross-validating them. This process generally is known as "triangulation" [15].

When data of different kinds and sources converge and are found congruent, the results have greater credibility than when they are based on only one method or source [15,33,49,76]. However, when the data seem to diverge, in line with the assumption that things make sense and the importance of focusing on puzzles or discrepancies, an explanation must be sought to account for all of them [77].

Feedback or Member Checking

This is the single most important way of ruling out the possibility of misinterpreting the meaning of what participants say and do or what the researcher observed, and the perspective the participants have on what is going on. Feedback, or member checking, involves systematically gathering feedback about one's conclusions from participants in the setting studied [47] and from others familiar with the setting. The researcher checks that the interpretation makes sense to those who know the setting especially well. In addition, this is an important way of identifying the researcher's biases [5] and affords the possibility for collecting additional important data.

Searching for Discrepant Evidence and Negative Cases

Identifying and analyzing discrepant data and negative cases is a key part of the logic of validity testing in qualitative research. Instances that cannot be accounted for by a particular interpretation or explanation can point up important defects in that account. There are strong pressures to ignore data that do not fit prior theories or conclusions, and it is important to rigorously examine *both* supporting and discrepant data. In particularly difficult cases, the only solution may be to report the discrepant evidence and allow readers to draw their own conclusions [23].

Example

We illustrate how issues of reliability and validity can be addressed by drawing on Kaplan and Duchon's study.

In the clinical laboratory information system evaluation, Kaplan had a systems designer's working knowledge of computer hardware and software, and of terminology in clinical settings, and in particular, with order entry and results reporting systems for a clinical laboratory. She was aware that this background influenced her study. As the primary field researcher, she could listen to, and participate in, discussions among laboratory staff and have a better understanding of them. In designing the study, Kaplan, an information systems specialist, sought colleagues with backgrounds different from hers. Duchon, a specialist in organizational behavior, was unfamiliar with clinical laboratories and with information systems. Each of these two researchers had to be convinced of the other's interpretations. Further, the study's sponsors and participants were aware of the researchers' backgrounds, which also were reported in publications so that others would be able to consider for themselves what effects the researchers' backgrounds might have.

Kaplan and Duchon collected data from multiple sources using several different methods. This provided them with rich data that led to puzzles and discrepancies that required resolution. Resolving these resulted in significant insights. For example, Kaplan and Duchon explored the puzzle presented by interviewees repeatedly saying the computer system would not change laboratory technologists' jobs but that it would change what technologists did. Kaplan and Duchon developed hypotheses and tentative theories to explain how the interviewees might not see a contradiction in their statements.

They also cross-validated their results by comparing their data. Qualitative and quantitative data at first seemed not to agree. The quantitative data initially indicated no differences among laboratories in their response to the computer system, yet differences were evident in the qualitative data. Discrepancies also occurred in only the qualitative data because technologists in the same laboratory disagreed over whether the computer system was a benefit. Rather than assuming that some technologists simply were wrong, or that either the qualitative or quantitative data were in error, an explanation was needed to allow for all these responses.

Resolving these puzzles and reconciling all the data contributed to a much richer final interpretation that resulted in a theory of how views of one's job and views of a computer system are related. Study results were made available to laboratory managers for comment, and presented to laboratory directors for discussion, thus creating opportunities for feedback and member checking of the researchers' interpretations. Further feedback was obtained by presenting the theory to staff from the laboratories studied as well as to knowledgeable individuals from other, related settings.

Units and Levels of Analysis

Often qualitative evaluation research focuses on individuals and then groups individuals in familiar ways, for example, by occupation or location. Important differences among the individuals may be obscured by grouping them together in this way. For example, in the Kaplan and Duchon study, individual technologists could be categorized based on how they conceptualized their jobs, and also the individual laboratories within the institution could be so categorized. Simply considering the category "laboratory technologist" would have lost these findings and revealed little of interest in how laboratory technologists responded to the new laboratory information system. Further, there are alternatives to taking individuals as units of analysis. Researchers can study how communities pursue their goals through using information technology [78] or conduct evaluations that cross organizational, geographic, or political boundaries through virtual health care [79]. Research designs might employ different degrees of granularity and different units and levels of analysis, and investigate how changes ripple across them [6].

Conclusion

We have presented an overview of qualitative research and how it can be used for evaluating computer information systems. This chapter has covered techniques for data collection and analysis, and discussed how and why such methods may be used. We have suggested research designs and data collection and analysis approaches that meet methodological guidelines useful when developing an evaluation plan: (1) focus on a variety of technical, economic, people, organizational, and social concerns; (2) use multiple methods; (3) be modifiable; (4) be longitudinal; and (5) be formative as well as summative [80–82].

We believe that qualitative methods are useful because they provide means of answering questions that cannot be answered solely by other methods. The strengths of qualitative methods relate primarily to the understanding of a system's specific context of development and use, the ways developers and users perceive the system, and the processes by which the system is accepted, rejected, or adapted to a particular setting. We believe that these are crucial issues for the development, implementation, and evaluation of computer information systems. Consequently, qualitative methods can make an important contribution to research and evaluation of computer information systems.

Additional Reading

Qualitative Methods

Patton [10] is an excellent introduction to qualitative research methods. It also is one of the best works on qualitative approaches to evaluation. More advanced discussion of theory and methods of qualitative research can be found in Hammersley and Atkinson [8] and in Denzin and Lincoln [9].

Specific techniques for qualitative data analysis are presented in Miles and Huberman [7], Coffey and Atkinson [65], and Strauss and Corbin [46]. A useful guide to both data analysis and writing of qualitative research is Wolcott [58].

Rogers's [24] work on the adoption of innovations is relevant to the introduction of computer information systems.

Information Systems Research Theory and Methodological Frameworks

Useful discussions of theoretical perspectives in information systems research can be found in several papers. Kling [83], Kling and Scacchi [4], Lyytinen [84], and Markus and Robey [29] present theoretical frameworks that are relevant to studies of the social aspects of computing. The paradigms of information systems development Hirschheim and Klein [37] discuss also are applicable to research approaches and, in fact, were derived from such a framework. Kaplan [43] illustrates the influences of theoretical stance using a medical information system as an example. Mumford, Fitzgerald, Hirschheim, and Wood-Harper [85]; Nissen, Klein, and Hirschheim [86]; Lee, Liebenau, and DeGross [11]; and Kaplan, Truex, Wastell, Wood-Harper, and De Gross [13] reflect trends in information systems research methods, including the development of qualitative research methods in this area.

Evaluation Studies of Computing Systems

Lundsgaarde, Fischer, and Steele [35] conducted an exemplary evaluation of a medical information system that combines both qualitative and quantitative methods. The study's primary results are summarized in Fischer, Stratman, and Lundsgaarde [36]. Kaplan and Duchon [16] give a detailed account of how a medical system evaluation actually progressed, including issues pertaining to combining qualitative and quantitative methods. Kaplan [30,31] reports qualitative methods and findings of the study, and Kaplan and Duchon [32] include quantitative results.

Both and Kaplan [2] and Kaplan and Shaw [6] cite a number of excellent qualitative studies. Kaplan explains the advantages of using qualitative methods for evaluating computer applications, while Kaplan and Shaw provide a comprehensive critical review of evaluation in medical informatics.

Turkle [87,88] and Zuboff [89], though not concerned with applications of computers in medicine, each superbly illustrate the kind of observations and analysis possible by using qualitative methods. Walsham [90] provides discussion and examples of an interpretive approach to studying information systems.

Glossary

Analytical memo (or memo, for short): Broadly defined, any reflective writing the researcher does about the research, ranging from a marginal comment on a transcript, or a theoretical idea incorporated into field-notes, to a full-fledged analytical essay.

Case study: An empirical inquiry that investigates a phenomenon within a specific natural setting and uses multiple sources of evidence.

Coding: Segmenting the data into units and rearranging them into categories that facilitate insight, comparison, and the development of theory.

Context: The cultural, social, and organizational setting in which a study is conducted, together with the history of and influences on the project and the participants in it. Context also includes the relationships between the evaluation sponsor, the researchers, and those who work in or influence the setting.

Contextual analysis or narrative analysis: Analyzing the relationships between elements in a particular text, situation, or sequence of events.

Display: Any systematic visual presentation of data or theory; elaborated as a method of qualitative data analysis by Miles and Huberman [7].

Ethnography: A form of qualitative research that involves the researcher's relatively long-term and intensive involvement in the setting studied, that employs participant observation and/or open-ended interviewing as major strategies, and that attempts to understand both the cultural perspective of the participants and the influence of the physical and social context in which they operate.

Field notes: Detailed, descriptive records of observations.

Field research: See *fieldwork*.

Fieldwork or field research: The researcher's direct engagement in the setting studied.

Formative evaluation: Evaluation of a developing or ongoing program or activity. The evaluation is aimed at improving the program or activity while it is being developed or implemented. See *summative evaluation*.

Grounded theory: A theory that is inductively derived from, and tested against, qualitative data during the course of the research; also, an approach to qualitative research that emphasizes this method of theory development [45,46].

Induction: A process by which generalizations are made from many particular instances found in the data.

Iteration: Repetition of a series of steps, as in a repeating cycle of data collection, hypothesis formulation, hypothesis testing by more data collection, additional hypothesis formulation, etc.

Member checking: Getting feedback from participants in the study to check the researchers' interpretation.

Narrative analysis: See *contextual analysis.*

Open-ended interviewing: A form of interviewing that does not employ a fixed interview schedule, but allows the researcher to follow the respondent's lead by exploring topics in greater depth and also by pursuing unanticipated topics.

Open-ended questions: Interview or survey questions that are to be answered in the respondent's own words, rather than by selecting pre-formulated responses.

Participant observation: A form of observation in which the researcher participates in the activities going on in a natural setting and interacts with people in that setting, rather than simply recording their behavior as an outside observer.

Qualitative research: A strategy for empirical research that is conducted in natural settings, that uses data in the form of words (generally, though pictures, artifacts, and other non-quantitative data may be used) rather than numbers, that inductively develops categories and hypotheses, and that seeks to understand the perspectives of the participants in the setting studied, the context of that setting, and the events and processes that are taking place there.

Rich data: Data that are detailed, comprehensive, and holistic.

Robustness: Interpretations, results, or data that can withstand a variety of validity threats because they hold up even if some of the underpinnings are removed or prove incorrect.

Summative evaluation: Evaluation that is aimed at assessing the value of a developed program for the purpose of administrative or policy decisions. This evaluation often is done by testing the impact of the program after it has been implemented. See *formative evaluation.*

Triangulation: The cross-checking of inferences by using multiple methods, sources, or forms of data for drawing conclusions.

Validity: The truth or correctness of one's descriptions, interpretations, or conclusions.

Validity threat: A way in which one's description, interpretation, or conclusion might be invalid, also known as "rival hypothesis" or "alternative explanation."

References

[1] A.F. Dowling, Jr. Do hospital staff interfere with computer system implementation? Health Care Management Review 5 (1980) 23–32.

[2] B. Kaplan, Evaluating informatics applications—some alternative approaches: Theory, social interactionism, and call for methodological pluralism, International Journal of Medical Informatics 64 (2001) 39–56.

[3] B. Kaplan, Evaluating informatics applications—clinical decision support systems literature review, International Journal of Medical Informatics 64 (2001) 15–37.

[4] R. Kling and W. Scacchi, The web of computing: Computer technology as social organization, in: M.C. Yovitz, editor *Advances in Computers*, Vol. 21 (Academic Press, New York, 1982), pp. 2–90.

[5] J.A. Maxwell, *Qualitative Research Design: An Interactive Approach* (Sage Publications, Thousand Oaks, CA, 1996).

[6] B. Kaplan and N.T. Shaw, People, organizational, and social issues: Future directions in evaluation research, Methods of Information in Medicine 43 (2004) 215–231.

[7] M.B. Miles and A.M. Huberman, *Qualitative Data Analysis: An Expanded Sourcebook* (Sage Publications, Beverly Hills, CA, 1994).

[8] M. Hammersley and P. Atkinson, *Ethnography: Principles in Practice* (Routledge, London, 1995).

[9] N. Denzin and Y. Lincoln, *Handbook of Qualitative Research* (Sage Publications, Thousand Oaks, CA, 2000).

[10] M.Q. Patton, *Qualitative Research and Evaluation Methods* (Sage Publications, Thousand Oaks, CA, 2001).

[11] A.S. Lee, J. Liebenau, and J.I. DeGross, *Information Systems and Qualitative Research: IFIP Transactions* (Chapman and Hall, London, 1997).

[12] J.A. Maxwell, Realism and the role of the researcher in qualitative psychology, in: M. Kiegelmann, editor, *The Role of the Researcher in Qualitative Psychology* (Verlag Ingeborg Huber, Tuebingen, Germany, 2002), pp. 11–30.

[13] B. Kaplan, D.P. Truex III, D. Wastell, A.T. Wood-Harper, and J.I. DeGross, *Relevant Theory and Informed Practice: Looking Forward from a 20 Year Perspective on IS Research* (Kluwer Academic Publishers, London, 2004).

[14] T.D. Cook and C.S. Reichardt, *Qualitative and Quantitative Methods in Evaluation Research* (Sage Publications, Beverly Hills, 1979).

[15] T.D. Jick, Mixing qualitative and quantitative methods: Triangulation in action, in: J.V. Maanen, editor, *Qualitative Methodology* (Sage Publications, Beverly Hills, CA, 1983), pp. 135–148.

[16] B. Kaplan and D. Duchon, Combining qualitative and quantitative approaches in information systems research: A case study, Management Information Systems Quarterly 12 (1988) 571–586.

[17] L.H. Kidder and M. Fine, Qualitative and quantitative methods: When stories converge, in: M.M. Mark and R.L. Shotland, editors, *Multiple Methods in Program Evaluation* (Jossey-Bass, San Francisco, 1987), pp. 57–75.

[18] J.A. Maxwell, P.G. Bashook, and L.J. Sandlow, Combining ethnographic and experimental methods in educational research: A case study, in: D.M. Fetterman and M.A. Pitman, editors, *Educational Evaluation: Ethnography in Theory, Practice, and Politics* (Sage Publications, Beverly Hills, CA, 1986), pp. 121–143.

[19] J.C. Greene and V.J. Caracelli, *Advances in Mixed-Method Evaluation: The Challenges and Benefits of Integrating Diverse Paradigms. New Directions for Evaluation*, Vol. 74 (Summer 1997) (Jossey-Bass, San Francisco, 1997).

[20] A. Tashakkori and C. Teddlie, *Mixed Methodology: Combining Qualitative and Quantitative Approaches* (Sage Publications, Thousand Oaks CA, 1998).

[21] J.A. Maxwell and D. Loomis, Mixed methods design: An alternative approach, in: A. Tashakkori and C. Teddlie, editors, *Handbook of Mixed Methods in Social and Behavioral Research* (Sage Publications, Thousand Oaks, CA, 2002), pp. 241–271.

[22] A. Tashakkori and C. Teddlie, *Handbook of Mixed Methods in Social and Behavioral Research* (Sage Publications, Thousand Oaks, CA, 2002).

[23] H. Wolcott, *Writing Up Qualitative Research* (Sage Publications, Thousand Oaks, CA, 1990).

[24] E.M. Rogers, *Diffusion of Innovations* (The Free Press, New York, 2003).

[25] B. Kaplan, Computer Rorschach test: What do you see when you look at a computer? Physicians & Computing 18 (2001) 12–13.

[26] T. Cook, Randomized experiments in education: A critical examination of the reasons the educational evaluation community has offered for not doing them, Educational Evaluation and Policy Analysis 24 (2002) 175–199.

[27] W.R. Shadish, T.D. Cook, and D.T. Campbell, *Experimental and Quasi-Experimental Designs for Generalized Causal Inference* (Houghton Mifflin, Boston, 2002).

[28] J.A. Maxwell, Causal explanation, qualitative research, and scientific inquiry in education, Educational Researcher 33 (2004) 3–11.

[29] M.L. Markus and D. Robey, Information technology and organizational change: Causal structure in theory and research, Management Science 34 (1988) 583–598.

[30] B. Kaplan, Impact of a clinical laboratory computer system: Users' perceptions, in: R. Salamon, B.I. Blum, and J.J. Jørgensen, editors, *Medinfo 86: Fifth Congress on Medical Informatics*, North-Holland, Amsterdam (1986) 1057–1061.

[31] B. Kaplan, Initial impact of a clinical laboratory computer system: Themes common to expectations and actualities, Journal of Medical Systems 11 (1987) 137–147.

[32] B. Kaplan and D. Duchon, A job orientation model of impact on work seven months post-implementation, in: B. Barber, D. Cao, D. Qin, and G. Wagner, editors, *Medinfo 89: Sixth Conference on Medical Informatics*, North-Holland, Amsterdam (1989) pp. 1051–1055.

[33] R.K. Yin, *Case Study Research: Design and Methods* (Sage Publications, Thousand Oaks, CA, 1984).

[34] E.M. Rogers, *Diffusion of Innovations* (The Free Press, New York, 1983).

[35] H.P. Lundsgaarde, P.J. Fischer, and D.J. Steele, *Human Problems in Computerized Medicine* (The University of Kansas, Lawrence, KS, 1981).

[36] P.J. Fischer, W.C. Stratman, and H.P. Lundsgaarde, User reaction to PROMIS: Issues related to acceptability of medical innovations, in: J.G. Anderson and S.J. Jay, editors, *Use and Impact of Computers in Clinical Medicine* (Springer, New York, 1987), pp. 284–301.

[37] R. Hirschheim and H.K. Klein, Four paradigms of information systems development, Communications of the ACM 32 (1989) 1199–1216.

[38] B. Kaplan. User acceptance of medical computer applications: A diffusion approach, in: B.I. Blum, editors, *Proceedings of the Symposium on Computing Applications in Medical Care*, Silver Spring, IEEE Computer Society Press (1982), pp. 398–402.

[39] B. Kaplan, The computer as Rorschach: Implications for management and user acceptance, in: R.E. Dayhoff, editor, *Proceedings Symposium Computing Application Medical Care*, Silver Spring, IEEE Computer Society Press (1983), pp. 664–667.

[40] B. Kaplan, The influence of medical values and practices on medical computer applications, in: J.G. Anderson and S.J. Jay, editors, *Use and Impact of Computers in Clinical Medicine* (Springer, New York, 1987), pp. 39–50.

[41] C. Sicotte, J. Denis, and P. Lehoux, The computer-based patient record: A strategic issue in process innovation, Journal of Medical Systems 22 (1998) 431–443.

[42] C. Sicotte, J. Denis, P. Lehoux, and F. Champagne, The computer-based patient record: Challenges toward timeless and spaceless medical practice, Journal of Medical Systems 22 (1998) 237–256.

[43] B. Kaplan, Models of change and information systems research, in: H.-E. Nissen, H.K. Klein, and R. Hirschheim, editors, *Information Systems Research: Contemporary Approaches and Emergent Traditions* (North Holland, Amsterdam, 1991), pp. 593–611.

[44] B. Kaplan, D.P. Truex III, D. Wastell, and A.T. Wood-Harper, Young Turks, Old Guardsmen, and the conundrum of the broken mold: A progress report on twenty years of IS research, in: B. Kaplan, D.P. Truex III, D. Wastell, A.T. Wood-Harper, and J.I. De Gross, editors, *Information Systems Research: Relevant Theory and Informed Practice* (Kluwer Academic Publishers, Boston, Dordrecht, London, 2004) pp. 1–18.

[45] B.G. Glaser and A.L. Strauss, *The Discovery of Grounded Theory: Strategies for Qualitative Research* (Aldine, New York, 1967).

[46] A. Strauss and J.M. Corbin, *Basics of Qualitative Research: Techniques and Procedures for Developing Grounded Theory* (Sage Publications, Thousand Oaks, CA, 1998).

[47] E.G. Guba and Y.S. Lincoln, *Fourth Generation Evaluation* (Sage Publications, Newbury Park, CA, 1989).

[48] B. Kaplan, National Health Service reforms: Opportunities for medical informatics research, in: K.C. Lun, P. Deglulet, T.E. Piemme, and O. Reinhoff, editors, *Medinfo 92: Seventh Conference on Medical Informatics*, Amsterdam, Elsevier Science Publishers (1992), pp. 1166–1171.

[49] T.V. Bonoma, Case research in marketing: Opportunities, problems, and a process, Journal of Marketing Research 22 (1985) 199–208.

[50] D.E. Forsythe, B. Buchanan, J. Osheroff, and R. Miller, Expanding the concept of medical information: An observational study of physicians' information needs, Computers and Biomedical Research 25 (1992) 181–200.

[51] J. Osheroff, D. Forsythe, B. Buchanan, R. Bankowitz, B. Blumenfeld, and R. Miller, Physicians' information needs: Analysis of clinical questions posed during patient care activity, Annals of Internal Medicine 14 (1991) 576–581.

[52] B. Kaplan, Objectification and negotiation in interrupting clinical images: Implications for computer-based patient records, Artificial Intelligence in Medicine 7 (1995) 439–454.

[53] D. Fafchamps, C.Y. Young, and P.C. Tang, Modelling work practices: Input to the design of a physician's workstation, in: P.D. Clayton, editor, *Proceedings*

Symposium Computing Application Medical Care, New York, McGraw Hill (1991), pp. 788–792.

[54] R.A. Krueger and M.A. Casey, *Focus Groups: A Practical Guide for Applied Research* (Sage Publications, Thousand Oaks, CA, 2000).

[55] J.M. Nyce and W.I. Graves, The construction of knowledge in neurology: Implications for hypermedia system development, Artificial intelligence in Medicine 29 (1990) 315–322.

[56] B. Kaplan, Development and acceptance of medical information systems: An historical overview, Journal of Health and Human Resources Administration 11 (1988) 9–29.

[57] M.H. Agar, *The Professional Stranger: An Informal Introduction to Ethnography* (Academic Press, New York, 1980).

[58] H. Wolcott, *Writing Up Qualitative Research* (Sage Publications, Thousand Oaks, CA, 2001).

[59] E. Mishler, *Research Interviewing: Context and Narrative.* (Harvard University Press, Cambridge, MA, 1986).

[60] J.P. Gee, S. Michaels, and M.C. O'Connor, Discourse analysis, in: M.D. LeCompte, W.L. Millroy, and J. Preissle, editors, *The Handbook of Qualitative Research in Education*, Vol. 227–291 (Academic Press, San Diego, 1992).

[61] C.K. Riessman, *Narrative Analysis* (Sage Publications, Thousand Oaks, CA, 1993).

[62] G. Psathas, *Conversation Analysis: The Study of Talk-in-Interaction* (Sage Publications, Thousand Oaks, CA, 1955).

[63] I.E. Seidman, *Interviewing as Qualitative Research: A Guide for Researchers in Education and the Social Sciences* (Teachers College Press, New York, 1998).

[64] F. Erickson, Ethnographic microanalysis of interaction, in: M.D. LeCompte, W.L. Millroy, and J. Preissle, editors, *The Handbook of Qualitative Research in Education* (Academic Press, San Diego, 1992), pp. 201–225.

[65] A. Coffey and P. Atkinson, *Making Sense of Qualitative Data* (Sage Publications, Thousand Oaks, CA, 1996).

[66] E. Weitzman and M. Miles, *Computer Programs for Qualitative Data Analysis* (Sage Publications, Thousand Oaks, CA, 1995).

[67] E. Weitzman, Software and qualitative research, in: N. Denzin and Y. Lincoln, editors, *Handbook of Qualitative Research* (Sage Publications, Thousand Oaks, CA, 2000), pp. 803–820.

[68] P. Eckert, *Jocks and Burnouts: Social Categories and Identity in the High School* (Teachers College Press, New York, 1989).

[69] J. Kirk and M.L. Miller, *Reliability and Validity in Qualitative Research* (Sage Publications, Thousand Oaks, CA, 1986).

[70] M.A. Eisenhart and K.R. Howe, Validity in educational research, in: M.D. LeCompte, W.L. Millroy, and J. Preissle, editors, *The Handbook of Qualitative Research in Education* (Academic Press, San Diego, 1992), pp. 643–680.

[71] J.A. Maxwell, Understanding and validity in qualitative research, Harvard Educational Review 62 (1992) 279–300.

[72] J.A. Maxwell, Using qualitative methods for causal explanation, Field Methods 16(3), (August 2004), pp. 243–264.

[73] H.S. Becker, Field work evidence, in: H.S. Becker, editor, *Sociological Work: Method and Substance* (Aldine, Chicago, 1970), pp. 39–62.

[74] E. Bredo and W. Feinberg, Part two: The interpretive approach to social and educational research, in: E. Bredo and W. Feinberg, editors, *Knowledge and Values in Social and Educational Research* (Temple University Press, Philadelphia, 1982), pp. 115–128.

[75] M.H. Agar, *Speaking of Ethnography* (Sage Publications, Beverly Hills, CA, 1986).

[76] I. Benbasat, D.K. Goldstein, and M. Mead, The case research strategy in studies of information systems, MIS Quarterly 11 (1987) 369–386.

[77] M.G. Trend, On the reconciliation of qualitative and quantitative analyses: A case study, in: T.D. Cook and C.S. Reichardt, editors, *Qualitative and Quantitative Methods in Evaluation Research* (Sage Publications, Beverly Hills, CA, 1979), pp. 68–86.

[78] B. Kaplan, L. Kvasny, S. Sawyer, and E.M. Trauth, New words and old books: Challenging conventional discourses about domain and theory in information systems research, in: M.D. Myers, E.A. Whitley, E. Wynn, and J.I. De Gross, editors, *Global and Organizational Discourse About Information Technology* (Kluwer Academic Publishers, London, 2002), pp. 539–545.

[79] B. Kaplan, P.F. Brennan, A.F. Dowling, C.P. Friedman, and V. Peel, Towards an informatics research agenda: Key people and organizational issues, Journal of the American Medical Informatics Association 8 (2001) 234–241.

[80] B. Kaplan, A model comprehensive evaluation plan for complex information systems: Clinical imaging systems as an example, in: A. Brown and D. Remenyi, editors, *Proceedings 2nd European Conference on Information Technology Investment Evaluation*, Henley on Thames, Birmingham, England, Operational Research Society (1995), pp. 14–181.

[81] B. Kaplan, Organizational evaluation of medical information systems, in: C.P. Friedman and J.C. Wyatt, editors, *Evaluation Methods in Medical Informatics* (Springer, New York, 1997), pp. 255–280.

[82] B. Kaplan, Addressing organizational issues into the evaluation of medical systems, Journal of the American Medical Informatics Association 4 (1997) 94–101.

[83] R. Kling, Social analyses of computing: Theoretical perspectives in recent empirical research, ACM Computing Surveys 12 (1980) 61–110.

[84] K. Lyytinen, Different perspectives on information systems: Problems and solutions, ACM Computing Surveys 19 (1987) 5–46.

[85] E. Mumford, G. Fitzgerald, R. Hirschheim, and A.T. Wood-Harper. *Research Methods in Information Systems* (North Holland, Amsterdam, 1985).

[86] H.-E. Nissen, H.K. Klein, and R. Hirschheim. *Information Systems Research: Contemporary Approaches and Emergent Traditions* (North Holland, Amsterdam, 1991).

[87] S. Turkle, *The Second Self: Computers and the Human Spirit* (Simon & Schuster, New York, 1984).

[88] S. Turkle, *Life on the Screen: Identity in the Age of the Internet* (Simon & Schuster, New York, 1995).

[89] S. Zuboff, *In the Age of the Smart Machine: The Future of Work and Power* (Basic Books, New York, 1988).

[90] G. Walsham, *Interpreting Information Systems in Organizations* (Wiley, Chichester, 1993).

3
Multiple Perspectives: Evaluating Healthcare Information Systems in Collaborative Environments

MADHU REDDY and ERIN BRADNER

Introduction

Patient care teams play a critical role in health care. A wide variety of practitioners—nurses, pharmacists, social workers, physicians, and others—work together on a day-by-day, hour-by-hour, and even minute-by-minute basis to provide patient care [1–6]. Although these teams vary depending on their roles and responsibilities, they have become an important and integral feature of medical care. Consequently, we must ensure that we design information systems to appropriately support patient care teams. In this chapter, we argue that good system design requires us not only to develop information systems with teams in mind but also to evaluate them within the context of a team.

Healthcare System Development

Many current healthcare information systems are developed with a focus on the individual user [7,8]. However, these same systems are often utilized in teams to support collaboration [9,10]. For instance, the electronic patient record (EPR) is viewed by most people as a repository for patient information. Individual healthcare workers can access the EPR to find out details about the patient's condition. Although it does serve as a patient information repository, the EPR also helps support coordination among team members by providing them with information about what other team members have done for the patient [11]. Clinical systems such as the EPR have played a more collaborative role than originally anticipated by their designers. Yet, evaluations of healthcare technology usually focus on how well it supports the individual user, for instance, focusing on the suitability and effectiveness of the user interface for single-user interaction [12]. With a few exceptions [4,5,10], evaluating how well these systems support collaboration is often ignored. For clinical systems, we must not only evaluate how well they store the information but also how well they support the collaborative features of team members' work.

Evaluation Techniques

Evaluating information systems within a team setting is often difficult because of the multiple perspectives present in a team. For instance, in a study of an electronic patient record system in a surgical intensive care unit (SICU) [13], the first author examined a patient care team of residents, fellows, attendings, pharmacists, and nurses. Each team member brought different backgrounds, perspectives, and skills to the team. These different skills and perspectives had implications for the adoption and use of the patient record system in the unit. To understand how the system was used in the unit, the first author needed to examine how the different members utilized the system and had to evaluate it from as many different perspectives on the team as possible.

However, this type of evaluation is not easy because of the need to understand the technology from diverse perspectives. To address this challenge, healthcare researchers have used a wide variety of techniques and methods for evaluating information systems. These evaluation methods include *qualitative* techniques such as observations and interviews [14–16] and *quantitative* techniques such as surveys [17,18]. Although much of our discussion in this chapter focuses on qualitative evaluation techniques, we do not claim that these are the only techniques or even always the most appropriate for evaluating information systems. The suitable evaluation technique depends on the nature and scope of the particular study. In many instances, quantitative methods have played an important role in understanding information systems use in teams [19–21].

While quantitative techniques have provided important insights into information systems, our experiences as well as others [9,22] have shown that qualitative methods provide us some of the best approaches to trying to answer the "how" and "why" questions of evaluation studies [23]. These questions bring to the forefront the important role that information systems play in supporting team activity. For instance, the question "How can an information system make team coordination more effective?" is difficult to answer without examining the different ways that team members coordinate with each other and the type of work activities that require coordination. Qualitative techniques allow researchers to try to answer these questions in greater detail.

The main goal of this chapter is to discuss how to evaluate information systems used in patient care teams. We will provide the reader with examples of information systems evaluation and methods, drawing from the first author's field study of EPR use in an intensive care unit. The reader should, at the end of this chapter, have a better understanding of how to evaluate information systems used in teams. The chapter is outlined as follows. In the next section, we discuss teams and the importance of context. In the section on the SICU team, we provide a brief field study of a technology use within a team. In the section following that, we present qualitative methods to evaluating information systems in teams. We then conclude with some comments about studying information systems use in team settings.

Teams and Context of Use

In this section, we discuss teams and technology use. First, we provide an introduction to teams. We then discuss healthcare teams. Finally, we discuss the importance of context in evaluating information systems.

Teams

Individuals rarely work independently in modern organizations. Instead, the dominant setting for work in these environments is interdisciplinary or multifunctional teams; people collaborating with others to accomplish their tasks. These teams play a vital role in an organization's ability to implement its goals.

The term "team" has been defined in a variety of different ways. Some researchers consider the term to be interchangeable with "group," especially "work groups" [24,25]. Hackman [25] defines three essential attributes for a work group:

1. Work groups are *real groups*. They are intact social systems, with boundaries, interdependence among members, and differentiated member roles.
2. They have one or more tasks to perform. The group produces some outcome for which members have collective responsibility and whose acceptability is potentially assessable.
3. They operate in an organizational context. The group, as a collective, manages relations with other individuals or groups in the larger social system in which the group operates.

Similarly, the classic self-managed, or autonomous, manufacturing team is six to 20 people organized around complementary tasks, with self-contained output [26]. Teams have been characterized in a variety of different ways: as an intellectual collective [27], a basic unit of performance [28], and a continuing work unit [29]. In organizations, five types of teams are said to exist: work teams, project teams, parallel teams (a.k.a. task forces), management teams, and ad hoc networks [29].

Although defining teams is difficult, one approach is to consider the dichotomies often used to classify groups (Table 3.1). Our working definition of teams is small groups in which participation is mandated by management. In teams, formal roles are prescribed by the organizational structure (managers don't stop being managers when they work on a team). Informal roles, such as team peacemaker, are emergent. Finally, time

TABLE 3.1. Properties and dichotomies commonly used to classify groups.

Dimensions	Examples
Setting	*Work:* Work group; occupational group; task force; team.
	Social: gang; religious group; club; sport team.
	Other: therapy group; political committee; jury.
Properties	Size (number of members)
	Amount of physical interaction among members
	Level of cohesion
	Extent of formalization of norms
	Extent of formalization of roles
	Extent of formalization of task
Dichotomies	Formal-informal
	Primary-secondary
	Voluntary-involuntary
	Small-large

matters in teams [30]. Teams have a task; that task is planned and carried out over a period of time.

Management guru Peter Drucker [31] argues that the strength of teams lies in their adaptability:

Teams are adaptable. They are highly receptive to experimentation, to new ideas and to new ways of doing things. They are the best means available for overcoming insulation and parochialism.

Nevertheless, it is this adaptability that poses challenges for designing information systems to support teams. For example, the adaptability enabled by the integration of multiple perspectives on a healthcare team can be difficult to define and capture in the design of an EPR system.

Teams in Health Care

Within most healthcare organizations, teams can be split into two broad categories: nonclinical and clinical. Nonclinical teams focus on the business and other nonclinical aspects of the organizations such as patient billing and patient admissions and discharge. In contrast, clinical or patient care teams are responsible for making the patient care decisions [4]. The clinical teams consist of a wide range of workers—physicians, nurses, pharmacists, physical therapists, and others—who provide patient care. Although physicians, nurses, pharmacists, and other members may have different concerns, work, and motivations [32], their primary goal as a team is to improve the patient's condition. These teams range from the well-known patient care team in hospitals portrayed in popular American television shows such as *ER* to seldom-mentioned home healthcare teams [33]. However, whether clinical teams are well-known or not, they are central to providing care for the patient. In many organizations, there are often teams that contain both types of personnel. For instance, teams dealing with technology implementation issues in hospitals often have both clinical and nonclinical personnel [34].

We focus on clinical teams in this chapter. Clinical teams play a crucial role in patient care and are of particular interest to researchers interested in developing and evaluating healthcare information systems.

Technology and Context of Use

Medical work is an inherently collaborative activity. Baggs and associates [1,2] found that poor collaboration between physicians and nurses in an ICU setting resulted in poor patient outcomes. To provide appropriate patient care, team members must interact frequently with each other. Information systems play a vital role in supporting this interaction. For instance, an information system such as the electronic patient record—as a repository of collected data, observations, and plans—is central to supporting teamwork. Team members routinely use the record to exchange patient care information. Physicians read nursing observations about the patient in the record and write orders for nurses to carry out. Therapists may read both nursing and physician notes before writing a therapy plan. The ability to exchange information through the record supports collaboration and co-ordination among healthcare team members.

When evaluating information systems used in teams, it is important to understand the *context* in which the technology is utilized [35]. Most evaluations focus only on the interaction between the user and the system; they tend to ignore the environment around the system. The lack of contextual understanding of the system could lead to inaccurate evaluations of a system. Orlikowski's [36] examination of an organizational adoption of *Lotus Notes*™ points to the importance of context. If she had not examined the organizational structure and found that disincentives for information sharing exist, then individuals looking at the low adoption levels of the information sharing tool *Lotus Notes* could have blamed the system itself for the failure, not the organizational context. Thus, Orlikowski's examination of the organizational context of the system allowed her to more accurately evaluate the system. Forsythe's comments about the importance of context further highlights its importance in evaluation studies. She [37] argues that:

The lack of contextual features also raises questions about whether important components of meaning are missing from the analysis.

Without examining the context, researchers would have a difficult time understanding the true reasons for a system's success or failure. Kaplan and Duchon [21] note that "the stripping of context buys 'objectivity' and testability at the cost of a deeper understanding of what actually is occurring." Therefore, removing the context of the system could make it easier to evaluate some aspects of the system. Yet, conversely, it would make it more difficult for researchers to examine issues such as the system's "fit" with its environment when evaluating the system.

Understanding the context of use is an important component to evaluating information technology use in teams. This requires evaluators to understand the team's daily work activities in order to understand how a particular technology will be used by team members. One way to accomplish this is via the ethnographic field study method. In the next section, we provide an example of a field study from our research.

SICU Team: A Field Study of Information Systems Use

This study took place in the surgical intensive care unit (SICU) of an 840-bed urban teaching hospital [5,11,38]. The SICU provides intensive care-monitoring, invasive and noninvasive, for patients requiring special attention after a surgical procedure. It consists of two 10-bed units each of which has the same technologies, staffing, and physical layout. Information technology plays a crucial role in this SICU. An EPR system—CareVue—mediates much of the work among unit staff, especially physicians, nurses, and pharmacists. The staff has used CareVue for more than 9 years and is well acquainted with its functionality [39]. Originally implemented in the SICU, the system is now in use in eight of the other nine ICUs in the hospital.

To collect data, the first author observed work of the SICU patient care team over a seven-month period. He collected data through more than 30 interviews and observations. The interviews were taped and transcribed. He also collected and analyzed CareVue application and internal communications, including written policies, procedures, and meeting notes.

SICU Team

Although the SICU had a wide variety of workers, the core of the SICU team consisted of:

- Three surgical residents.
- Two surgical fellows (to supervise the residents).
- Surgical attending—a surgical faculty member headed the team.
- SICU pharmacist—a pharmacist was assigned to the SICU team.
- Nurses—the SICU had 50 critical care nurses.

The primary goal of the SICU team is to stabilize patients as quickly as possible so they can be safely transferred out of the unit. Effective and timely coordination between physicians, nurses, and pharmacists is critical, otherwise the patient will suffer. In one observed example, a nurse failed to notify the physician that the patient's sodium was rising to dangerous levels. If the physician had been notified quickly, he would have been able to give the patient medication to lower the sodium. However, the physician only found out about the sodium levels six hours later, by which time the patient's condition had deteriorated so far that the physician had to intubate the patient to protect her airways. As the example highlights, team members work under constant time pressure that can affect patient care. Therefore, on a daily basis, the physicians, nurses, and pharmacists must successfully coordinate their activities to ensure appropriate patient care.

SICU Team Work

The SICU team has both formal and informal responsibilities. Formally, the SICU team must visit all the patients in the unit two times a day—morning and afternoon rounds. Informally, team members must continuously collaborate with each other to ensure that patients receive appropriate medication. To provide a better understanding of how CareVue is integrated into the work practices of the SICU, we briefly present two team work examples: morning rounds and medication administration.

Morning Rounds

SICU morning rounds play an important role in the unit's patient care process. The goal of morning rounds is to discuss and decide on a plan of care for that day for each patient. During morning rounds, the SICU team visits each patient. The team begins by viewing x-rays of all the SICU patients. After examining the x-rays, the team "rounds" on each patient. Each of the three residents is responsible for a certain number of patients in the unit. During rounds, the residents "present" their patients to the team. As a resident outlines the patient's current condition, vital signs, and other information, the fellow and other team members view the patient's record on the CareVue workstation. They do this both to verify the resident's information and to gather other pertinent information. As one fellow stated, "It is much easier for me to find the information in the system than to wait for them [residents] to give it to me." After the resident presents, the fellow examines the patient. The team then discusses the patient's condition and decides on the plan of care for the day. After all the decisions are made, a resident writes a progress note in the patient's CareVue record.

Medication Administration

Ordering and administering medication requires collaboration between physicians, nurses, and pharmacists. In routine situations, most surgeons use a standard set of drugs. However, for complex cases, nurses and pharmacists often provide information that help physicians tailor the medication prescription. Since nurses are constantly by the bedside, they can inform physicians about the patient's physical and mental state. This information can help physicians to decide whether a current drug and dosage are appropriate. If physicians need to prescribe a drug for a problem with which they are not familiar, pharmacists can provide a list of appropriate medications.

Nurses must collaborate directly with both physicians and pharmacists. When ordered to give an unfamiliar drug, nurses commonly ask the physician why it is being given, especially when the drug causes discomfort or pain to the patient. Most physicians want the nurse to understand the plan of care and will answer such questions readily. The nurses also ask the pharmacist questions concerning the medication and dosage administration. For certain kinds of drugs, such as pain relievers, it is the nurse who observes the patient's response most directly, and whose opinion is usually given high regard by physicians for subsequent pain medication orders.

CareVue: Supporting Collaboration

During morning rounds and medication administration, SICU team members must continuously interact with each other in order to provide appropriate patient care. CareVue plays an important role in supporting this collaboration among team members. In the following section, we describe how CareVue supports collaboration during the medication administration process.

Awareness

One important way that CareVue supports collaboration among team members is by providing "awareness." Dourish and Bellotti [40] define awareness as "the understanding of the activities of others which provides a context for your own activity." Individuals can more efficiently coordinate their work if they know about one another's activities. Bricon-Souf and colleagues [41] argue that one way to support successful collaboration is to share information about users' work activities. An EPR can provide users with this awareness, if it is designed to incorporate:

• Knowledge of others' work activities
• Knowledge of an individual's own work activities

CareVue's presentation of medication information supports awareness. All healthcare providers need information about the patient's medication; however, the exact information they need varies with their roles. CareVue provides a different view of the data to different team members (Figure 3.1). These customized views of shared information allow team members to remain aware of what other team members are doing in the medication process. Physicians (Figure 3.1A) can see what medications have been

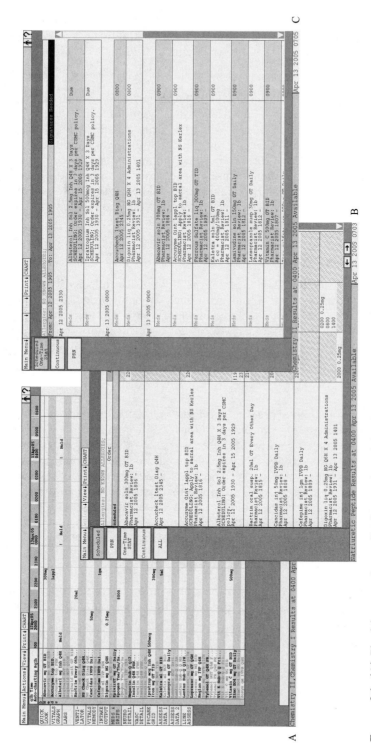

FIGURE 3.1. (A) Physicians use the medication section of the CareVue Flowsheet to check on patient medications. It provides them with the dosage and administration time. (B) Nurses and pharmacists use the Medication Administration Record (MAR) to provide them with the more detailed information on each medication. (C) Nurses also use the nursing Medication Worklist to keep track of their work activities. It lists the medications for a patient and when they need to be given.

administered and are scheduled to be administered by the nurse. Since physicians need to quickly survey the status of the treatment, the Flowsheet provides them with quick information about the nurses' past and future work actions regarding patient medication. If physicians have any questions about these actions, they can look elsewhere in CareVue or contact the patient's nurse.

Nurses and pharmacists use a different visual interface, the Medication Administration Record (MAR) (Figure 3.1B). The MAR provides additional details about each drug and keeps nurses and pharmacists aware of each other's activities regarding the medications. When a pharmacist approves each medication, he adds an electronic signature to the MAR that is visible to the nurse. Thus, the nurse is aware that the pharmacist has checked the drug for appropriateness, route, and dosage. To administer medications effectively and on time, nurses use another view of the MAR, the Medication Worklist (Figure 3.1C). The Worklist provides a time-ordered list of the medications, dosages, and administration times for all drugs due to be administered on the current nursing shift. The Worklist allows nurses to know what actions the other team members expect from them in the near future. For convenience, nurses can chart drugs as "given" or "held" directly on the Worklist. Such information instantly appears in the other members' views. CareVue's ability to transform information into different views that are understandable to each member helps the members remain constantly aware of each other's activities.

Clinical systems are not simply information repositories of patient data but rather are an integral part of the collaboration among healthcare team members. This field study described how an EPR supported team activities such as medication administration. The system kept team members informed about each other's activities, allowing them to coordinate their work more effectively. Evaluating the system to see how effectively it supported "awareness" required using qualitative methods that allowed us to examine not only the system but the environment (e.g., work) surrounding the system. In the next section we discuss in more detail qualitative research methods.

Qualitative Methods

Qualitative methods are the leading technique for investigating organizational and technological settings in research on collaboration (e.g., [42,43,44]). In health care, these methods have also been widely used to study technology use in teams (e.g., [5,45,46]). Using qualitative methods requires the system evaluators to become ethnographers—observing work environments, artifacts, and human interaction to form an understanding of the culture of a given technology setting in order to accurately evaluate the system.

Data Collection

Using ethnographic techniques such as observations and interviews, researchers have examined a wide variety of social phenomenon in situ [47,48]. Phenomena that are most amenable to qualitative research are those that have multifaceted interdependencies that make it difficult to separate the independent and dependent variables; this is especially true in complex settings where technical, organizational, and social factors intersect (e.g., [36,49]). Ethnographic techniques used by researchers include observations, interviews, and artifact collection.

- *Observations.* In qualitative field study, the researcher must engage in direct observation of the study environment (i.e., the field). The researcher attempts to be a faithful witness to the working lives of people being studied [47,48]. Observations are logged while the researcher is *looking, listening* and *asking* questions (*ibid.*). The ratio of each activity is dictated by the environment and events being observed. The researcher must strive to faithfully document his observations as they occur, avoiding injecting his opinion or bias. For example, for the field study described in the previous section, the first author directly observed work in the SICU for seven months; he was given permission to don a white coat and carry a clipboard while shadowing different members of the patient care team. In the early stages of his observations, he hung around the unit during the day taking field notes about worker–worker interactions, worker–system interactions, and general work practices. He observed both day-shift and night-shift work. He also attended regular meetings organized and attended by the CareVue operations team.
- *Interviews.* Compared to observation, interviewing trades breadth for depth with regard to understanding each team member's roles, responsibilities, and perspectives. Interviews are commonly conducted using a semistructured list of topics for discussion. The list is used as a guide for conversation, not as a questionnaire that is read verbatim [47,48]. The researcher must strive to avoid leading questions. At times, she must also be willing to permit the interview subject to recast the interview questions in a language and context that is relevant to the subject. The degree to which an interview subject *recasts* the interview questions provides data about him and about the work environment that can be used to refine the questions for subsequent interviews. To better understand patient care team members' jobs as well as their views about CareVue, the first author conducted a number of interviews at his field site. The interviews lasted between a half-hour and forty-five minutes in length. The interviews were driven by a previously prepared set of questions; however, this set of questions was only a guide to topics of interest. In many cases, the interviews took different and interesting turns that provided the author with greater insight into people's work practices. The interviews were tape-recorded and transcribed for later data analysis.

- *Artifact collection.* Artifacts are physical objects in the environment that are significantly meaningful to the members of the work team. For example, in the field study described above, the first author collected documents recording the policies and procedures of the SICU. He also collected screenshots of the various CareVue software interfaces used by members of the patient care teams.

The data collection techniques provided the tools to gather rich, informative data. However, the data are meaningless unless they are appropriately analyzed.

Analysis

Qualitative data are characteristically text-based and voluminous. Transcripts from interviews and notes from observations of a modest study often constitute hundreds of pages of text. The question becomes, how does one distill meaningful patterns, or theories, from this unstructured body of text? The researcher does not distill the data; instead he creates and distills analytical categories that describe meaningful uniformities in the data. Theories about the data emerge through an iterative process of comparing and delimiting categories [50,51]. This approach to data analysis is known as *grounded theory.* Applied to information systems in health care, grounded theory dictates that the abstract principles formulated to describe a healthcare setting must be grounded in the data and thus must be the product of inductive rather than deductive reasoning. A detailed discussion of grounded theory is beyond the scope of this chapter, yet an understanding of the philosophy and techniques is warranted.

The ethnographic approach to the analysis of qualitative data involves reviewing the data and creating a classification scheme to describe (i.e., *code*), all relevant observations. The creative researcher can generate innumerable descriptive categories to code her data. How does she know when she is finished coding her data? Glaser and Strauss [51] provide these two heuristics: *parsimony* and *scope.* The researcher achieves parsimony of categories through careful comparison of each category to all others to verify that each category is unique. The researcher achieves parsimony of theory through integrating categories into cohesive conceptual clusters. Integrating categories is a natural byproduct of the constant comparison of categories. The researcher achieves scope when she delineates the boundaries of the categories (e.g., what the category does and does not apply to).

For example, in analyzing interviews with patient care teams, the data may reveal that both physicians and nurses need to track the administration of medication. When the data document a nurse or physician making a mental note of the next time a particular medication must be administered, this might be categorized as "awareness of medication administration schedule." Yet, when the data document a physician scanning records for the frequency and synchronicity of administration of multiple medications to assess the possibility of a drug interaction, this might be compared and then integrated with the "schedule" category and labeled "awareness of co-administration of medications." Various additional variables about medication administration, such as the route a nurse must use to deliver the drug or the physician's personal preference for one particular drug over another may be contained in the data that are not categorized. They are not categorized to maintain parsimony of the categories and to focus the scope of the analysis on the awareness of medication administration schedule rather than execution of medication administration (e.g., route) or medication preferences.

By constraining the scope of the analysis in this manner the researcher may theorize about the effectiveness of various EPR interfaces on collaboration—in our example, the data would reveal that an interface that provides a separate administration schedule for each drug may be sufficient for the nurse but may be entirely inappropriate for the physician. Thus the researcher's theories about the effectiveness of an EPR interface emerge through the parsimonious use of descriptive categories, through the integration of categories, and by scoping the analysis to observations that pertain to information awareness.

Themes

Here we ask the reader to recall several key themes discussed in the CareVue field study. We consider these themes to be a few of the universal properties of collaborating in teams that are germane to the evaluation of information systems. These themes include *workflow dependencies, awareness, multiple perspectives on information*, and *shared artifacts*. We will briefly discuss each of the themes for purposes of providing specific questions to ask when evaluating information systems use in teams.

Dependencies

Some degree of workflow dependencies exist in all team work. The factory assembly line is the canonical example of highly interdependent team work. Factory automation is evaluated based on the effectiveness by which it isolates and orders the dependencies between factory workers along an assembly line. The dependencies of a patient care team are less visible due to the intellectual nature of the work, nevertheless they are present. The medication administration process highlights the interdependences that exist among members of a patient care team. The physicians order the medications but do not have the ability to continuously monitor the effects of the medication on the patient. The nurses can monitor the patient but cannot order the medications that are needed by the patient. Finally, the pharmacist cannot order the medications nor monitor the patient but has the detailed knowledge of particular medications needed by both the physicians and nurses. Therefore, each team member depends on the other members in order to successfully carry out the medication administration process.

To expose and analyze dependencies on a patient care team, a researcher may ask questions regarding how work is ordered, reordered, communicated, delegated, and controlled for quality. Questions may include: How is a patient's presenting condition assessed and documented? How is the presenting condition communicated to the team? How is a patient diagnosed? Once a diagnosis is made, how is the plan of care documented and shared with the team? How is the quality of care assessed?

Awareness

Members of work teams must share detailed information about their activities and knowledge with each other in order to coordinate their work. Often, awareness is achieved through peripherally monitoring the conversations or behaviors of others in collocated workspaces; for example, air traffic controllers routinely monitor the pilot–controller conversations of their teammates in the control tower [42]. On first examination, peripheral auditory monitoring may remain undetected by the researcher—since it is peripheral and auditory—and it may even seem inconsequential. Yet consider the consequences of implementing an information system that converts conversations in an air traffic control tower from a verbal format that is easily monitored by all occupants of the tower to a textual format. According to data from ethnographic studies of air traffic controllers, doing so would likely slow the detection of incidents when conflicting flight instructions are given to pilots.

Similarly, shared awareness among members of patient care teams is vital to maintaining high quality care. Patients suffer when awareness breaks down. In his evaluation of the CareVue EPR system, the first author observed an incident reported above in which a nurse noted that patient's sodium was rising to dangerous levels, yet failed to notify the physician. If the physician had been alerted quickly (i.e., if there were a shared awareness among the nurse and physician of this condition) the physician would have medicated the patient to lower the sodium. Unfortunately, the physician learned about the rising sodium levels only after the patient's condition had deteriorated so far that he had to intubate the patient. Likewise, shared awareness about the time and route a medication is administered is crucial to delivering quality patient care.

Thus, when evaluating information systems in healthcare settings the researcher must carefully probe issues of awareness among team members. Research questions may include: How is information about a patient (vital statistics, medical administration, patient complaints, history, etc.) formally documented in the system? How is this information formally shared among members of the team (consider how it is verbally shared as well as how and when it is printed from the system)? How is this information informally shared: via impromptu conversation, marginalia in written records, special numeric codes sent via numeric pagers, and so forth? To what extent does the system accommodate informal observations and annotations? For what periods of time do different kinds of information remain relevant? To what extent does the credibility of the information provider affect the way information is documented and used? What happens when awareness breaks down? How does the information system under evaluation help or hinder information sharing?

Multiple Perspectives on Information

The discussion of CareVue's Flowsheet in the field study provides a nice example of multiple perspectives on information in an EPR interface [5]. Recall that in CareVue, physicians can see not only nurses' past medication administration but also future medication administration activities. Nurses see a time-ordered list of the medications, dosages, and administration times for all drugs due to be administered on the current nursing shift. These two different views provide the team members with different information required to carry out their responsibilities, while preserving the uniformity of the underlying medication data.

When evaluating the appropriateness of an information system vis-à-vis multiple perspectives on information, the researcher might ask the following questions: What are the information needs of each member of the work team: How are these needs similar across the formal work role and how are they unique? What, if any, information can be shared in a universal format (by what media, in what level of detail)? What information must be tailored to specific work role and why? What are the consequences of one member of the team viewing, editing, or deleting information intended for the other members?

Shared Artifacts

In the context of this discussion of information systems evaluation in healthcare settings, a shared artifact is any meaningful object that is manipulated by multiple members of a work team to aid in patient care. For example, in the ICU unit studied by the first author, a whiteboard at the nurses' station constituted a shared artifact that warranted study. This whiteboard was used by the entire team to track who was assigned to which patient and where each patient was located on the ward. Although every member of the patient care team read information from the board, only the clinical partner (an aide to the nurses), was normally permitted to edit the information on the board. This use of a whiteboard has implications if the assignment information is ported to electronic format such as an EPR. It would dictate that the patient assignment and room location would be read-only to all members of the team; permitting all members of the team to have editing privileges would conceivably undermine the ability of the clinical partner to maintain accurate information.

Thus, to understand artifacts that have implications for EPR and related healthcare systems, the researcher must ask questions such as: From what physical objects do team members obtain vital information? How is this information vital to caring for the patient, coordinating work, documenting work, and so on? How do different team members in different work roles use artifacts similarly? How do they use them differently? What are the consequences of one member using a given artifact in a manner customarily intended for another member?

Summary

Evaluating information systems used in teams requires researchers to understand not only the technical aspects of the system but also the work and interactions of team members who use the system. Researchers using methods such as grounded theory combined with qualitative data collection techniques of observations, interviews, and artifact collection have gained tremendous insight into technology use in teams. Yet, there is still much work to be done. To ensure that information systems effectively support collaboration in teams, we must rigorously evaluate these systems using methods appropriate to studying teams in the healthcare setting.

Additional Readings

There are a number of books and articles that provide useful insight into teams, evaluation of information systems, grounded theory, and other issues we have discussed in the chapter.

Further information about teams can be found in:

Jon R. Katzenbach and Douglas K. Smith, *The Wisdom of Teams: Creating the High-Performance Organization* (HarperCollins Publishers, 1993).

Ed. R. Hackman, *Groups that Work (and Those That Don't): Creating Conditions for Effective Teamwork* (Jossey-Bass Publications, 1990).

Two good examples of ethnographic field studies are:

Julian E. Orr, *Talking About Machines: An Ethnography of a Modern Job* (Cornell University Press, 1996).

Richard Harper, *Inside the IMF: An Ethnography of Documents, Technology, and Organisational Action* (Academic Press, 1998).

For more details about grounded theory, please read:

Barney G. Glaser. and A.L. Strauss, *The Discovery of Grounded Theory: Strategies for Qualitative Research* (Aldine, 1967).

A. Strauss and J. Corbin, *Basics of Qualitative Research: Grounded Theory Procedures and Techniques* (Sage Publications, 1990).

References

[1] J.G. Baggs and M.H. Schmitt, Collaboration between nurses and physicians, Image Journal Nurs. Sch. 20(3) (1988) 145–149.

[2] J.G. Baggs, Intensive care unit use and collaboration between nurses and physicians, Heart Lung 18(4) (1989) 332–338.

[3] J.G. Baggs, S.A. Ryan, C.E. Phelps, et al., The association between interdisciplinary collaboration and patient outcomes in a medical intensive care unit, Heart Lung 21(1) (1992) 18–24.

[4] P.N. Gorman, J. Ash, M. Lavelle, et al., Bundles in the wild: Managing information to solve problems and maintain situation awareness, Library Trends 49(2) (2000) 266–289.

[5] M. Reddy, P. Dourish, and W. Pratt, Coordinating heterogeneous work: Information and representation in medical care, in: *Proceedings of the European Conference on Computer Supported Cooperative Work (ECSCW'01)*. Bonn, Germany (2001), pp. 239–258.

[6] E. Coiera and V. Tombs, Communication behaviours in a hospital setting: An observational study, BMJ 316(7132) (1998) 673–676.

[7] J.J. Cimino, Linking patient information systems to bibliographic resources, Methods of Information in Medicine 2 (1996) 122–126.

[8] W.M. Detmer, G.O. Barnett, and W.R. Hersh, MedWeaver: Integrating decision support, literature searching, and Web exploration using the UMLS Metathesaurus, in: *Proceedings of the AMIA Annual Fall Symposium (AMIA'97)* (1997), pp. 490–494.

[9] M. Berg, C. Langenberg, Ivd. Berg, et al., Considerations for sociotechnical design: Experiences with an electronic patient record in a clinical context, International Journal of Medical Informatics 52 (1998) 243–251.

[10] M. Berg, Patient care information systems and health care work: A sociotechnical approach, Int J Med Inf 55(2) (1999) 87–101.

[11] M. Reddy, W. Pratt, P. Dourish, et al., Sociotechnical requirements analysis for clinical systems, Methods Inf. Med. (42) (2003) 437–444.

[12] S.J. Nelson, D.D. Sherertz, and M.S. Tuttle, Issues in the development of an information retrieval system: The Physician's Information Assistant, in: *Proceedings of the 7th World Congress on Medical Informatics (Medinfo'92)*, Amsterdam, Netherlands, North-Holland (1992), pp. 371–375.

[13] M. Reddy, W. Pratt, P. Dourish, et al., Asking questions: Information needs in a surgical intensive care unit, in: *Proceedings of American Medical Informatics Association Fall Symposium (AMIA'02)*, San Antonio, TX (2002), pp. 651–655.

[14] B. Kaplan and J.A. Maxwell. Qualitative research methods for evaluating computer information systems, in: J.G. Anderson, C.E. Aydin, and S.J. Jay, editors, *Evaluating Health-care Information Systems: Methods and Applications* (Sage Publications, Thousand Oaks, CA, 1994), pp. 45–68.

[15] D.A. Travers and S.M. Downs, Comparing the user acceptance of a computer system in two pediatric offices: A qualitative study, in: *Proceedings of the American Medical Informatics Association Symposium*, Los Angeles, CA (2000), pp. 853–857.

[16] C. Heath and P. Luff, Documents and professional practice: "Bad" organisational reasons for "good" clinical records, in: *Proceedings of the ACM Conference on Computer-Supported Cooperative Work (CSCW'96)*, Boston, MA (1996), pp. 354–363.

[17] J. Ash, Factors affecting the diffusion of the computer-based patient record, Journal of the American Medical Informatics Association Supplement, *AMIA Proceedings* (1997), pp. 682–686.

[18] C.R. Weir, R. Crocket, S. Gohlinghorst, et al., Does user satisfaction relate to adoption behavior?: An exploratory analysis using CPRS implementation, in: *Proceedings of the American Medical Informatics Association*, Los Angeles, CA (2000), pp. 913–917.

[19] R.E. Kraut, M.D. Miller, and J. Siegel, Collaboration, in performance of physical tasks: Effects on outcomes and communication, in: *Proceedings of the ACM Conference on Computer Supported Cooperative Work (CSCW'96)*, Boston, MA, ACM Press (1996), pp. 57–66.

[20] K. McKeown, D. Jordan, S. Feiner, et al., A study of communication in the cardiac surgery intensive care unit and its implications for automated briefing, in: *Proceedings of the American Medical Informatics Association*, Los Angeles, CA (2000), pp. 570–574.

[21] B. Kaplan and D. Duchon, Combining qualitative and quantitative methods in information systems research: A case study, MIS Quarterly (1988) 571–586.

[22] G. Symon, K. Long, and J. Ellis, The coordination of work activities: Cooperation and conflict in a hospital context, Computer Supported Cooperative Work 5(1) (1996) 1–31.

[23] J. Ash and M. Berg, Report of conference track 4: Sociotechnical issues of HIS, International Journal of Medical Informatics 69 (2003) 305–306.

[24] D.R. Ilgen, Teams embedded in organizations: Some implications, American Psychologist 54(2) (1999) 129–139.

[25] R. Hackman, editor, *Groups that Work (and Those That Don't): Creating Conditions for Effective Teamwork.* (Jossey-Bass Publications, San Francisco, 1990).

[26] E. Savoie, Tapping the power of teams, in: R.S. Tindale, L. Health, J. Edwards, et al., editors, *Theory and Research on Small Groups* (Plenum Press, New York, 1998).

[27] J. Galegher and R.E. Kraut, Technology for intellectual teamwork: Perspectives on research and design, in: J. Galegher, R.E. Kraut, and C. Egido, editors, *Intellectual Teamwork: Social and Technological Foundations of Cooperative Work* (Lawrence Erlbaum Associates, Hillsdale, NJ, 1990), pp. 1–20.

[28] J. Katzenbach and D. Smith, *The Wisdom of Teams* (Harvard Business School Press, Boston, MA, 1993).

[29] D. Mankin, S. Cohen, and T. Bikson, *Teams and Technology* (Harvard Business School Press, Boston, MA, 1996).

[30] J.E. McGrath, Time matters in groups, in: J. Galegher, R.E. Kraut, and C. Egido, editors, *Intellectual Teamwork: Social and Technological Foundations of Cooperative Work* (Lawrence Erlbaum Associates, Hillsdale, 1990), pp. 23–61.

[31] P. Drucker, *Management: Tasks, Responsibilities, Practices* (Harper Collins, New York, 1973).

[32] A. Strauss, S. Fagerhaugh, B. Suczek, et al., *Social Organization of Medical Work* (University of Chicago, 1985).

[33] D. Pinelle and C. Gutwin, Designing for loose coupling in mobile groups, in: *Proceedings of the ACM Conference on Supporting Group Work (Group'03)*, Sanibel Island, FL, ACM (2003), pp. 75–84.

[34] B.L. Goddard, Termination of a contract to implement an enterprise electronic medical record system, JAMIA 7(6) (2000) 564–568.

[35] P. Dourish, What we talk about when we talk about context, Personal and Ubiquitous Computing 8(1) (2004) 19–30.

[36] W.J. Orlikowski, Learning from notes: Organizational issues in groupware implementation, in: *Proceedings of the ACM Conference on Computer-Supported Cooperative Work Conference (CSCW '92)*, Toronto, Canada (1992), pp. 362–369.

[37] D.E. Forsythe, B.G. Buchanan, J.A. Osheroff, et al., Expanding the concept of medical information: An observational study of physicians' information needs, Computers and Biomedical Research 25(2) (1992) 181–200.

[38] M. Reddy and P. Dourish, A finger on the pulse: Temporal rhythms and information seeking in medical care, in: *Proceedings of the ACM Conference on Computer Supported Cooperative Work (CSCW'02)*, New Orleans, LA; New York, ACM (2002), pp. 344–353.

[39] M.M. Shabot, The HP CareVue clinical information system, International Journal of Clinical Monitoring Computing 14(3) (1997) 177–184.

[40] P. Dourish and V. Bellotti, Awareness and coordination in shared workspaces, in: *Proceedings of the ACM Conference on Computer Supported Cooperative Work (CSCW'92)*, Toronto, Canada, ACM Press (1992), pp. 107–114.

[41] N. Bricon-Souf, J.M. Renard, and R. Beuscart, Dynamic workflow model for complex activity in intensive care unit, Medinfo 9(pt. 1) (1998) 227–231.

[42] R. Bentley, J.A. Hughes, D. Randall, et al., Ethnographically-informed systems design for air traffic control, in: *Proceedings of the ACM Conference on Computer-Supported Cooperative Work (CSCW 92)*, Toronto, Canada, ACM Press (1992), pp. 123–129.

[43] J. Bowers, G. Button, and W. Sharrock, Workflow from within and without, in: *Proceedings of the 4th European Conference on Computer Supported Cooperative Work (ECSCW'95)*, Stockholm, Sweden, Dordrecht: Kluwer (1995), pp. 51–66.

[44] E. Bradner, W.A. Kellogg, and T. Erickson, The adoption and use of "Babble": A field study of chat in the workplace, in: *Proceedings of the the the 6th European Conference on Computer Supported Cooperative Work (ECSCW'99)*, Copenhagen, Denmark (1999), pp. 139–158.

[45] J.E. Bardram, "I love the system—I just don't use it," in: *Proceedings of the CM Conference on Group Work (GROUP'97)*, Phoenix, AZ, ACM Press (1997), pp. 251–260.

[46] M. Pettersson, D. Randall, and B. Helgeson, Ambiguities, awareness and economy: A study of emergency service work, in: *Proceedings of the ACM Conference on Computer Supported Cooperative Work (CSCW'02)*, New Orleans, LA (2002), pp. 286–295.

[47] B. Malinowski, Baloma: Spirits of the dead in the Trobriand Islands, Journal of the Royal Anthropological Institute 46 (1916) 354–430.

[48] J. Lofland and L.H. Lofland, *Analyzing Social Settings*, 3rd ed. (Wadsworth, 1995).

[49] D.W. McDonald, and M.S. Ackerman, Just talk to me: A field study of expertise location, in: *Proceedings of the ACM Conference on Computer Supported Cooperative Work (CSCW'98)*, Seattle, WA (1998), pp. 315–324.

[50] A. Strauss and J. Corbin, *Basics of Qualitative Research: Grounded Theory Procedures and Techniques* (Sage Publications, Newbury Park, CA, 1990).

[51] Barney G. Glaser and A.L. Strauss, The Discovery of Grounded Theory: Strategies for Qualitative Research (Aldine, Chicago, 1967).

4
Survey Methods for Assessing Social Impacts of Computers in Healthcare Organizations

Carolyn E. Aydin

Introduction

This chapter provides a guide to the use of survey methods in evaluating the potential impacts of computerized information systems on the functioning of healthcare organizations and the work life of the individuals within them. In any setting, the impacts of computing go beyond the efficiency or cost-effectiveness of a system to the ways in which the technology interacts with the organization's ongoing routine policies and practices [1–4]. Because the delivery of healthcare requires coordination and cooperation between numerous different occupations and departments, changes in how these groups perform their work and interact with one another can have important consequences for the organization as a whole. Furthermore, the emphasis on cost efficacy, quality improvement, and patient safety has increased the demand for computer systems to improve patient safety, reduce costs, and provide new and better information to administrators and healthcare providers. In the long term, new computer technology has the potential to change the experience and process of work as well as the structure and delivery of medical care.

The chapter draws from studies of healthcare computing, as well as from research on computing in other types of organizations, to suggest potential areas for investigation and appropriate measures. The examples described were selected to illustrate specific evaluation issues and methods and are not meant to comprise a comprehensive review of the literature. The discussion includes the evaluation of immediate system outcomes as well as some of the work-oriented long-term impacts of new systems. Although other methodologies are mentioned, the present chapter focuses primarily on quantitative survey methods to measure system impacts.

When the first edition of this book was published in 1994, much of the research on computers in healthcare had focused on the efficiency of the systems themselves, with little attention directed toward their potential social impacts. Although research on information systems in other settings had traditionally been problem-oriented as well, there was also a significant body of research on the social impacts of computer technology [5–6]. Some of these issues have more recently begun to appear in healthcare literature as well. While the field is constantly changing, the studies cited here provide researchers and system evaluators with a starting point to conduct further literature reviews for the newest studies on the topics discussed, as well as an appendix with selected instruments (including several new to this edition) available for use as appropriate to each setting or system.

Survey Research

Survey research, one of the most common methods used for evaluating information system impacts, involves gathering information from a sample of a population using standardized instruments [7]. For scientific purposes, the intent of survey research also includes generalization to a population of individuals extending beyond the organization under study. In evaluation research, however, the sample may not be randomly selected and the population may be limited to individuals within a specific organization. Even in the case of convenience samples within a single organization, however, investigators need to take steps to ensure an adequate and representative response from individuals comprising the groups in question.

A survey or questionnaire is the primary data collection method within survey research [7]. In designing any project, questionnaires should never be developed from scratch when appropriate instruments already exist [8]. The use of a standard measure with established validity and reliability allows comparison of scores with other settings and spares the investigator the time-consuming process of developing a new measure [9]. (*Validity* may be defined as the extent to which the measure actually captures the concept it purports to measure, whereas *reliability* refers to the extent to which it is free from measurement error.)

The survey instruments described in the present chapter are drawn primarily from literature on information systems, organizations and organizational development, and work attitudes and values. The examples selected for inclusion either have been developed specifically for healthcare organizations or are widely used in other organizational settings with documented reliability and validity. In most cases, the instrument is included in its entirety in the chapter appendix. In other instances, references are provided to enable the investigator to obtain the instrument. This chapter is divided into sections detailing measurement strategies for: (1) user reactions to information systems and the implementation process; (2) characteristics of users that may influence their attitudes toward the system and system implementation; and (3) assessments of social impacts of computers organized into the following six dimensions: decision making, control, productivity, social interaction, job enhancement, and work environment [5].

User Reactions to Computers and Implementation: General Measures of User Satisfaction

Assessing user satisfaction with a new computer system and the system implementation process constitutes a first step in information system evaluation. A user satisfaction survey should not be seen as a definitive evaluation; it provides a starting point for analyzing system impacts and identifying possible areas of conflict and dissatisfaction [9]. Research has shown that user involvement in the computer implementation process improves both use of and satisfaction with information systems (see Kraemer and Dutton [6] for summary information). Thus questions about the level of involvement in implementation and satisfaction with computer training are often included in user satisfaction measures. Furthermore, users who hold realistic expectations about an information system prior to implementation also tend to use the system more and be more satisfied with it [6]. However, those with unrealistically high expectations prior to system implementation may become disillusioned with the system when the final product fails to meet their expectations, emphasizing the importance of an ongoing evaluation strategy that measures user attitudes both before and after system implementation [10,11].

User Information Satisfaction Scale

Baroudi and Orlikowski's [9] short form of Ives, Olson, and Baroudi's [12] User Information Satisfaction Scale is one of the few measures in the information systems literature that meets strict criteria for a well-developed survey instrument [8]. The scale includes 13 paired items measuring user satisfaction with: (1) the data processing staff and services, (2) the information product, and (3) their own knowledge and involvement (see Instrument 1 in the Appendix).

The User Information Satisfaction Scale, widely used in settings outside of healthcare, is intended to provide the investigator with a tool to detect problems with user satisfaction and facilitate investigation of specific trouble spots pinpointed by the individual scale items. The investigator may want to compare the responses of individuals in different groups or departments on different scale components or specific items to assess how well the new computer system meets the needs of different user groups. In addition, comparative data from surveys conducted in a number of different settings are available.

Because it was designed to save time, the questions on the survey are brief. For clarity, it may be necessary to modify the questionnaire for the specific computer system or organization. The investigator may also wish to add additional items, although the changes may compromise the established validity and reliability of the instrument [9].

End-User Computing Satisfaction

Doll and Torkzadeh's measure of End-User Computing Satisfaction [13] is another of the few measures in the information systems literature meeting strict criteria for a well-developed survey instrument [8]. The concept of end-user computing addresses applications in which the information users being surveyed actually use the computer terminal themselves. Thus, the measure focuses on issues such as ease of use and satisfaction with a specific computer application rather than involvement in implementation and relations with data processing staff [13]. The measure provides Likert-type scaling as an alternative to semantic differential scaling and includes the following five factors: (1) content, (2) accuracy, (3) format, (4) ease of use, and (5) timeliness (see Instrument 2).

Doll and Torkzadeh also address the issue of user involvement in system development in the end-user computer environment [14]. The authors hypothesize that successful involvement depends not only on the amount of involvement but also on the user's actual desire for involvement. They suggest asking system users questions describing both (1) the amount of time *actually spent* participating in specific development activities, and (2) the amount of time they wanted to spend in development activities, on a 5-point scale ranging from "a little" to "a great deal" (p. 1163) [14].

Implementation Attitudes Questionnaire

Schultz and Slevin took a different approach, developing a comprehensive attitude measurement instrument by examining general research on organizations to determine which variables would be relevant to the implementation of information systems in the organizational environment [15]. Their final instrument, based on factor analysis results, includes seven areas of impact (see Instrument 3). The questionnaire also includes five dependent variables measuring the respondent's likelihood of using the system and evaluation of the system's worth. Robey describes the results of several studies using the Schultz and Slevin instrument [15,16].

Innovation Process

A different approach to analysis of computer implementation in healthcare is to focus on the innovation process. Both Snyder-Halpern and Hebert and Benbasat, whose instruments have been added to the appendix to this chapter, explore different aspects of the innovation process. Snyder-Halpern's Organizational Information Technology/Systems Innovation Readiness Scale (OITIRS), included as Instrument 4, focuses on the readiness of the organization for clinical information technology [17,18]. Hebert and Benbasat, on the other hand, use a research model adapted from Moore and Benbasat that borrows from both Rogers's adoption of innovations and Fishbein and Ajzen's theory of reasoned action [19–22]. This theoretical framework forms the basis of their survey addressing potential use of bedside terminals by nursing staff (see Instrument 5, "Point of Care Technology").

Adding Other Measures

The investigator can also include components of the implementation process not covered by the scales described above. Aydin and Rice [23], for example, used items developed by Taylor and Bowers [24] to assess (1) work group communication (i.e., discussions with co-workers and management about ways to apply or adapt the system) and (2) organizational policies (i.e., the extent to which the organization supports the system by allowing individuals time to experiment and learn more about it). (See Instrument 6.) Such organizational policies and communication support can influence the extent to which individuals develop their own methods for using the system in the process of adoption and implementation (i.e., "reinvention") [21,25].

Single-Item Measures

Baroudi and Orlikowski also suggest that there may be instances in which it is appropriate to employ a single-item measure of user satisfaction [9]. Although single-item measures have been criticized for possible measurement error and lack of discriminatory power (e.g., Zmud and Boynton [8]), research also shows that single-item global measures may be more inclusive and convenient than the summation of many facet responses [9,26].

Following this line of reasoning, Rice and Aydin used a single-item measure in their evaluation of computerization in a student health clinic [27,28]. Based on Schultz and Slevin's [15] conclusion that an individual's cost-benefit evaluation was one of the most useful measures of perceived system success, respondents were asked to indicate their level of agreement (on a 7-point scale ranging from "strongly disagree" to "strongly agree") with the following question: "The new information system is worth the time and effort required to use it." In addition to the single-item measure, two additional questions were added after the computer was implemented asking respondents to rate the extent to which the system increased (1) the ease of performing the department's work and (2) the quality of the department's work (see Instrument 7). The three items together comprise a short global scale combining a general cost-benefit evaluation with an evaluation of the system's contribution to a department's work [10,29].

Measuring User Adaptation

Kjerulff, Counte, Salloway, and Campbell adopted a different approach to user satisfaction by developing three instruments to assess employee attitudinal and behavioral adaptation to computerization. Employees themselves completed the Use Scale and the Change Scale while supervisors completed the Behavioral Scale for each employee using the computer (see Instrument 8) [30]. Study results described the relationship of these measures to other standardized measures such as cognitive structure, role conflict, and role ambiguity [31]. (see Cook, Hepworth, Wall, and Warr for additional job measures such as role conflict and ambiguity) [32]. Findings for the Use Scale, for example, indicated that greater difficulty in using the system was reported by employees who faced more ambiguity in their jobs, had a negative orientation toward change and little desire for routine or structure, and a history of working at a number of different hospitals.

Level of System Use

Level of system use can also indicate user satisfaction with an information system, especially when system use is discretionary [33–35]. Even with mandatory systems, however, user satisfaction with the system may determine how well they use it. How frequently an individual uses the system can also affect attitudes toward the system. Nonusers or infrequent users, for example, may not be familiar enough with a new system to realize its strengths and shortcomings. Frequent users, however, may report changes in their daily work such as an increased workload or new communication with other workers to discuss system functions and issues [23].

Measuring system use often requires system-specific questionnaire items. Schultz and Slevin, for example, asked prospective users to indicate the probability that they would use the computer system (see dependent variables on Instrument 3 in the appendix) [15]. Anderson, Jay, Schweer, and Anderson asked physicians to respond to items such as: "How frequently do you *personally* use MIS to retrieve patient lists?" and "How frequently do you *personally* use MIS to enter medical orders?" using the following scale: 5 = "several times a day," 4 = "daily," 3 = "several times a week," 2 = "weekly," 1 = "less than weekly, but occasionally," and 0 = "never" [36,37]. Aydin and Ischar asked nurses "When medications are entered on the computer for the patients you are assigned to care for, what percent of these are entered within two hours after the order is written?" on a scale of 0%, 10%, 20%, and so on [38]. In 1998, Cork et al. reviewed available measures of physician use of, knowledge about, and attitudes toward computers [39]. System use can also be monitored through online tracking of how frequently individuals log onto the system and/or how long they use it each time they log on [33–35]. Online tracking can also provide measures of communication relationships among users or how individuals used common features of the system (see Chapter 5 of this book).

Provider–Patient Interactions

A frequently voiced theme of physician or healthcare providers when considering implementation of an electronic medical record has been the concern that computers will have a detrimental effect on the provider–patient rapport, depersonalizing the interaction [40]. (See Chapter 10.) Some research has addressed this issue from both the provider and patient perspective. Results showed that, while patients did not perceive any loss of communication or rapport with providers, recent studies report that both providers and patients were concerned about confidentiality about the electronic medical record. Instrument 9 in the appendix addresses a selection of these patient–provider issues.

Situation-Specific User Satisfaction Measures

Kaplan and Duchon's investigation of a computer system's impact on work in clinical laboratories illustrates another approach to measuring user satisfaction [41,42]. Rather than using a general satisfaction measure, Kaplan and Duchon designed an instrument to measure specific expectations, concerns, and perceived changes related to the impact of the computer system on laboratory work. Although the items may not be applicable to all systems, the questionnaire (Instrument 10) should guide investigators in developing similar situation-specific measures. The survey form also included open-ended items such as: "What important changes do you think the computer system has caused?" and "In what ways has the computer system affected how the labs and technologists are treated by others in the Medical Center?" Kaplan and Duchon used the instrument in combination with both standardized measures of other job dimensions (see the section on job enhancement below) and qualitative measures of system impacts.

Combining Standardized Survey Items

Many researchers combine scales from standard measures with established reliability and validity such as those published in the appendix to this chapter to create a survey that meets the needs of their specific study. Aydin et al. used this approach to develop a survey to provide pre- and postmeasures of user acceptance of the WatchChild obstetrical and fetal monitoring system. Instrument 11 in the appendix was developed as a pre-measure and distributed and collected during WatchChild training [43]. Results showed positive responses to most items and the postmeasure (Instrument 12) was very short, focusing only on the most essential items from Instrument 11. The source for each of the items in Instrument 11 was as follows:

Survey item 1: Instrument 7 in appendix.

Survey items 2–14: "Performance and visibility" (coefficient alpha = .95, mean response = 3.97). Adapted from Instrument 3 in appendix.

Survey items 15–17, 20–23: "Support" (coefficient alpha = .86, mean response = 3.83). Adapted from Instrument 3 in appendix.

Survey items 18–19: "Resistance" (mean response = 3.1). Adapted from Instrument 3 in appendix.

Survey item 24: "Service Outcome." Adapted from Instrument 10 in appendix.

Survey items 25–26: "Negative Intentions" (coefficient alpha = −.90). Adapted from Instrument 10 in appendix. Positive item (26) reversed to create scale.

Survey items 27–31: "Personal Hassles" (coefficient alpha = .85, mean response = 2.77). Adapted from Instrument 10 in appendix.

Survey items 32–34, 41: Developed specifically for this study. Used as single items, not scale.

Survey items 35–39: "End User Satisfaction" (coefficient alpha = .93, mean response = 4.16). Adapted from Instrument 2 in appendix.

Characteristics of Individual Users

The characteristics of individual users can help system implementers predict individual attitudes toward an information system. Individual attributes are those such as age, occupation, education, job tenure, previous computer experience, prior attitudes toward computers in general, and personality variables such as cognitive style, learning style, orientation toward change, or cognitive structure. Outcomes, however, are not always predictable. Age, job tenure, and previous computer experience, for example, have been shown to lead to both positive and negative attitudes in different settings. For example, although individuals who have worked in an organization for many years often find change difficult, Counte et al. found individuals who had a history of working in a larger number of hospitals had greater difficulty in using a new system [31]. Although less computer experience may predict negative attitudes, the lack of standardization between computer systems may also make it difficult for experienced computer users to adapt to a new system. Measuring these background factors enables the investigator to either eliminate them or document their influence when investigating reasons for computer-related problems and issues.

Personality Factors

This section addresses user personality traits and the implementation of information systems. Whereas copyright restrictions do not permit publication of the measures themselves, specific references are provided at the end of the chapter to obtain copies of the measures.

Cognitive Style/Learning Style

Beginning in the 1970s, a number of investigators began to focus on traits such as cognitive style as an issue in the design of information systems [44–46]. "Cognitive styles represent characteristic modes of functioning shown by individuals in their perceptual and thinking behavior" (p. 967) [47]. Most models distinguish between an individual's analytical, systematic approach to problem solving and a more intuitive, global approach as the two main types of cognitive style. Overall, this line of research has had limited success, with generally inconclusive findings regarding information systems design and use [48–50]. Meta-analytical findings indicate that the impact of cognitive style on implementation success is relatively small, with a stronger impact on user attitudes than on user performance [51].

In the healthcare arena, for example, Aydin found a relationship between cognitive style, as measured by the short form of the Myers-Briggs Type Indicator, and self-reported use of a newly implemented order entry system [52,53]. Results showed "feeling types" reported that they used the computer less than did "thinking types." Subsequent studies, however, found no relationship between cognitive style and self-reported use [10,38,52].

Cognitive style or learning style may, however, be important in the design of effective training for computer users [49]. Bostrom, Olfman, and Sein recommend giving the Kolb Learning Style Inventory to potential trainees and using the results to ensure accommodating the mix of individuals in the group [49,54]. Summers makes a similar recommendation for educating nurses [55]. A series of experiments on field-dependence/independence (i.e., the degree to which an individual can isolate or differentiate patterns from a complex field) also resulted in recommendations for information system components to make disembedding easier to perform [48]. Chapter 6 of this book addresses recent cognitive approaches to evaluation in detail.

Orientation Toward Change/Cognitive Structure

Approaching personality traits from a different perspective, Counte et al. asked users to complete two personality subscales from the Jackson Personality Research Form: orientation toward change and cognitive structure [31,56,57]. The first subscale measures general acceptance of change; the second measures a need for order and structure in one's life [31,56].

Results showed that employees who had a negative orientation toward change of any kind and little desire for routine or structure in their daily lives had greater difficulty in using the new computer system. Since personality is, by definition, not highly subject to change, the authors concluded that individuals who are less adaptable may need more time and support during training and implementation [56].

Social Impacts of Computers

The preceding sections of this chapter have covered instruments to assess user satisfaction with a computer system, as well as some of the individual traits and attitudes that may help predict user satisfaction. The following sections suggest ways to measure the impacts on work life that may be experienced by computer users. Impacts are divided into the six dimensions cited by Kraemer and Danziger (p. 594) [5] as the most commonly identified impacts of computing on work:

1. *Decision making*—the capacity to formulate alternatives, estimate effects, and make choices
2. *Control*—the power relations between different actors
3. *Productivity*—the ratio of inputs to outputs in the production of goods and services
4. *Social interaction*—the frequency and quality of interpersonal relationships among co-workers
5. *Job enhancement*—the skill variety and job domain
6. *Work environment*—the affective and evaluative orientations of the worker toward the setting of work

Since much of the research has been conducted outside of healthcare, each section begins with a brief summary of findings in other settings, followed by examples of research in healthcare along with suggestions for measurement and additional research.

Decision Making

Kraemer and Danziger (p. 594) define *decision making* as "the capacity to formulate alternatives, estimate effects, and make choices" [5]. Results of research in other settings indicate that, although computers provide workers with higher quality and more accessible information for decision and action, expert systems that actually make decisions or aid human decision makers remain elusive. In healthcare, decision support systems may aid in diagnostic decision making as well as interpret, alert, and make therapeutic suggestions. Langton, Johnston, Haynes, and Mathieu (p. 629), in their review of prospective studies that use control groups, assert that very little of the literature focuses on evaluating their "effects on real patients when used by clinicians in everyday practice" [58].

One area in which the medical decision-making capabilities of computers have received considerable attention, however, involves computerization in inpatient, particularly intensive care unit (ICU), settings [59]. Specifically, studies have focused on the *clinical* impacts of systems that provide clinicians with reminders, pharmacy and laboratory alerts, infectious disease monitoring, perioperative antibiotic use, and utilization assessment [61–67]. The success of such systems, documented by the studies cited above as well as much subsequent research, has led to the current emphasis on the importance of clinical reminders and alerts for patient safety.

Understanding the impact of computers on decision making goes beyond expert systems, however. One of the most important purposes of computerized order entry and results reporting, for example, is to provide the clinician with faster and more accessible information for clinical decision making [34,68,69]. Thus the assessment of user satisfaction with the availability of information for decision making could be supplemented by measures such as the actual elapsed time between when the order is written and when the results are available to the physician for clinical decisions on patient care. One medical center, for example, documented an average delay of 107 minutes between the time a physician wrote a TPN (total parenteral nutrition) order and the time the order was entered in the computer by the unit clerk [70]. This delay was eliminated with the implementation of physician order entry. The success of the change depended, however, on physician acceptance of order entry, which may be lacking in other institutions and remains an issue in medical informatics. In 1994, Sittig and Stead reviewed the "state of the art" of computer-based physician order entry and the *Journal of the American Informatics Association* focused the entire March/April 2004 issue on "Perspectives on Computerized Physician Order Entry (CPOE) and Patient Care Information Systems" [71,72].

In addition to the timing of information, the amount of information available can affect the decision-making ability of healthcare professionals [73]. Radiologists, for example, emphasize the importance of knowing physicians' reasons for requesting specific tests to ensure that the appropriate test has actually been ordered and to assist in their interpretation of results. An important factor in radiologists' acceptance of the PROMIS system was the ability of PROMIS to provide the radiologist with the complete patient record on demand, enhancing their decision-making capability [73].

The complex division of tasks between departments, however, may increase the difficulty of implementing systems to transmit information from one department to another. Order entry for radiology, for example, may require that the individual entering the radiology order in the computer include the reason for the test as well. The physician, who may not enter his or her own orders, also may not have included the reason for ordering the test on the written order form. If the physician is no longer accessible when the clerk enters the order, the clerk may simply hazard a guess to fill the space so the computer will accept the order. In this case, the system has the capability to meet the radiologists' needs, but the organization of tasks and the unwillingness or inability of the physician and clerk to provide the required information may result in errors in tests performed and interpretation of films [74].

Several items designed to measure the decision-making aspects of a system are included in the Schultz and Slevin measure (see Instrument 3, especially Factor 1). (The instrument was originally pilot tested with a computer system for making advertising budgeting decisions.) User satisfaction measures may also reflect decision-making issues if radiologists, for example, indicate dissatisfaction with the information provided by the system. Follow-up to uncover specific problems then could include an audit of system use, interviews, and observation of individuals as they work with the new computer system.

Control

Kraemer and Danziger define several aspects of control that warrant consideration, including: (1) control of the individual's work by others, (2) the individual's ability to alter the behavior of others, (3) constraints imposed by the job itself such as time pressures, and (4) an increased sense of mastery over one's own work [5]. The control aspects of computerization need not be conceived of as "zero sum," however, but can result in increased control by all groups [75,76].

Research in settings outside of healthcare has shown that computing has had minimal impact in control over people in the work situation, perhaps because few systems to monitor employee work are actually implemented and monitoring capabilities are seldom used [5]. In the healthcare arena, computer systems that have the capability to either monitor or control physician ordering patterns have the potential to shift more control to institution administrators. In the example described above in which physicians began entering their own TPN orders in the computer, evaluation results showed a significant increase in physician compliance with hospital policies on the type and duration of orders. In fact, the computer was diplomatically referred to as a "teaching tool" and guidelines were printed on the computer screen where the physicians made their selections, but the end result was enforcement of physician compliance with medical center policies [70].

In a similar vein, computerized order entry and results reporting provide an opportunity for both peer review and quality assurance operations, as well as a "teaching tool" to encourage the use of practice guidelines [77]. How frequently these capabilities are actually used, however, remains an open question. Evaluation of these aspects of computerization may involve examination of organization policies on the use of computer information; interviews and surveys of key officials, physicians, and other administrators; and audits of changes in compliance with institutional policies and guidelines.

The adoption of a centralized system such as order entry and/or results reporting might also be considered to enhance administrative control over all departments in the organization simply because, whatever system is selected, it is likely to involve compromises on the part of individual departments to meet the needs of the organization as a whole. In fact, Aydin, using interviews with key administrators and system users, found that pharmacy departments perceived a loss of control over both the database of physician orders on which they depended to perform their work, as well as their department's revenues, when nurses were assigned the tasks of order entry and computerized charting of medications [78]. To regain at least some control, the pharmacy department in one hospital agreed to accept what they considered to be a "nursing system" only after hospital administration agreed to let them resume the pharmacy's expanded consultative role that had been eliminated during budget cuts. In another hospital, the pharmacy used system audits to demonstrate nursing errors in order entry and convince administrators that it would be cost effective to assign pharmacy order entry to pharmacy technicians instead of to nursing, effectively shifting control of the orders database back to the pharmacy department [79].

Both interviews and observation of the meetings that occur during system adoption and the implementation process can provide important evaluation information on shifts in control and the negotiations that occur between the respective groups. In addition, evaluation surveys distributed both before and after system implementation might include situation-specific questions regarding the amount of control an individual or department has over specific aspects of the work situation. For example, individuals might be asked: "For each of the following decisions, please indicate how much say you actually have in making these decisions" on a scale of "no say at all" to "a very great deal" [80]. The question would be followed by a series of items such as "decisions about changing how you do your work," as well as situation-specific items that might be affected by computerization. Schultz and Slevin also include several items measuring impacts of computerization on control (see Instrument 3, especially Factor 1).

Finally, the use of computers also has the potential to shift the power relationship between physicians and patients. Although little research has addressed this aspect of computerization, there are at least two possible scenarios [81]. On one hand, the physician may consolidate his or her position as an expert by becoming better informed but releasing only decisions to the patient. On the other hand, the computer may be used to share information with patients and involve them in decision making about their healthcare [81]. Survey instruments designed to measure patient perceptions of the consultation process may be used to address potential shifts in the power relationships between patients and healthcare professionals (see Instrument 9) [82,83].

Productivity

Research on changes in productivity accompanying computerization in settings outside of healthcare indicates that there has been little displacement of workers with the increased productivity made possible by computers. Rather, the same number of workers tends to handle more work, with productivity gains from increased quality of work and reduced errors in information handling [5]. Most studies agree that the quantity of work has substantially increased, with more mixed results on the quality of work.

In the healthcare arena, nursing research, in particular, has focused on the impacts of computers on the time and quality of nursing work [84]. In general, results show that computers save nurses time in performing clerical activities such as filling out requisition slips and assembling charts [85]. Computers that manage the flow of information between nursing and ancillary departments save time for nurses, whereas systems that emphasize online charting and not communications may not save time [86]. Also interesting, however, is the finding that the extra time available after computerization is not usually spent in direct patient care as hypothesized but is channeled into other areas, such as professional growth activities, inservice education, and management planning, or spread out across other nursing activities [85,87]. In studies outside of nursing, Counte, Kjerulff, Salloway, and Campbell measured how individuals using an Admission, Discharge, and Transfer (ADT) system apportioned their time on the job before and after computer implementation [88]. Respondents were employees in all hospital departments, most in clerical positions or lower-level supervisors, who were trained to use the system. Findings showed that system implementation decreased the amount of time employees spent helping other departments acquire information while, as expected, increasing the time spent on data processing (see Instrument 13). Andrews, Gardner, Metcalf, and Simmons also addressed work patterns, quality and content of charting, and productivity in their evaluation of a respiratory care computer system [89]. Survey questions included asking therapists to compare the amount of time spent charting before and after computerization, as well as a number of other questions comparing manual and computerized charting (see Chapter 15 of this book).

Computers also have the potential to increase the quality of information work by reducing errors. In considering nursing work, however, Hendrickson and Kovner note that few studies have been conducted to examine this effect [86]. Instruments 3, 7, and 10 in the appendix include some questions addressing respondent perceptions of changes in quality and service attributable to computerization in both general and laboratory settings.

Getting data into the computer in a timely, accurate, and efficient manner also remains an overriding issue in the implementation of medical information systems and especially the computerized medical record [90,91]. Issues surrounding the accuracy of order entry, for example, illustrate some important concerns. With computerized order entry, a clerk with limited expertise may enter orders in the database by selecting from menu options that may not match the exact terminology used by the physician [74,90]. Audit data can enable system implementers to determine the need for additional training of individual employees or entire groups. In one hospital, audit results indicated that initially 60% to 70% of the medication orders entered required changes by the pharmacy, a figure that was later reduced through training provided to clerical employees by the pharmacy department [78]. Concerns for patient safety have led to a renewed emphasis on the universal implementation of computerized physician order entry (CPOE) systems to eliminate errors attributable to employees with less knowledge entering physician orders.

Another essential measure of the productivity of today's hospitals is patient length of stay. Kjerulff (p. 244) [87] cites an experimental study in which two intensive care units were carefully matched for staffing and patient characteristics. Results showed that patients on the computerized unit had shorter lengths of stay with computerized data providing "better blood management." Although length-of-stay data should provide readily available outcome measures in most institutions, well-designed studies are needed to control for patient acuity and other variables in determining the impacts of computerization on patient care.

Social Interaction

Social interaction is defined by Kraemer and Danziger (p. 594) as the "frequency and quality of interpersonal relationships among coworkers" [5]. Research on computer impacts has documented increased interdependence and communication between individuals and work groups connected by computers. Individuals use electronic mail to send information that would not have been sent or received without electronic mail and individuals who share common databases meet face-to-face as often as before computerization to discuss the shared system [5].

Some of the evidence cited above comes from research in healthcare organizations. Aydin [78], for example, showed that dependence on a common database and shared tasks can increase interdependence and cooperation between departments (see also Connelly et al. [92], Pryor et al. [69]). Anderson and Jay used network analysis to study social interactions between healthcare professionals as predictors of system use (see Chapter 8 of this book) [93]. Results showed that physicians' location in a communication network had a significant effect on the adoption and utilization of a hospital information system independently of background and practice characteristics. In a smaller organization, Aydin and Rice focused specifically on the communication aspects of implementing a new clinic scheduling system [23]. Findings showed that workers created new contacts and learned more about the work of computer users in other parts of the organization. These increases in communication also have implications for productivity when combined with findings that indicate that the more co-workers an individual talks to about the new technology, the more productive he or she is likely to be using the new system [94].

New patterns of communication between workers may not all be positive, however. New task arrangements can also create new problems or continue old conflicts in new guises. Kaplan highlighted interdepartmental issues in her study of the implementation of a laboratory computer system [95]. Although respondents agreed that the computer system made results available more quickly, some laboratory workers felt a loss of contact with physicians, nurses, and patients. In addition, some physicians and nurses refused to use the terminals for results inquiry. Laboratory workers felt that these physicians and nurses expected to get test results by telephone and resented being referred to terminals or to a central processing area for their information.

Both survey research and network methods, as well as interviews and audits of system use, can be used to evaluate changes in social interaction accompanying computerization. Schultz and Slevin (1975) and Kaplan and Duchon both include questionnaire items to explore impacts of computerization on changes in communication patterns and issues (see Instruments 3 and 10) [15,42,96]. Instrument 13 also includes communication in the list of work role activities being evaluated, and Instrument 14 provides an example of a questionnaire used to collect information on respondent contacts for network analysis (see Chapter 8). Instrument 15 provides a sample measure to document changes in the frequency of telephone contacts between departments. In addition, documentation of changes in interdependence may be measured by asking employees (both before and after computer implementation) questions such as: "How much do you have to depend on each of the following people to obtain the information needed to do your work?" The question is followed by a list of individuals or departments involved in the computerization process and response categories ranging from 1 to 4, "not at all" to "very much" [97].

Job Enhancement

Job enhancement, in contrast to the broader concept of work environment addressed below, focuses specifically on job content, particularly the variety of different tasks and level of skills for a given job [5]. One of the early debates related to computerization concerned whether the use of computers would reduce or expand the task variety and skills associated with specific jobs. Attewell and Rule, for example, note that although some investigators argue that low-level clerical jobs can largely be replaced by new technologies, others argue that even the lowest stratum of white-collar workers may benefit from retraining schemes to upgrade their jobs [75].

According to Kraemer and Danziger, most of the research indicates that, particularly for jobs that involve diverse skills, computing has enhanced workers' perceptions of their job domain [5].

Research on job design usually focuses on five specific components [98]:

1. *Skill variety*—the degree to which a job requires a range of activities and abilities to perform the work
2. *Task identity*—the degree to which a job requires the completion of a relatively whole and identifiable piece of work
3. *Task significance*—the degree to which a job has a significant impact on other people's lives
4. *Autonomy*—the degree to which a job provides freedom and discretion in scheduling work and determining methods
5. *Feedback about results*—the degree to which a job provides employees with clear and direct feedback about task performance

Hackman and Oldham developed the Job Diagnostic Survey (included in Cook et al. [32]) to measure these core job dimensions [99]. A shorter and easier-to-use questionnaire designed to measure the same dimensions was developed by Lawler, Mohrman, and Cummings (see Instrument 16) [98].

Research on computers in settings outside of healthcare has frequently focused on changes in these job dimensions (e.g., word processing [100]). In some studies, computerization has been accompanied by attempts at work redesign specifically intended to create enriched jobs high on each of the five dimensions. Other studies simply measure whether the implementation of computers has had an impact on the dimensions of workers' jobs.

Griffin studied the long-term effects of computerization and work redesign on the jobs of tellers in 38 member banks of a large bank holding corporation [101]. Survey data were collected at four time periods: prior to implementation, 6 months after implementation, 24 months after implementation, and 48 months after implementation. Results showed different patterns for the different measures, underscoring the importance of evaluating the impacts of computerization and job changes at multiple points in time. Job satisfaction, for example, increased between Time 1 and Time 2, but returned to levels similar to Time 1 at Times 3 and 4. Individuals also perceived changes in their jobs (i.e., changes in task variety, autonomy, feedback, significance, and identity) at Time 2 and these perceptions did not diminish over the study period. Performance scores also followed a different pattern, showing no significant increase until Time 3 and maintaining that level at Time 4.

In the healthcare arena, the emphasis on cost efficacy and the need to streamline work processes and retain highly trained employees resulted in a renewed interest in job-design issues. Evaluating the impact of computerization on the skills of healthcare workers, however, must also consider existing job content. With the exception of some clerical workers and other particularly routine jobs, many healthcare occupations involve highly varied and skilled work. For these individuals, using a computer comprises one task in a workday filled with diverse tasks. Although healthcare professionals sometimes voice resentment at being required to take time away from patient care to learn to use a computer system (e.g., Aydin and Rice [10,23]), deskilling or routinization is not usually an issue.

Research on computerization in healthcare settings has, however, addressed the issue of job redesign, using the measures described above [27,96]. Neither study, however, showed that computerization had an impact on the core job dimensions of the employees under study. Further research on job dimensions in healthcare settings should probably focus on employees for whom using the computer constitutes a major part of their job. In the Rice and Aydin study, in particular, computer use constituted only one task in the busy workday of most employees [27]. Kaplan and Duchon, however, also suggest that the lack of findings related to core job dimensions may reflect the fact that standard job characteristic measures do not take into account differences in how individuals holding ostensibly the same jobs actually view their work [96].

Work Environment

The quality of the work environment focuses on broader and more evaluative responses to work, going beyond the specific dimensions examined under job enhancement to include issues such as general job satisfaction, job stress, time pressures, and the like [5]. Research results in general do indicate that computing may increase stress and time pressure for some workers. In most studies, however, results show that computing has increased workers' job satisfaction and interest in their work. Karasek and Theorell provide a detailed analysis of job-design issues and their relationship to the health and well-being of individual workers [102].

In an example of comprehensive longitudinal research on the impacts of computerization, Kraut, Dumais, and Koch investigated the specific job dimensions described above, as well as the overall impact of computerization on the work lives of customer service representatives in a large public utility [103]. Results showed that computerization can have complex and profound effects on job effectiveness and employment.

The information system investigated by Kraut et al. was designed to provide recent billing information and to allow interactive updating of customers' accounts, but no intentional attempt was made to redesign jobs or to alter the range of tasks or the interactions with customers [103]. (Similar systems are in use in billing departments in healthcare institutions.) Along with the introduction of the computer system, however, other changes were made that altered the office layout, disrupting familiar seating arrangements and changing the social organization of the department. Overall, results showed that the service representatives liked their jobs less after computerization. Contact with work colleagues became less frequent and less satisfying, but there was also less job pressure and service representatives believed their overall workload had been reduced. Workers also modified the technology by finding innovative ways to use the new system as well as ways to use the system for clandestine note-passing strongly discouraged by supervisors.

Kaplan and Duchon [42,96] with their study of the laboratory computer system; Counte et al. [31,56] studying clerical employees involved in the admission, discharge, and transfer of patients; and Aydin and Rice [10,23] with their study of computerization in a student health clinic, have all conducted comprehensive longitudinal studies aimed at uncovering changes in the work life of healthcare workers following the implementation of a new computer system. (See Chapter 15 in this book and references [11] and [69].) Results of each study reflect both the approach taken by the investigators and actual impacts of computerization in the specific healthcare context.

Counte et al., for example, focused on individual differences to explain reactions of employees to computerization [31,56]. Long-term results indicated that both personality traits and attitudes toward computers were important predictors of individual reactions. Results of studies by both Kaplan and Duchon and Aydin and Rice focused on work group issues as well as individual differences in predicting adaptation to computerization [10,23,42,96]. Findings showed that, although employees cited both additional work and improvements in quality following computerization, departmental membership was an important predictor of individual reactions. In the laboratory, Kaplan and Duchon found that technologists in some laboratories focused on work increases, whereas in other laboratories they emphasized improved information flow [42,95,96]. In the student health clinic, Aydin and Rice found that attitudes toward the computer system and new communication with other departments about the system varied both by department and by occupation [10,23]. One of the most important predictors was the way in which work was organized within the individual departments and the negotiated assignment of the new tasks that accompanied computerization. In comprehensive studies such as these, general job satisfaction surveys can supplement the measures already described in providing important information on employee reactions to change (see Instrument 17). Another approach to the some of the same concepts can be found in the organizational culture literature, with Scott et al. providing a review of the available instruments to measure organizational culture in healthcare [104].

Summary

In summary, the survey methods described in this chapter comprise an essential dimension in a multimethod approach to evaluating the impacts of computers on the functioning of healthcare organizations and the work life of the individuals within them. The chapter and the instruments included in the chapter appendix should provide investigators with standardized instruments, as well as guidance and examples for questionnaire design where no standardized measure exists. Although not intended as a complete review of the literature, this chapter also provides investigators with an overview of topics to consider when planning any investigation of the social impacts of computers in healthcare organizations.

Additional Readings

Introduction

The references listed below were included as Additional Readings in the first edition of this book and remain valuable resources for survey research concepts and instruments for assessing the social impacts of computers in healthcare organizations. In addition, the website www.isworld.org/ surveyinstruments/surveyinstruments.htm also provides researchers with a repository of actual survey instruments used in information systems, either in full text or via links or citations.

Organizational Change and Information Systems

Markus provides an excellent analysis of the changes that occur in organizations with the introduction of information systems [1].

Survey Research

See Kraemer for a collection of detailed reviews and discussions of survey methods in information systems research [7]. This volume also includes Zmud and Boynton's archive of over 100 instruments (although the scales themselves are not included) and Kraemer and Dutton's assessment of survey research in management information systems as well as other references on topics discussed throughout this chapter [6,8]. Cook, Hepworth, Wall, and Warr review nearly 250 scales for measuring work attitudes, values, and perceptions and include the most widely used instruments in their entirety [32].

User Reactions and Characteristics of Individual Users

Kraemer—see above review [7].

Nelson reviews the literature on individual reactions to systems and suggests a framework that includes additional measures such as job satisfaction, organizational commitment, involvement, and performance [105].

Alavi and Joachimsthaler's meta-analysis of the information systems literature provides important information on the relative importance of different variables with suggestions for future research [51].

Social Impacts of Computers

Kraemer and Danziger provide a framework for the social impacts of computers and review the results of research [5].

Cummings and Huse is an excellent organization development textbook that addresses many of the organizational change issues involved in the implementation of an information system [98].

Hendrickson and Kovner review the literature and make recommendations for future research [86].

Karasek and Theorell provide a detailed analysis of job design issues and their relationship to the health and well-being of individual workers [102].

References

[1] M.L. Markus, *Systems in Organizations* (Pitman, Boston, 1984).

[2] R.E. Rice, Computer-mediated communication and organizational innovation, Journal of Communication 37 (1987) 64–94.

[3] L. Sproull and S. Kiesler, *Connections* (MIT Press, Cambridge, 1991).

[4] S. Zuboff, *In the Age of the Smart Machine* (Basic Books, New York, 1988).

[5] K.L. Kraemer and J.N. Danziger, The impacts of computer technology on the worklife of information workers, Social Science Computer Review 8 (1990) 592–613.

[6] K.L. Kraemer and W.H. Dutton, Survey research in the study of management information systems, in: K.L. Kraemer, editor, *The Information Systems Research Challenge: Survey Research Methods* (Harvard Business School, Boston, MA, 1991), pp. 3–57.

[7] K.L. Kraemer, editor, *The Information Systems Research Challenge: Survey Research Methods* (Harvard Business School, Boston, MA, 1991).

[8] R.W. Zmud and A.C. Boynton, Survey measures and instruments in MIS: Inventory and appraisal, in: K.L. Kraemer, editor, *The Information Systems Research Challenge: Survey Research Methods* (Harvard Business School, Boston, MA, 1991), pp. 149–180.

[9] J.J. Baroudi and W.J. Orlikowski, A short-form measure of user information satisfaction: A psychometric evaluation and notes on use, Journal of Management Information Systems 4 (1988) 44–59.

[10] C.E. Aydin and R.E. Rice, Social worlds, individual differences, and implementation: Predicting attitudes toward a medical information system, Information and Management 20 (1991) 119–136.

[11] H.P. Lundsgaarde, R.M. Gardner, and R.L. Menlove, Using attitudinal questionnaires to achieve benefits optimization, in: *Proceedings of the 13th Annual Symposium on Computer Applications in Medical Care* Washington, DC, Computer Society of the IEEE (1989), pp. 703–707.

[12] B. Ives, M.H. Olson, and J.J. Baroudi, The measurement of user information satisfaction, Communications of the ACM 26 (1983) 785–793.

[13] W.J. Doll and G. Torkzadeh, The measurement of end-user computing satisfaction, MIS Quarterly 12 (1988) 259–274.

[14] W.J. Doll and G. Torkzadeh, A discrepancy model of end-user computing involvement, Management Science 35 (1989) 1151–1171.

[15] R.L. Schultz and D.P. Slevin, Implementation and organizational validity: An empirical investigation, in: R.L. Schultz and D.P. Slevin, editors, Implementing operations research/management science, New York, American Elsevier (1975), pp. 153–182.

[16] D. Robey, User attitudes and management information system use, Academy of Management Journal 22 (1979) 527–538.

[17] R. Snyder-Halpern, Indicators of organizational readiness for clinical information technology/systems innovation: A Delphi study, Ijmedinf 63 (2001) 179–204.

[18] R. Snyder-Halpern, Development and pilot testing of an Organizational Information Technology/Systems Innovation Readiness Scale (OITIRS), in: *Proceedings of the AMIA 2002 Annual Symposium* Washington DC (2002), pp. 702–706.

[19] M. Hebert and I. Benbasat, Adopting information technology in hospitals: The relationship between attitudes/expectations and behavior, Hospital and Health Services Administration 39 (1994) 369–383.

[20] G.C. Moore and I. Benbasat, Development of an instrument to measure the perceived characteristics of adopting an information technology innovation, Information Systems Research 2 (1991) 192–222.

[21] E.M. Rogers, *Diffusion of Innovations*, 3rd ed. (The Free Press, New York, 1983).

[22] M. Fishbein and I. Ajzen, Belief, attitude, intention and behaviour: An introduction to theory and research, (Addison-Wesley, Reading, MA, 1975).

[23] C.E. Aydin and R.E. Rice, Bringing social worlds together: Computers as catalysts for new interactions in healthcare organizations, J Health Soc Behav 33 (1992) 168–185.

[24] J.C. Taylor and D.G. Bowers, *Survey of Organizations: A Machine Scored Standardized Questionnaire Instrument* (Institute for Social Research, University of Michigan, Ann Arbor, MI, 1972).

[25] B.M. Johnson and R.E. Rice, Reinvention in the innovation process: The case of word processing, in: R.E. Rice and Associates, editors, *The New Media* (Sage, Beverly Hills, 1984), pp. 157–183.

[26] V. Scarpello and J.P. Campbell, Job satisfaction: Are all the parts there? Personnel Psychology 36 (1983) 577–600.

[27] R.E. Rice and C.E. Aydin, *Summary Report: Student Health Service Information System Study* (Annenberg School for Communication, University of Southern California, Los Angeles, 1988).

[28] R.E. Rice and C.E. Aydin, Attitudes toward new organizational technology: Network proximity as a mechanism for social information processing, Administrative Science Quarterly 36 (1991) 219–244.

[29] F.D. Davis, Perceived usefulness, perceived ease of use, and user acceptance of information technology, M1S Quarterly September 13 (1989) 319–340.

[30] K.H. Kjerulff, J.A. Counte, J.C. Salloway, and B.C. Campbell, Understanding employee reactions to a medical information system, in: *Proceedings of the 5th Annual Symposium on Computer Applications in Medical Care* Los Angeles, CA, IEEE Computer Society Press (1981), pp. 802–805.

[31] M.A. Counte, K.H. Kjerulff, J.C. Salloway, and B.C. Campbell, Implementation of a medical information system: Evaluation of adaptation, HCM Review Summer 8 (1983) 25–33.

[32] J.D. Cook, S.J. Hepworth, T.D. Wall, and P.B. Warr, *The Experience of Work* (Academic Press, New York, 1981).

[33] G. Hendrickson, R.K. Anderson, P.D. Clayton, J. Cimino, G.M. Hripcsak, S.B. Johnson, M. McCormack, S. Sengupta, S. Shea, R. Sideli, and N. Roderer, The integrated academic information management system at Columbia-Presbyterian Medical Center, MD Comput 9 (1992) 35–42.

[34] C. Safran, W.V. Slack, and H.L. Bleich, Role of computing in patient care in two hospitals, MD Comput 6 (1989) 141–148.

[35] W. Slack, Editorial: Remembrance, thanks, and welcome, MD Comput 6 (1989) 183–185.

[36] J.G. Anderson, S.J. Jay, H.M. Schweer, and M.M. Anderson, Why doctors don't use computers: Some empirical findings, J R Soc Med 79 (1986) 142–144.

[37] C.E. Aydin, Survey methods for assessing social impacts of computers in healthcare organizations: 8. Perceived desirability of computer applications in medical care, in: J.G. Anderson, C.E. Aydin, and S.J. Jay, editors, *Evaluating Healthcare Information Systems: Methods and Applications* (Sage Publications, Thousand Oaks, CA, 1994), pp. 108–111.

[38] C.E. Aydin and R. Ischar, Predicting effective use of hospital computer systems: An evaluation, in: J.G. Anderson, C.E. Aydin, and S.J. Jay, editors, *Evaluating Healthcare Information Systems: Methods and Applications* (Sage Publications, Thousand Oaks, CA, 1994), 245–259.

[39] R.D. Cork, W.M. Detmer, and C.P. Friedman, Development and initial validation of an instrument to measure physician use of, knowledge about, and attitudes toward computers, Journal of the American Medical Informatics Association 5 (1998) 164–176.

[40] C.S. Gadd and L.E. Penrod, Dichotomy between physicians' and patients' attitudes regarding EMR use during outpatient encounters, in: *Proceedings of the AMIA 2000 Annual Symposium*, Washington DC (2000), pp. 275–279.

[41] B. Kaplan and D. Duchon, Combining qualitative and quantitative methods in information systems research: A case study, MIS Quarterly 12 (1988) 571–586.

[42] B. Kaplan and D. Duchon, A qualitative and quantitative investigation of a computer system's impact on work in clinical laboratories. Unpublished manuscript (1987).

[43] C.E. Aydin, K. Gregory, L. Korst, J. Polaschek, and T. Chamorro, Panel: Making it happen: Organizational changes required to implement an electronic medical record in a large medical center, in: *AMIA'99 Annual Symposium*, Washington, DC (November 6–10, 1999).

[44] P.G.W. Keen and M.S.S. Morton, *Decision Support Systems: An Organizational Perspective* (Addison-Wesley, Reading, MA, 1978).

[45] R.H. Kilmann and I.I. Mitroff, Qualitative versus quantitative analysis for management science: Different forms for different psychological types, Interfaces 6 (1976) 17–27.

[46] R.O. Mason and I.I. Mitroff, A program for research on management information systems, Management Science 19 (1973) 475–487.

[47] R.W. Zmud, Individual differences and MIS success: A review of the empirical literature, Management Science 25 (1979) 966–979.

[48] I. Benbasat, Laboratory experiments in information systems studies with a focus on individuals: A critical appraisal, in: I. Benbasat, editor, *The*

Information Systems Research Challenge: Experimental Research Methods (Harvard Business School, Boston, 1989), pp. 33–48.

[49] R.P. Bostrom, L. Olfman, and M.K. Sein, The importance of learning style in end-user training, MIS Quarterly (March 1990).

[50] G.P. Huber, Cognitive style as a basis for MIS and DSS designs: Much ado about nothing? Management Science 29 (1983) 567–579.

[51] M. Alavi and E.A. Joachimsthaler, Revisiting DSS implementation research: A meta-analysis of the literature and suggestions for researchers, MIS Quarterly 16 (1992) 95–116.

[52] C.E. Aydin, The effects of social information and cognitive style on medical information system attitudes and use. In: W.W. Stead, editor, *Proceedings of the 11th Annual Symposium on Computer Applications in Medical Care*, New York, Institute of Electrical and Electronics Engineers (1987), pp. 601–606.

[53] I.B. Myers and M.H. McCaulley, *Manual: A Guide to the Development and Use of the Myers-Briggs Type Indicator* (Consulting Psychologists Press, Palo Alto, CA, 1985).

[54] D.A. Kolb, *The Learning Style Inventory Technical Manual* (McBer, Boston, MA, 1976).

[55] S. Summers, Attitudes of nurses toward hospital computerization: Brain dominance model for learning, in: R.A. Miller, editor, *Proceedings of the 14th Annual Symposium on Computer Applications in Medical Care* Los Alamitos, CA, IEEE Computer Society Press (1990), pp. 902–905.

[56] M.A. Counte, K.H. Kjerulff, J.C. Salloway, and B.C. Campbell, Adapting to the implementation of a medical information system: A comparison of short-versus long-term findings, Journal of Medical Systems 11 (1987) 11–20.

[57] D. Jackson, *Personality Research Form Manual* (Research Psychologists Press, Goshen, NY, 1967).

[58] K.B. Langton, M.E. Johnston, R.B. Haynes, and A. Mathieu, A critical appraisal of the literature on the effects of computer-based clinical decision support systems on clinician performance and patient outcomes, in: M.E. Frisse, editor, *Proceedings of the 16th Annual Symposium on Computer Applications in Medical Care* (McGraw-Hill, New York, 1993), pp. 626–630.

[59] M.M. Shabot and R.M. Gardner, *Decision Support Systems for Critical Care* (Springer-Verlag, New York, 1993).

[60] K.E. Bradshaw, R.M. Gardner, and T.A. Pryor, Development of a computerized laboratory alerting system, Comput Biomed Res 22 (1989) 575–587.

[61] R.S. Evans, R.A. Larsen, J.P. Burke, R.M. Gardner, F.A. Meier, J.A. Jacobson, M.T. Conti, J.T. Jacobson, and R.K. Hulse, Computer surveillance of hospital-acquired infections and antibiotic use, JAMA 256 (1986) 1007–1011.

[62] R.S. Evans, R.M. Gardner, A.R. Bush, J.P. Burke, J.A. Jacobson, R.A. Larsen, F.A. Meier, and H.R. Warner, Development of a computerized infectious disease monitor (CIDM), Comput Biomed Res 18 (1985) 103–113.

[63] R.M. Gardner and R.S. Evans, Computer-assisted quality assurance, Group Practice Journal 41 (1992) 8–11.

[64] R.M. Gardner, R.K. Hulse, and K.G. Larsen, Assessing the effectiveness of a computerized pharmacy system, in: *Proceedings of the 14th Annual Symposium on Computer Applications in Medical Care* Los Alamitos, CA, IEEE Computer Society Press (1990), pp. 668–672.

[65] R.A. Larsen, R.S. Evans, J.P. Burke, S.L. Pestotnik, R.M. Gardner, and D.C. Classen, Improved perioperative antibiotic use and reduced surgical wound infections through use of computer decision analysis, Infect Control Hosp Epidemiol 10 (1989) 316–320.

[66] M.M. Shabot, H.S. Bjerke, M. LoBue, and B.J. Leyerle, Quality assurance and utilization assessment: The major by-products of an ICU clinical information system, in: P.D. Clayton, editor, *Proceedings of the 15th Annual Symposium on Computer Applications in Medical Care* New York, McGraw-Hill (1992), pp. 554–558.

[67] D.M. Rind, C. Safran, R.S. Phillips, W.V. Slack, D.R. Calkins, T.L. Delbanco, and H.L. Bleich, The effect of computer-based reminders on the management of hospitalized patients with worsening renal function, in: P.D. Clayton, editor, *Proceedings of the 15th Annual Symposium on Computer Applications in Medical Care* New York, McGraw-Hill (1992), pp. 28–32.

[68] D.P. Connelly, G.R. Werth, D.W. Dean, B.K. Hultman, and T.R. Thompson, Physician use of an NICU laboratory reporting system, in: M.E. Frisse, editor, *Proceedings of the 16th Annual Symposium on Computer Applications in Medical Care* New York, McGraw-Hill (1993), pp. 8–12.

[69] T.A. Pryor, R.M. Gardner, P.D. Clayton, and H.R. Warner, The HELP system, Journal of Medical Systems 7 (1983) 87–102.

[70] TPN audits: MD order entry. Department of Nursing, University of California, Irvine Medical Center. Unpublished report (1990).

[71] D.F. Sittig and W.W. Stead, Computer-based physician order entry: The state of the art, Journal of the American Medical Informatics Association 1 (1994) 108–23.

[72] Journal of the American Medical Informatics Association 2 (2004) 95–126.

[73] P.J. Fischer, W.C. Stratmann, H.P. Lundsgaarde, and D J. Steele, User reaction to PROMIS: Issues related to acceptability of medical innovations, in: *Proceedings of the 4th Annual Symposium on Computer Applications in Medical Care* Washington, DC, IEEE (1980), pp. 1722–1730.

[74] T. Chamorro, Knowledge as transference in automating hospital operations. Nursing Information Systems, Cedars-Sinai, Medical Center, Los Angeles, CA. Unpublished report (1992).

[75] P. Attewell and J. Rule, Computing and organizations: What we know and what we don't know, Communications of the ACM 27 (1984) 1184–1192.

[76] L. Thompson, M. Sarbaugh-McCall, and D.F. Norris, The social impacts of computing: Control in organizations, Social Science Computer Review 7 (1989) 407–417.

[77] T.M. Shuman, Hospital computerization and the politics of medical decision-making, in: R. L. Simpson and I.H. Simpson, editors, *Research in the Sociology of Work*, Vol. 4 (JAI, Greenwich, CT, 1988), pp. 261–287.

[78] C.E. Aydin, Occupational adaptation to computerized medical information systems, J Health Soc Behav 30 (1989) 163–179.

[79] P.A. Kidder, J.M. Muraszko, and R. Shane, Utilization of pharmacy technicians for computer medication order entry. Paper presented at the *1992 Annual Meeting of the American Society of Hospital Pharmacists*, Washington, DC (1992).

[80] M. Moch, C. Cammann, and R.A. Cooke, Organizational structure: Measuring the distribution of influence, in: S.E. Seashore, E.E. Lawler III, P.H. Mirvis, and C. Cammann, editors, *Assessing Organizational Change* New York, (John Wiley & Sons, 1983).

[81] M. Fitter, Evaluation of computers in primary healthcare: The effect on doctor-patient communication, in: H.E. Peterson and W. Schneider, editors, *Human-Computer Communications in Health Care* (Elsevier, Amsterdam, 1986), pp. 67–80.

[82] G. Brownbridge, G.A. Herzmark, and T.D. Wall, Patient reactions to doctors' computer use in general practice consultations, Soc Sci Med 20 (1985) 47–52.

[83] G. Brownbridge, R.J. Lilford, and S. Tindale-Biscoe, Use of a computer to take booking histories in a hospital antenatal clinic, Medical Care 26 (1988) 474–487.

[84] K.E. Bradshaw, D.F. Sittig, R.M. Gardner, T.A. Pryor, and M. Budd, Computer-based data entry for nurses in the ICU, MD Comput 6 (1989) 274–280.

[85] N. Staggers, Using computers in nursing. Comput Nurs 6 (1988) 164–170.

[86] G. Hendrickson and C.T. Kovner, Effects of computers on nursing resource use, Comput Nurs 8 (1990) 16–22.

[87] K.H. Kjerulff, The integration of hospital information systems into nursing practice: A literature review, in: M.J. Ball, K.J. Hannah, Jelger U. Gerdin, and H. Peterson, editors, *Nursing Informatics* (Springer Verlag, New York, 1988).

[88] M.A. Counte, K.H. Kjerulff, J.C. Salloway, and B.C. Campbell, Implementing computerization in hospitals: A case study of the behavioral and attitudinal impacts of a medical information system, Journal of Organizational Behavior Management 6 (1984) 109–122.

[89] R.D. Andrews, R.M. Gardner, S.M. Metcalf, and D. Simmons, Computer charting: An evaluation of a respiratory care computer system, Respiratory Care 30 (1985) 695–707.

[90] C.J. McDonald, W.M. Tierney, J.M. Overhage, D.K. Martin, and G.A. Wilson, The Regenstrief Medical Record System: Twenty years of experience in hospitals, clinics, and neighborhood health centers, MD Comput 9 (1992) 206–217.

[91] Q.E. Whiting-O'Keefe, A. Whiting, and J. Henke, The STOR clinical information system, MD Comput 5 (1988) 8–21.

[92] J. Ouellett, G. Sophis, S. Duggan, L. Driscoll, and S. Priest, Automating a multiple-day medication administration record, Nursing Management 22 (1991) 30–35.

[93] J.G. Anderson and S.J. Jay, Computers and clinical judgment: The role of physician networks, Soc Sci Med 20 (1985) 969–979.

[94] M.J. Papa, Communication network patterns and employee performance with new technology, Communication Research 17 (1990) 344–368.

[95] B. Kaplan, Initial impact of a clinical laboratory computer system, Journal of Medical Systems 11 (1987) 137–147.

[96] B. Kaplan and D. Duchon, A job orientation model of impact on work seven months post-implementation, in: *Proceedings of Medinfo 89: Sixth World Congress on Medical Informatics* Amsterdam, North Holland (1989), pp. 1051–1055.

[97] A.H. Van de Ven and D.L. Ferry, *Measuring and Assessing Organizations* (Wiley, New York, 1980).

[98] T.G. Cummings and E.F. Huse, *Organization Development and Change*, 4th ed. (West, St. Paul, 1989).

[99] J.R. Hackman and G.R. Oldham, Development of the Job Diagnostic Survey, Journal of Applied Psychology 60 (1975) 159–170.

[100] B.M. Johnson and R.E. Rice, *Managing Organizational Innovation* (Columbia University Press, New York, 1987).

[101] R. Griffin, Effects of work redesign on employee perceptions, attitudes, and behaviors: A long-term investigation, Academy of Management Journal 34 (1991) 425–435.

[102] R. Karasek and T. Theorell, Healthy work: Stress, Productivity, and the Reconstruction of Working Life (Basic Books, New York, 1990).

[103] R. Kraut, S. Dumais, and S. Koch, Computerization, productivity, and quality of work-life, Communications of the ACM 32 (1989) 220–238.

[104] T. Scott, R. Mannion, H. Davies, and M. Marshall, The quantitative measurement of organizational culture in healthcare: A review of available instruments, HSR 38 (2003) 923–945.

[105] D. Nelson, Individual adjustment to information-driven technologies: A critical review, MIS Quarterly 14 (1990) 79–98.

APPENDIX: SURVEY INSTRUMENTS

SURVEY INSTRUMENTS

1. Short-Form Measure of User Information Satisfaction
2. End-User Computing Satisfaction
3. Implementation Attitudes Questionnaire
4. Organizational Information Technology/Systems Innovation Readiness Scale (OITIRS)
5. Point of Care Technology
6. Scales Adapted from Survey of Organizations
7. Examples of Short Global User Satisfaction Measures
8. Instruments to Assess Employee Adaptation
9. Patient Survey
10. Laboratory Computer Impact Study
11. WatchChild Obstetrical System Pre-Implementation Survey
12. WatchChild Obstetrical System Post-Implementation Survey
13. Work Role Activities
14. Network Survey
15. Communication Between Departments
16. Job Design Questionnaire
17. Job Satisfaction

1. Short-Form Measure of User Information Satisfaction

The purpose of this study is to measure how *you* feel about certain aspects of the computer-based information products and services that are provided to you in your present position.

On the following pages you will find different factors, each related to some aspect of your computer-based support.[a] You are to rate each factor on the descriptive scales that follow it, based on your evaluation of the factor.

The scale positions are defined as follows:

adjective X:___:___:___:___:___:___: ___:adjective Y
            (1) (2) (3) (4) (5) (6) (7)

(1) Extremely X   (5) Slightly Y
(2) Quite X   (6) Quite Y
(3) Slightly X   (7) Extremely Y
(4) Neither X or Y; Equally X or Y; Does not apply

The following example illustrates the scale positions and their meanings:

My vacation in the Bahamas was:restful:___:___:___: :___:___: X :hectic
healthy: X :___:___: :___:___::unhealthy

According to the responses, the person's vacation was extremely hectic and quite healthy.

Instructions

1. Check each scale in the position that describes your evaluation of the factor being judged.
2. Check every scale; do not omit any.
3. Check only one position for each scale.
4. Check in the space, not between spaces.

This   Not this
:_X_::__X__:

5. Work rapidly. Rely on your first impressions.

Thank you very much for your cooperation.

Answer based on your own feelings:

1. Relationship with the EDP[a] staff

   dissonant:___:___:___:___:___:___:___:harmonious
        bad:___:___:___:___:___:___:___:good

2. Processing of requests for changes to existing systems

       fast:___:___:___:___:___:___:___:slow
   untimely:___:___:___:___:___:___:___:timely

3. Degree of EDP training provided to users

   complete:___:___:___:___:___:___:___:incomplete
        low:___:___:___:___:___:___:___:high

4. Users' understanding of systems

insufficient:___:___:___:___:___:___:sufficient
complete:___:___:___:___:___:___:incomplete

5. Users' feelings of participation

positive:___:___:___:___:___:___:negative
insufficient:___:___:___:___:___:___:sufficient

6. Attitude of the EDP staff

cooperative:___:___:___:___:___:___:belligerent
negative:___:___:___:___:___:___:positive

7. Reliability of output information

high:___:___:___:___:___:___:low
superior:___:___:___:___:___:___:inferior

8. Relevancy of output information (to intended function)

useful:___:___:___:___:___:___:useless
relevant:___:___:___:___:___:___:irrelevant

9. Accuracy of output information

inaccurate:___:___:___:___:___:___:accurate
low:___:___:___:___:___:___:high

10. Precision of output information

low:___:___:___:___:___:___:high
definite:___:___:___:___:___:___:uncertain

11. Communication with EDP staff

dissonant:___:___:___:___:___:___:harmonious
destructive:___:___:___:___:___:___:productive

12. Time required for new systems development

unreasonable:___:___:___:___:___:___:reasonable
acceptable:___:___:___:___:___:___:unacceptable

13. Completeness of output information

sufficient:___:___:___:___:___:___:insufficient
adequate:___:___:___:___:___:___:inadequate

Scoring

The values for each item range from −3 to +3 with 0 indicating neutrality. Each scale is scored by taking the average of the two items. (Some items are reverse scored to prevent respondents from marking down one column of the questionnaire.) The total score is determined by summing the scores on the 13 scales. Three subtotals (information product, EDP staff and services, and knowledge/involvement) are the averages of their component scales. The total score can range from +39 to −39 and the subtotals from +3 to −3. All of the reliabilities (Cronbach's alpha) are above .80 and the total score has a reliability of .89.

[a]*Note*: Computer-based support includes the following: in-house computer, timesharing, service bureau, access to a remote computer, use of computer-generated reports.

Source: Reprinted with permission from J.J. Baroudi, and W.J. Orlikowski. A short-form measure of user information satisfaction: A psychometric evaluation and notes on use, Journal of Management Information Systems 4 (1988) 44–59.

2. End-User Computing Satisfaction

Scale

1 = Almost never
2 = Some of the time
3 = Almost half of the time
4 = Most of the time
5 = Almost always

The 12-item End-User Computing Satisfaction measure includes the following five components (Cronbach's Alpha for the 12-item scale = .92):

Factor 1: CONTENT (coefficient alpha = .89)
   C1: Does the system provide the precise information you need?
   C2: Does the information content meet your needs?
   C3: Does the system provide reports that seem to be just about exactly what you need?
   C4: Does the system provide sufficient information?
Factor 2: ACCURACY (coefficient alpha = .91)
   A1: Is the system accurate?
   A2: Are you satisfied with the accuracy of the system?
Factor 3: FORMAT (coefficient alpha = .78)
   F1: Do you think the output is presented in a useful format?
   F2: Is the information clear?
Factor 4: EASE OF USE (coefficient alpha = .85)
   E1: Is the system user-friendly?
   E2: Is the system easy to use?

Factor 5: TIMELINESS (coefficient alpha = .82)
   T1: Do you get the information you need in time?
   T2: Does the system provide up-to-date information?

Source: Adapted from W.J. Doll, and G. Torkzadeh. The measurement of end-user computing satisfaction, MIS Quarterly 12 (1988) 259–274.

3. Implementation Attitudes Questionnaire

You are asked to read each statement carefully and to circle one of the words from each following line that describes most clearly how you feel about the statement. For example:

I find the computer system interesting.

Strongly disagree   Disagree   Uncertain   Agree   Strongly agree
                                                    X

This would indicate that you agree with the statement.

Please keep in mind that what is important is your own opinion. The computer system is presently being considered for implementation. Remember, this questionnaire is asking for *your opinion about the computer system.*

Each item implies "after the implementation," that is, this questionnaire is concerned with how you feel about each statement as it applies to the situation *after the computer system is operational.*

Each item implies that changes will occur *after the computer system is in use.* For example, the statement

"My job will be more satisfying."

implies

"My job will be more satisfying *"after the computer system is in use."*

Note: The original questionnaire included 67 items. The items listed below were interpretable in 7 factors. An additional 10 items did not load significantly on a factor or were not interpretable.

Factor List

Factor 1: PERFORMANCE—Effect on Job Performance and Performance Visibility
   My job will be more satisfying.
   Others will better see the results of my efforts. It will be easier to perform my job well.

The accuracy of information I receive will be improved by the computer system.

I will have more control over my job.

I will be able to improve my performance.

Others will be more aware of what I am doing.

The information I will receive from the computer system will make my job easier.

I will spend less time looking for information.

I will be able to see better the results of my efforts.

The accuracy of my forecast will improve as a result of using the computer system.

My performance will be more closely monitored.

The division/department will perform better.

Factor 2: INTERPERSONAL—Interpersonal Relations, Communication, and Increased Interaction and Consultation with Others

I will need to communicate with others more.

I will need the help of others more.

I will need to consult others more often before making a decision.

I will need to talk with other people more.

I will need the help of others more.

Factor 3: CHANGES—Changes Will Occur in Organizational Structure and People I Deal With

The individuals I work with will change.

The management structure will be changed.

The computer system will not require any changes in division/department structure.

I will have to get to know several new people.

Factor 4: GOALS—Goals Will Be More Clear, More Congruent to Workers, and More Achievable

Individuals will set higher targets for performance.

The use of the computer system will increase profits.

This project is technically sound.

Company goals will become more clear.

My counterparts in other divisions/departments will identify more with the organization's goals.

The patterns of communication will be more simplified.

My goals and the company's goals will be more similar than they are now.

The aims of my counterparts in other divisions/departments will be more easily achieved.

My personal goals will be better reconciled with the company's goals.

Factor 5: SUPPORT/RESISTANCE—Computer System Has Implementation Support—Adequate Top Management, Technical, and Organizational Support—and Does Not Have Undue Resistance

Top management will provide the resources to implement the computer system.

People will accept the required change.
Top management sees the computer system as being important.
Implementing the computer system will be difficult.
Top management does not realize how complex this change is.
People will be given sufficient training to utilize the computer system.
This project is important to top management.
There will be adequate staff available to successfully implement the computer system.
My counterparts in other divisions/departments are generally resistant to changes of this type.
Personal conflicts will not increase as a result of the computer system.
The developers of the computer system will provide adequate training to users.

Factor 6: CLIENT—System Developers Understand the Problems and Work Well with Their Clients

The developers of these techniques don't understand our problems.
I enjoy working with those who are implementing the computer system.
When I talk to those implementing the computer system, they respect my opinions.

Factor 7: URGENCY—Need for Results, Even with Costs Involved; Importance to Me, Boss, Top Management

The computer system costs too much.
I will be supported by my boss if I decide not to use this model.
Decisions based on the computer system will be better.
The results of the computer system are needed now.
The computer system is important to me.
I need the computer system.
It is important that the computer system be used soon.
This project is important to my boss.
The computer system should be put into use immediately.
It is urgent that the computer system be implemented.
The sooner the computer system is in use the better.
Benefits will outweigh the costs.

Dependent Variables

1. Please circle the number on the scale below that indicates the probability that you will use the computer system.

   0. .1 .2 .3 .4 .5 .6 .7 .8 .9 1.0

2. Please circle the number on the scale below that indicates the probability that others will use the computer system.

   0. .1 .2 .3 .4 .5 .6 .7 .8 .9 1.0

3. Please circle the number on the scale below that indicates the probability that the computer system will be a success.

<u>0.   .1   .2   .3   .4   .5   .6   .7   .8   .9   1.0</u>

4. On the 10-point scale below indicate your evaluation of the worth of the computer system.

Not useful at all	Moderately useful		Excellent
1	2 3 4	5 6	7 8 9	10

5. Please circle the number on the scale below that indicates the level of accuracy you expect from the computer system.

Not useful at all	Moderately useful		Excellent
1	2 3 4	5 6	7 8 9	10

Source: Adapted from R.L. Schultz, and D.P. Slevin. Implementation and organizational validity: An empirical investigation, in: R.L. Schultz and D.P. Slevin, editors, *Implementing Operations Research/Management Science.* (American Elsevier, New York, 1975) 153–182. Scales were determined by factor analysis. (Used by permission.)

4. Organizational Information Technology/Systems Innovation Readiness Scale (OITIRS)

Directions: Listed below are a series of statements about the *readiness* of your organization to implement the _____ **(insert name of IT/S innovation)**. For each statement, please *circle* the number of the *one* response that *best reflects* your personal opinion. A *"no opinion"* option is provided for those statements about which you have limited information. Thank you for responding to each statement.

KEY: SD = Strongly Disagree   **SA** = Strongly Agree   **NO** = No Opinion

In this organization:	SD	NO	SA
1. Funding is adequate for completion of IT/S innovation implementation.	1 2 3 4 5 6 7 8		
2. Project teams have included both technical support staff and users.	1 2 3 4 5 6 7 8		
3. The project budget includes training/retraining costs.	1 2 3 4 5 6 7 8		
4. The project budget is consistent with the organization's strategic plan.	1 2 3 4 5 6 7 8		
5. There is a good ratio of full-time in-house to contract IS staff to support the project.	1 2 3 4 5 6 7 8		

6. Good quality vendor support for the IT/S   1 2 3 4 5 6 7 8
   innovation is typically available.
7. Most users have an adequate level of computer   1 2 3 4 5 6 7 8
   literacy.
8. Users are typically supportive of IT/S   1 2 3 4 5 6 7 8
   innovation.
9. User competencies are appropriately   1 2 3 4 5 6 7 8
   incorporated into job performance criteria.
10. Users are typically involved in IT/S projects.   1 2 3 4 5 6 7 8
11. Adequate training is available to support   1 2 3 4 5 6 7 8
    users.
12. A core group of users is available to support   1 2 3 4 5 6 7 8
    implementation.
13. Current work practices are adequately   1 2 3 4 5 6 7 8
    supported by existing information systems.
14. There is a good fit between organizational   1 2 3 4 5 6 7 8
    and IS strategic plans.
15. Research and development activities to learn   1 2 3 4 5 6 7 8
    about new technology are supported.
16. IT/S project implementation time frames are   1 2 3 4 5 6 7 8
    usually adequate.

In this organization: **SD   NO   SA**
17. Development of information systems is based   1 2 3 4 5 6 7 8
    on current market trends.
18. There are good quality vendor contracts.   1 2 3 4 5 6 7 8
19. There is a lot of knowledge about IS operational   1 2 3 4 5 6 7 8
    and capital budget trends.
20. Historically, the strategic and IS goals have   1 2 3 4 5 6 7 8
    been integrated.
21. In the past, IS staff have been included in   1 2 3 4 5 6 7 8
    decision-making processes.
22. Administrators are very knowledgeable about IT/S   1 2 3 4 5 6 7 8
    innovation based on their past experience.
23. There is a lot of knowledge about the ongoing   1 2 3 4 5 6 7 8
    development needs of IS support staff.
24. Knowledge is available about how IT/S innovations   1 2 3 4 5 6 7 8
    are being used by other organizations.
25. Adequate communication mechanisms exist to   1 2 3 4 5 6 7 8
    support shared communication across all
    organizational levels.
26. Effective mechanisms are in place to evaluate   1 2 3 4 5 6 7 8
    IT/S innovations.
27. The most appropriate individuals are involved in   1 2 3 4 5 6 7 8
    the development of the IS strategic plan.

28. IS needs are routinely incorporated into the organization's business processes.   1 2 3 4 5 6 7 8

29. Process improvement mechanisms are used effectively to identify work process redesign needs.   1 2 3 4 5 6 7 8

30. IS decision makers are adequately represented on key organizational committees.   1 2 3 4 5 6 7 8

31. There is a willingness to act on work process improvement recommendations.   1 2 3 4 5 6 7 8

32. There is satisfaction with the contribution that IS has made to the organization.   1 2 3 4 5 6 7 8

33. There is an openness to different perspectives about IS.   1 2 3 4 5 6 7 8

34. There is an emphasis on the importance of collaborative interdisciplinary teams to support IT/S innovation.   1 2 3 4 5 6 7 8

In this organization: **SD   NO   SA**

35. There is a willingness to engage in the IT/S innovationprocess.   1 2 3 4 5 6 7 8

36. Individuals have a positive attitude toward IT/S innovation.   1 2 3 4 5 6 7 8

37. The business structure supports involvement of IS in strategic planning.   1 2 3 4 5 6 7 8

38. Formal communication mechanisms exist to support user and IS support staff communication.   1 2 3 4 5 6 7 8

39. The IS department reporting structure adequately supports IS staff.   1 2 3 4 5 6 7 8

40. The IS strategic plan is an effective guide for the organization's IT/S innovation processes.   1 2 3 4 5 6 7 8

41. The IS department effectively manages the organization's shared databases.   1 2 3 4 5 6 7 8

42. Formal policies and procedures are available to guide IS processes.   1 2 3 4 5 6 7 8

43. IS initiatives are usually addressed as part of the organization's overall strategic planning.   1 2 3 4 5 6 7 8

44. Board members are actively engaged in key IS committees.   1 2 3 4 5 6 7 8

45. Sufficient funds are available to support IS planning activities.   1 2 3 4 5 6 7 8

46. The top-ranking IS executive is regularly included in senior executive meetings.   1 2 3 4 5 6 7 8

47. Non-IS executives are routinely named as co-sponsors for IS projects.   1 2 3 4 5 6 7 8

48. Executives engage in mutual decision making   1 2 3 4 5 6 7 8
    with IS leaders regarding proposals and ideas.

Printed with permission from Rita Snyder-Halpern. Reliability for the 48-item subscale: Cronbach's alpha coefficients of .83 (resources), .79 (end-users), .84 (technology), .83 (knowledge), .79 (processes), .84 (values and goals), .80 (management structures), and .87 (administrative support).

Source: R. Snyder-Halpern, Development and pilot testing of an Organizational Information Technology/Systems Innovation Readiness Scale (OITIRS), in: *Proceedings of the AMIA 2002 Annual Symposium*, Washington DC (2002), pp. 702–706.

5. *Point of Care Technology*

What do you think? Please complete this questionnaire:

SECTION A: Your Views About Using the Point of Care System

In the following section you will be presented with a number of statements expressing different viewpoints about the *point of care system.*

Circle the number that indicates how much each statement reflects *your personal* viewpoint.

Example survey setup for each question:

Using the point of care system would enable me to accomplish tasks more quickly.

1	2	3	4	5	6	7
Strongly disagree			Neither agree nor disagree		Strongly agree	

Note: Questions 3, 8, 17, 18, 30, 33–38, 42, 43, 47, and 48 are answered on the following scale:

1	2	3	4	5	6	7
Extremely unlikely			Neither likely nor unlikely		Extremely likely	

1. Using the point of care system would enable me to accomplish tasks more quickly.
2. It would be easy to get the point of care system to do what I want it to do.
3. If the decision were totally up to me, I would decide to start using the point of care system in the future.
4. Using the point of care system would enable my work to be more controlled by others.

5. Using the point of care system would fit well with the way I like to work.
6. Using the point of care system would result in many aspects of my job becoming more repetitive and boring.
7. I would have no difficulty telling others about the results of using the point of care system.
8. I intend to use the point of care system frequently.
9. Using the point of care system would enable my job performance to be more closely monitored by others.
10. Nursing staff in my hospital who use the point of care system would have a high profile.
11. I would be able to communicate to others the consequences of using the point of care system.
12. My interaction with the point of care system would be clear and understandable.
13. Using the point of care system may adversely affect my health.
14. Using the point of care system would improve the quality of work I do.
15. Nursing staff in my hospital who use the point of care system would have more prestige than those who do not.
16. Although it may be helpful, using the point of care system would certainly *not* be compulsory in my job.
17. I intend to be a heavy user of the point of care system.
18. I would feel very positive about using the point of care system.
19. Introduction of the point of care system in my hospital may eventually result in the elimination of my job.
20. Learning to operate the point of care system would be easy for me.
21. Using the point of care system would enhance my effectiveness on the job.
22. The results of using the point of care system would be apparent to me.
23. Using the point of care system would fit into my work style.
24. I would have difficulty explaining why using the point of care system may or may not be beneficial.
25. Using the point of care system would give me greater control over my work.
26. Using the point of care system would be a status symbol in my hospital.
27. Using the point of care system would be completely compatible with my current situation.
28. Using the point of care system would unrealistically raise others' expectations about the amount of work that I can accomplish.
29. Overall, the point of care system would be easy for me to use.
30. My Nursing Manager would not require me to use the point of care system.
31. Using the point of care system would make it easier to do my job.
32. One final question in this section:

When I am faced with a task or decision of the sort that the point of care system is designed to support, I intend to use the system. . . . ___ % of the time.

Indicate a number between 0 and 100 where:
0 = I don't intend to use the system at all.
100 = I intend to use the system each and every time that I am faced with a task or decision of the sort that the system is designed to support.

SECTION B: Questions About Yourself

For each of the following statements, please circle the number that indicates how likely or unlikely each of the statements are. Note that you are being asked *how likely the statements are*, not whether you have discussed the topics. Remember that your *individual* opinions are important.

33. My *co-workers* think that I should use the point of care system in my job.
34. My *Nursing Manager* thinks that I should use the point of care system in my job.
35. My *Director of Nursing* thinks that I should use the point of care system in my job.
36. With respect to the Nursing Unit, I want to do what my *co-workers* think I should do.
37. With respect to the Nursing Unit, I want to do what my *Nursing Manager* thinks I should do.
38. With respect to the Nursing Unit, I want to do what my *Director of Nursing* thinks I should do.

In the following questions please circle the number that best indicates your response.

39. Does your *collective bargaining unit* (union) have any official position with respect to the use of information technology in the workplace? (Circle number)

    Yes . . . .   Go to Question 40
    No . . . .   Go to Question 41
    Don't Know . . . .   Go to Question 41

40. Do you think this *official position* is in favor of, or against, the use of information technology?
41. In general, how do you feel the *general membership* of your union view the use of information technology?
42. In general, how likely are you to follow or support *your union's* official policies?
43. In general, how likely are you to follow or support the *general membership's* viewpoints?

44. Does your *professional association* have any official position with respect to the use of information technology in the workplace? (Circle number)

Yes . . . .   Go to Question 45
No . . . .   Go to Question 46
Don't Know . . . .   Go to Question 46

45. Do you think this *official position* is in favor of, or against, the use of information technology?
46. In general, how do you feel the *general membership* of your professional association view the use of information technology?
47. In general, how likely are you to follow or support *your professional association's* official policies?
48. In general, how likely are you to follow or support the *general membership's* viewpoints?

Printed with permission. Three attitude factors (compatibility, relative advantage, and result demonstrability) and one subjective norm factor (Director of Nursing) were the strongest predictors of intent to use the point of care technology. "A score for subjective norm was calculated by multiplying the response to normative belief held by referents (i.e., "the degree to which [referent X] thinks I should use a bedside terminal") by the motivation to comply with that particular referent (i.e., "Generally speaking, I want to do what [referent X] thinks I should do")." (p. 377).

Source: M Hebert, and I. Benbasat. Adopting information technology in hospitals: The relationship between attitudes/expectations and behavior, Hospital and Health Services Administration 39 (1994) 369–383.

6. Scales Adapted from Survey of Organizations

This section asks about learning to use the system. Use the following codes to indicate your response:

1 = Strongly disagree   5 = Slightly agree
2 = Disagree   6 = Agree
3 = Slightly disagree   7 = Strongly agree
4 = Neutral

Please indicate the extent to which you agree with the following statements:

1. I attend regular meetings where we talk   1 2 3 4 5 6 7
   about how to use the system.
2. Organizational policies generally discourage   1 2 3 4 5 6 7
   me from developing new procedures or uses
   of the system

3. I receive praise for developing new ways
   to use the system to accomplish my job or
   to solve problems using the system:
   —from my supervisor   1 2 3 4 5 6 7
   —from my co-workers   1 2 3 4 5 6 7
4. I generally do not have time to learn or   1 2 3 4 5 6 7
   experiment with possible new procedures or
   uses of the system.
5. My co-workers and/or I develop new   1 2 3 4 5 6 7
   procedures or uses of the system.
6. Other people do not generally encourage me   1 2 3 4 5 6 7
   to experiment with new procedures or uses
   of the system.
7. I talk about ways to use the system to
   accomplish my job or solve problems:
   —with my supervisor   1 2 3 4 5 6 7
   —with my co-workers   1 2 3 4 5 6 7

Note: The variables were interpretable in 2 factors. Questions 1, 3, 5, and 7 comprise Factor 1—Work Group Communication About the Computer. Questions 2, 4, and 6 comprise Factor 2—Organizational Support for Implementation. Cronbach's coefficient alpha for Factor 1 when the variables were added = .88; Factor 2 = .61. See Aydin and Rice (references [10] and [23]) for details.

Source: Adapted from J.C. Taylor and D.G. Bowers. *Survey of Organizations: A Machine Scored Standardized Questionnaire Instrument*. (Institute for Social Research, University of Michigan, Ann Arbor, 1972).

7. Examples of Short Global User Satisfaction Measures

Single-Item Measure

Use the following codes to indicate your response:

1 = Strongly disagree   5 = Slightly agree
2 = Disagree   6 = Agree
3 = Slightly disagree   7 = Strongly agree
4 = Neutral

How much do you agree with the following statement about the system?

The new computer system is worth the time and effort required to use it.   1 2 3 4 5 6 7

Use the following code to indicate your response:

1 = Significantly decreased   5 = Slightly increased
2 = Decreased   6 = Increased
3 = Slightly decreased   7 = Significantly increased
4 = No change, no opinion

Overall, to what extent has the system changed these two aspects of *your own* department?

Ease of performing our department's work	1 2 3 4 5 6 7
Quality of our department's work	1 2 3 4 5 6 7

Note: Single-item measure test-retest reliability on same questionnaire in different context is .73. Cronbach's alpha for three items combined is .83.

Source: C.E. Aydin and R.E. Rice. Social worlds, individual differences, and implementation: Predicting attitudes toward a medical information system, Information and Management 20 (1991) 119–136.

8. *Instruments to Assess Employee Adaptation*

Use Scale

How frequently have you had problems with the MIS since implementation?

1. All day long every day
2. Several times a day
3. About once a day
4. Several times a week
5. Once a week or less

If you could do away with the MIS and go back to the old way of doing things, would you?

1. Yes
2. No

How frequently do you find it necessary to bypass the MIS and use the old way of doing things?

1. All day long every day
2. Several times a day
3. About once a day
4. Several times a week
5. Once a week or less

How frequently do you feel like hitting the MIS terminal or breaking a light pen?

1. All day long every day
2. Several times a day

3. About once a day
4. Several times a week
5. Once a week or less
6. Never

Change Scale

How has the MIS changed your job?
This MIS has made my job:

more difficult	1	7 easier
more interesting	1	7 less interesting
less stressful	1	7 more stressful
more fun	1	7 less fun
more pleasant	1	7 less pleasant

Behavioral Scale

Please rate the frequency with which this employee has exhibited the following behaviors with regard to the MIS (1 = never, 2 = occasionally, 3 = fairly frequently, 4 = very frequently):

1. Praising the MIS
2. Difficulty learning to use the MIS
3. Very cooperative with MIS personnel
4. Complaining about the MIS
5. A high level of proficiency learning to use the MIS
6. Lack of cooperation with the MIS personnel
7. Improved work performance
8. Increased absenteeism or tardiness
9. Using the MIS appropriately
10. Slowing work performance
11. Enjoying working on the MIS
12. Bypassing the MIS (i.e., using pre-MIS procedures to do things)

Scoring

Use Scale: Responses to the items were summed to derive a total score. Cronbach alpha was .79.

Change Scale: Responses to items 2 through 5 were reversed and then the five items were summed to derive a total change score. Cronbach alpha was .82.

Behavioral Scale: All of the negative items are reversed and a total score computed. Cronbach Alpha was .80.

Source: K.H. Kjerulff, M.A. Counte, J.S. Salloway, and B.C. Campbell. Understanding employee reactions to a medical information system, in:

Proceedings of the Fifth Annual Symposium on Computer Applications in Medical Care, Los Angeles, CA, IEEE Computer Society Press (1981), pp. 802–805.

9. *Patient Survey*

The Department of Preventive Medicine (Health Appraisal Clinic) is continually striving to meet your expectations for excellence in quality of care and service. You can help us understand how we might do better by filling out this survey. The following questions are designed to focus our attention on areas of concern to you. Questions concerning computers are included to help us determine how they may add or detract from the quality of the examination. Videotaping examinations allows us to learn about interactions during the exam that patient surveys and interviews alone cannot. The results of the survey will be confidential and anonymous. Thank you for helping us improve our service to you.

Please complete the survey by answering the following questions:

Age___   Sex M___F___   Length membership___ years
Do you have a regular doctor?   ___Yes   ___No
Highest education level: 6–12___   college___   postgrad___
Income level: ___under $20,000 ___under $50,000 ___greater than $50,000
I use a computer at home and/or work.   Yes___   No___

Please answer the following questions by placing a circle around the number that most closely fits. For example, if you strongly disagree with the statement, circle #1. If you strongly agree, circle #5. If you fall somewhere in between, circle #2 or #3 or #4. We are asking for you opinion; there are no right or wrong answers. Feel free to give us your honest opinion.

Strongly Disagree (1)	Disagree (2)	Neutral (3)	Agree (4)	Strongly Agree (5)

1. I am satisfied with my visit to the Health Appraisal Clinic.   1 2 3 4 5
2. The staff of the Health Appraisal Clinic treat me with courtesy and respect.   1 2 3 4 5
3. The Health Appraisal Clinic is a valuable part of my membership in the Health Plan.   1 2 3 4 5
4. I am satisfied with the "multiphasic" (first half) portion of the examination.   1 2 3 4 5
5. I am satisfied with the physical examination (second half).   1 2 3 4 5
6. The Health Appraisal Clinic is one of the reasons I will renew my membership in the Health Plan. 1 2 3 4 5

7. The examiner seemed to care about my problems.	1 2 3 4 5
8. The examiner gave me a chance to really say what was on my mind.	1 2 3 4 5
9. I really felt understood by the examiner.	1 2 3 4 5
10. The examiner accepted me as a person.	1 2 3 4 5
11. The examiner relieved my anxiety.	1 2 3 4 5
12. The examiner paid attention to me.	1 2 3 4 5
13. The examiner's attention was focused on the chart/computer.	1 2 3 4 5
14. It was easy to talk to the examiner.	1 2 3 4 5
15. The examiner answered all of my questions.	1 2 3 4 5
16. I am confident with the results of the history and physical examinations.	1 2 3 4 5
17. The examiner explained my health status in words that I could understand.	1 2 3 4 5
18. The examiner is good at explaining the reasons for medical tests.	1 2 3 4 5
19. After talking with the examiner, I have a good understanding of my health status.	1 2 3 4 5
20. I understood the examiner's plan for follow-up of my health related status (if needed).	1 2 3 4 5
21. The examiner gave me a thorough examination.	1 2 3 4 5
22. The examiner looked into all the problems I mentioned.	1 2 3 4 5
23. I am confident with the abilities of the examiner.	1 2 3 4 5
24. The examiner spent enough time with me.	1 2 3 4 5
25. The examiner seemed rushed during his/her examination of me.	1 2 3 4 5
26. It will be easy to follow the advice of the examiner.	1 2 3 4 5
27. I will follow the advice of the examiner completely.	1 2 3 4 5
28. The advice the examiner gave me is very important.	1 2 3 4 5
29. If I follow all the advice, my health is likely to improve.	1 2 3 4 5
30. It is important for me to get well and stay well.	1 2 3 4 5
31. I trust computers.	1 2 3 4 5
32. Computers can make mistakes.	1 2 3 4 5
33 The examiner seemed to have trouble using the computer.	1 2 3 4 5
34. I think the computer helps the examiner take care of me.	1 2 3 4 5
35 If given a choice, I would choose an examiner who uses a computer.	1 2 3 4 5

Sources: C.E. Aydin, J.G. Anderson, P.N. Rosen, V.J. Felitti, and H.C. Weng. Computers in the consulting room: Clinician and patient perspectives, Health Care Management Science 1 (1998) 61–74. Used with permission.

Survey items 7–14 (Affective Scale), 15–20 (Cognitive Scale), and 21–25 (Behavior Scale) were adapted from M.H. Wolf, S.M. Putnam, S.A. James, and W.B. Stiles. The medical interview satisfaction scale: Development of a scale to measure patient perceptions of physician behavior, Journal of Behavioral Medicine 1 (1978) 391–401. Items 7–12 and 14 were used as a 6-item scale. Item 13, the reversed item, did not scale with the others (i.e., after scoring was reversed the addition of this item to the scale reduced the Cronbach alpha coefficient significantly). Item 13 was used as a single item. Items 21–24 were used as 4-item scale. Item 25, the reversed item, did not scale with the others and was used as a single item. Items 26–30 (Acceptance of advice scale) were adapted from J. Kincey, P. Bradshaw, and P. Ley. Patients' satisfaction and reported acceptance of advice in general practice, Journal of the Royal College of General Practitioners 25 (1975) 558–566. Items 31–35 (Computer in exam room scale) were adapted from G. Brownbridge, E.J. Lilford, and S. Tindale-Biscoe. Use of a computer to take booking histories in a hospital antenatal clinic, Medical Care 26 (1988) 474–487. Items 31, 34–35 were used as 3-item scale. Items 32 and 33, the reversed items, did not scale with the others. Item 32 was not used; item 33 was used as a single item. Question 35 was also used as a single item in some analyses.

10. Laboratory Computer Impact Survey

The next set of questions asks about how things have changed since the introduction of the laboratory computer system. Please base your answers on what it is like now, not on how it was when the computer system was installed. Please answer as best as you can, even if you weren't here when the computer was installed.

External Communication (coefficient alpha = .62; mean response = 3.37)
>   The computer makes it easier to route samples to the appropriate laboratory.
>   Computerized lab records aid communication between the lab and other personnel.
>   The computer system improves the relationship between the labs and other medical personnel.

Service Outcomes (coefficient alpha = .84; mean response = 3.13)
>   We provide better service because of the computer.
>   We should have gotten a computer system a long time ago.
>   The computer helps make the labs better managed.
>   Overall, reports from my lab are more accurate now than before the computer was installed.
>   Test reports are more accurate because they have to be entered into the computer.

Because of the computer there is better interpretive information provided with test reports.

Personal Intentions (coefficient alpha = .53; mean response = 4.30)

I plan to avoid using the computer system as much as possible. I

I plan to use the computer system as much as possible.

Personal Hassles (coefficient alpha = .86; mean response = 2.68)

The number of phone calls I answer has increased.

Since the computer was installed my work is more satisfying than it used to be. I

The computer makes it harder to meet all the demands placed on me.

Because of the computer I now have more work to do.

The computer has changed my job from being a technologist to being a clerk.

My responsibilities have increased because of the computer.

Our work is slowed down because we have to do data entry.

We have to find ways around the computer in order to get our work done.

Increased Blame (coefficient alpha = .87; mean response = 2.71)

People call the lab now with more problems and questions that I wish I didn't have to deal with.

Since the computer was installed people in the labs are getting blamed for problems that aren't really their fault.

Doctors and nurses complain to us more now that we have the computer.

We now do a lot of work CPA (specimen intake) did.

We get blamed for CPA's mistakes.

The computer people run the labs now.

Doctors and nurses cooperate with us less than they did before the computer.

I don't think doctors and nurses like the computer system.

The computer system causes ill will toward the labs.

Response Scale: Range from 1 to 5: 1 = Strongly disagree, 3 = Neutral, 5 = Strongly agree. I indicates reverse scoring.

Note: Questions concerning personal intentions were adapted from Kjerulff et al., Predicting employee adaptation to the implementation of a medical information system, in: *Proceedings of the Sixth Annual Symposium on Computer Applications in Medical Care*, Silver Springs, MD, IEEE Computer Society (1982), pp. 392–397.

Source: B. Kaplan and D. Duchon. A qualitative and quantitative investigation of a computer system's impact on work in clinical laboratories (unpublished manuscript) (1987); B. Kaplan and D. Duchon, A job orientation model of impact on work seven months post-implementation, in: *Proceedings of Medinfo 89: Sixth World Congress on Medical Informatics*, Amsterdam, North-Holland (1989), pp. 1051–1055.

11. WatchChild Obstetrical System Pre-Implementation Survey

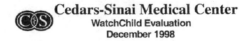

Cedars-Sinai Medical Center
WatchChild Evaluation
December 1998

This questionnaire asks you what you think it will be like using WatchChild as part of your job. You will be asked to answer the same questions again after you have had experience using the system. Your responses will help us evaluate how well WatchChild meets your needs. Your responses are anonymous and your opinions are important to us. *Please fill in the circle that indicates your response to each question. (Use blue or black ink or No. 2 pencil and darken the circle completely.)*

	Strongly Disagree		Neutral or Uncertain		Strongly Agree
1. WatchChild will be worth the time and effort required to use it.	○ 1	○ 2	○ 3	○ 4	○ 5
2. My job will be more satisfying.	○ 1	○ 2	○ 3	○ 4	○ 5
3. Others will better see the results of my efforts.	○ 1	○ 2	○ 3	○ 4	○ 5
4. It will be easier to perform my job well.	○ 1	○ 2	○ 3	○ 4	○ 5
5. The accuracy of iinformation I receive will be improved by WatchChild.	○ 1	○ 2	○ 3	○ 4	○ 5
6. I will have more control over my job.	○ 1	○ 2	○ 3	○ 4	○ 5
7. I will be able to improve my performance.	○ 1	○ 2	○ 3	○ 4	○ 5
8. Others will be more aware of what I am doing.	○ 1	○ 2	○ 3	○ 4	○ 5
9. The information I receive from WatchChild will make my job easier.	○ 1	○ 2	○ 3	○ 4	○ 5
10. I will spend less time looking for information.	○ 1	○ 2	○ 3	○ 4	○ 5
11. I will be better able to see the results of my effort.	○ 1	○ 2	○ 3	○ 4	○ 5
12. The accuracy of my charting will improve as a result of using WatchChild	○ 1	○ 2	○ 3	○ 4	○ 5
13. My performance will be more closely monitored.	○ 1	○ 2	○ 3	○ 4	○ 5
14. The Department will perform better.	○ 1	○ 2	○ 3	○ 4	○ 5
15. Top management will provide the resources to implement WatchChild.	○ 1	○ 2	○ 3	○ 4	○ 5
16. People will accept the required changes.	○ 1	○ 2	○ 3	○ 4	○ 5
17. Top management sees the computer system as being important.	○ 1	○ 2	○ 3	○ 4	○ 5
18. Implementing WatchChild will be difficult.	○ 1	○ 2	○ 3	○ 4	○ 5
19. Top management does not realize how complex this change is.	○ 1	○ 2	○ 3	○ 4	○ 5
20. People will be given sufficient training to utilize WatchChild.	○ 1	○ 2	○ 3	○ 4	○ 5
21. There will be adequate staff available to successfully implement WatchChild.	○ 1	○ 2	○ 3	○ 4	○ 5
22. Personal conflicts will not increase as a result of WatchChild.	○ 1	○ 2	○ 3	○ 4	○ 5
23. The developers of WatchChild will provide adequate training to users.	○ 1	○ 2	○ 3	○ 4	○ 5
24. We will provide better service because of WatchChild.	○ 1	○ 2	○ 3	○ 4	○ 5
25. I plan to avoid using WatchChild as much as possible.	○ 1	○ 2	○ 3	○ 4	○ 5
26. I plan to use WatchChild as much as possible.	○ 1	○ 2	○ 3	○ 4	○ 5
27. WatchChild will make it harder to meet all the demands placed on me.	○ 1	○ 2	○ 3	○ 4	○ 5
28. Because of WatchChild I will have more work to do.	○ 1	○ 2	○ 3	○ 4	○ 5
29. My responsibilities will increase because of WatchChild.	○ 1	○ 2	○ 3	○ 4	○ 5
30. My work will be slowed down because I will have to do data entry.	○ 1	○ 2	○ 3	○ 4	○ 5
31. I will have to find ways around WatchChild to get my work done.	○ 1	○ 2	○ 3	○ 4	○ 5
32. WatchChild will interfere with my relationships with my patients.	○ 1	○ 2	○ 3	○ 4	○ 5

48506

48506

	Strongly Disagree		Neutral or Uncertain		Strongly Agree
33. Having WatchChild will improve patient satisfaction with care.	○ 1	○ 2	○ 3	○ 4	○ 5
34. I am confident that I will be able to learn to use WatchChild.	○ 1	○ 2	○ 3	○ 4	○ 5

	Almost never	Some of the time	Almost half of the time	Most of the time	Almost Always
35. I am satisfied with the accuracy of the WatchChild system.	○ 1	○ 2	○ 3	○ 4	○ 5
36. WatchChild output is presented in a clear and useful format.	○ 1	○ 2	○ 3	○ 4	○ 5
37. The information is clear.	○ 1	○ 2	○ 3	○ 4	○ 5
38. The system is user-friendly.	○ 1	○ 2	○ 3	○ 4	○ 5
39. The system is easy to use	○ 1	○ 2	○ 3	○ 4	○ 5

40. How long have you worked in Women's Health at Cedars-Sinai? ○ 1 year or less   ○ 2-5 years ○ More than 5 years

41. Please evaluate the WatchChild training you have received so far.

○ Poor   ○ Fair   ○ Good   ○ Very Good   ○ Excellent

Position   ○ RN   Shift (Check only one) ○ Day   Primary Area: ○ Labor & Delivery
           ○ MD   ○ Night   (RNs only)   ○ Triage
           ○ NCT   ○ Not Applicable   Check only   ○ MFCU
           ○ Other   one   ○ Postpartum
                                                                         ○ Antepartum Testing
                                                                         ○ Generalist

Are you a WatchChild Superuser? ○ Yes   ○ No

Comments:

For office use only

○ ○ ○
① ① ①
② ② ②
③ ③ ③
④ ④ ④
⑤ ⑤ ⑤
⑥ ⑥ ⑥
⑦ ⑦ ⑦
⑧ ⑧ ⑧
⑨ ⑨ ⑨

48506

12. WatchChild Obstetrical System Post-Implementation Survey

55608

Cedars-Sinai Medical Center
WatchChild Evaluation
April 2000

This questionnaire asks you what it is like using WatchChild as part of your job. You were asked some of the same questions before you began using the system. Your responses help us evaluate how well WatchChild meets your needs. Your responses are anonymous and your opinions are important to us. *Please fill in the circle that indicates your response to each question. (Use blue or black ink or No. 2 pencil and darken the circle completely.)*

	Strongly Disagree		Neutral or Uncertain		Strongly Agree
1. WatchChild is worth the time and effort required to use it.	○ 1	○ 2	○ 3	○ 4	○ 5
2. Others now see the results or my efforts better.	○ 1	○ 2	○ 3	○ 4	○ 5
3. The information I receive from WatchChild makes my job easier.	○ 1	○ 2	○ 3	○ 4	○ 5
4. I avoid using WatchChild as much as possible.	○ 1	○ 2	○ 3	○ 4	○ 5
5. WatchChild makes it harder to meet all the demands placed on me.	○ 1	○ 2	○ 3	○ 4	○ 5
6. WatchChild interferes with my relationships with my patients.	○ 1	○ 2	○ 3	○ 4	○ 5

	Almost never	Some of the time	Almost half of the time	Most of the time	Almost Always
7. I am satisfied with the accuracy of the WatchChild system.	○ 1	○ 2	○ 3	○ 4	○ 5
8. WatchChild output is presented in a clear and useful format.	○ 1	○ 2	○ 3	○ 4	○ 5
9. The information is clear.	○ 1	○ 2	○ 3	○ 4	○ 5
10. The system is user-friendly.	○ 1	○ 2	○ 3	○ 4	○ 5
11. The system is easy to use.	○ 1	○ 2	○ 3	○ 4	○ 5

12. How long have you worked in Women's Health at Cedars-Sinai? ○ 1 year or less   ○ 2-5 years   ○ More than 5 years

Position   ○ RN   Shift (Check only one) ○ Day   Primary Area: ○ Labor & Delivery
            ○ MD   ○ Night   (RNs only)   ○ Triage
            ○ NCT   ○ Not Applicable Check only   ○ MFCU
            ○ Other   one   ○ Postpartum
                                                                               ○ Antepartum Testing
Are you a WatchChild Superuser? ○ Yes   ○ No   ○ Generalist

Comments:

For office use only

| ⓪①②③④⑤⑥⑦⑧⑨ |
| ⓪①②③④⑤⑥⑦⑧⑨ |
| ⓪①②③④⑤⑥⑦⑧⑨ |

55608

WatchChild2 4/2000

Sources: C.E. Aydin, K. Gregory, L. Korst, J. Polaschek, and T. Chamorro. Panel: Making it happen: Organizational changes required to implement an electronic medical record in a large medical center, in: *AMIA'99 Annual Symposium*, Washington, DC (November 6–10, 1999). Reprinted with permission: K. Gregory, Cedars-Sinai Medical Center.

13. Work Role Activities

Each subject is asked how they spent their time yesterday (in hours and minutes). They are also asked if that time period was a typical working day: Very typical, Somewhat typical, Not at all typical. The proportion of time on each activity is calculated by summing their total work time in minutes and dividing the reported minutes spent on each activity by that sum. Data are collected before and after implementation of a computer system: Before implementation, 6 months after implementation, 1 year after implementation.

Activities

Talking on the telephone
Filling out forms
Talking with patients and families
Extraneous paperwork
Helping other departments acquire information
Talking with co-workers
Data processing
Traveling around the hospital
Attendance at meetings

Sources: M.A. Counte, K.H. Kjerulff, J.C. Salloway, and B.C. Campbell. Implementing computerization in hospitals: A case study of the behavioral and attitudinal impacts of a medical information system, Journal of Organizational Behavior Management 6 (1984) 109–122. Printed with permission.

14. Network Survey

This question is a little different. Your answers will help describe how some jobs are related to other jobs. Again, we assure you that your answers will be kept completely confidential. Please indicate: *How frequently, on the average, do you have significant discussions with other SHS personnel about how you accomplish your work?* For each person, please circle the number that best indicates the frequency of those discussions:

0 = Not once in the past year
1 = Once a month or so
2 = Several times a month

3 = Every week
4 = Several times a week
5 = Every day
6 = Several times a day

The names and units of all personnel are listed in alphabetical order in the first two columns. For example:

Personnel	Unit	Never	Month	Times/Mo.	Week	Times/Wk.	Day	Times/Day
Jones, J.	Lab	0	1	2	3	4	5	6
Smith	Admin	0	1	2	3	4	5	6
West	Clinic	0	1	2	3	4	5	6
Etc.								

Source: R.E. Rice and C.E. Aydin. Attitudes toward new organizational technology: Network proximity as a mechanism for social information processing, Administrative Science Quarterly 36 (1991) 219–244.

15. Communication Between Departments

This survey asks you to think about communication between your area and other departments in the medical center. Please circle only one answer *on each line*. All responses will be *confidential*.

How often do you usually speak to someone from each of the following departments on the telephone?

	Many Times a Day	A Few Times a Day	Once a Day	A Few Times a Week	Once a Week	Never
Admitting	6	5	4	3	2	1
Radiology	6	5	4	3	2	1
Etc.						

(Add additional departments to list)

Note: Test-retest reliabilities for Admitting = .79, Radiology = .80, from beginning to end of 3-hour class on order entry.

Source: C.E. Aydin. Computerized order entry in a large medical center: Evaluating interactions between departments, in: J.G. Anderson, C.E. Aydin, and S.J. Jay, editors, *Evaluating Health Care Information Systems: Methods and Applications* (Sage Publications, Thousand Oaks, CA, 1994), pp. 260–275.

16. Job Design Questionnaire

Here are some statements about your job. How much do you agree or disagree with each?

1 = Strongly disagree   5 = Slightly agree
2 = Disagree   6 = Agree

3 = Slightly disagree   7 = Strongly agree
4 = Undecided

My job:

1. provides much variety   1 2 3 4 5 6 7
2. permits me to be left on my own to do   1 2 3 4 5 6 7
   my own work
3. is arranged so that I often have the opportunity   1 2 3 4 5 6 7
   to see jobs or projects through to completion
4. provides feedback on how well am doing as   1 2 3 4 5 6 7
   I am working
5. is relatively significant in our organization   1 2 3 4 5 6 7
6. gives me considerable opportunity for   1 2 3 4 5 6 7
   independence and freedom in how I do my work
7. gives me the opportunity to do a number of   1 2 3 4 5 6 7
   different things
8. provides me an opportunity to find out how well   1 2 3 4 5 6 7
   am doing
9. is very significant or important in the broader   1 2 3 4 5 6 7
   scheme of things
10. provides an opportunity for independent thought   1 2 3 4 5 6 7
    and action
11. provides me with a great deal of variety at work   1 2 3 4 5 6 7
12. is arranged so that I have the opportunity to   1 2 3 4 5 6 7
    complete the work I start
13. provides me with the feeling that I know whether   1 2 3 4 5 6 7
    I am performing well or poorly
14. is arranged so that I have the chance to do   1 2 3 4 5 6 7
    a job from the beginning to the end (i.e.,
    a chance to do the whole job)
15. is one where a lot of other people can be   1 2 3 4 5 6 7
    affected by how well the work gets done

Scoring

Skill variety: Questions 1, 7, 11
Task identity: Questions 3, 12, 14
Task significance: Questions 5, 9, 15
Autonomy: Questions 2, 6, 10
Feedback about results: Questions 4, 8, 13

A total score for each job dimension is computed by adding the responses for the three items for a total score ranging from 3 (low) to 21 (high).

Source: T.G. Cummings and E.F. Huse. *Organization Development and Change*, 4th ed. (West, St. Paul, MN, 1989), p. 92. Reprinted by permission of T. Cummings, University of Southern California.

17. Job Satisfaction

Use the following codes to indicate your response:

1 = Strongly dissatisfied
2 = Dissatisfied
3 = Neutral or No opinion
4 = Satisfied
5 = Strongly satisfied

How satisfied are you with:

The nature of the work you perform?	1 2 3 4 5
The person who supervises you—your organizational superior?	1 2 3 4 5
Your relations with others in the organization with whom you work—your co-workers?	1 2 3 4 5
The pay you receive for your job?	1 2 3 4 5
The opportunities that exist in this organization for advancement—with promotion?	1 2 3 4 5

Scoring

Sum into one global job satisfaction index.

Test-retest reliability over 14 days for individual items involving 36 secretaries ranged from .71 to .73; for overall sum, .83. Convergent validity correlations, compared to Job Descriptive Index (JDI) and Minnesota Importance Questionnaire (MSQ) for 308 public utility employees and 96 middle managers of a transport company were from .59 to .80. (See J.D. Cook, S.J. Hepworth, T.D. Wall, and P.B. Warr. *The Experience of Work* (Academic Press, New York, 1981), for details of JDI and MSQ.) Discriminant validity showed 100% of directional comparisons and Kendall's W showed .72 to .90 for patterns across different items by methods. Criterion validity showed nearly identical correlations as JDI to task structure, group cohesiveness, and supervisory consideration.

Source: C. Schriesheim and A. Tsui. Development and validation of a short satisfaction measure for use in survey feedback interventions. Paper presented at the Academy of Management Western Region Meeting (April 1981).

5
Using the Internet for Surveys and Research

Gunther Eysenbach

Introduction

This chapter gives an overview of the use of the Internet in the research process, with emphasis on using the Internet as a source for qualitative research and on using the Web for surveys. The Internet obviously also plays a role in literature research, finding methods, protocols and instruments, communicating with peers, and dissemination of results (i.e., electronic publishing). These topics are beyond the scope of this chapter.

Qualitative Research

The Internet is the most comprehensive archive of written material representing our world and peoples' opinions, concerns, and desires, at least those of the industrialized world. Physicians who surf the Internet for the first time are often stunned by what they learn on websites of patient self-support groups. This illustrates that material published on the Internet may be a valuable resource for researchers desiring to understand people and the social and cultural contexts within which they live, giving due emphasis to the meanings, experiences, and views of people.

With its myriad websites, blogs, chats, mailing lists, and discussion boards, the Internet is a rich source for qualitative research (e.g., identifying research issues, generating hypotheses, or for *needs assessment*). Systematic reviews (content analysis) of information posted by consumers and/ or health professionals on the Internet may help to identify health beliefs, common topics, motives, information, and emotional needs of patients and healthcare professionals, and point to areas where research is needed or where information systems can fill an information gap. Log-files of search terms used by consumers or health professionals [1] or questions asked in private e-mail conversations (e.g., between patients and providers) are another potential data source for an information system needs analysis.

In the context of iteratively developing a healthcare information system, developers may integrate discussion boards in the system for users to discuss the system and make suggestions for improvements. Qualitative analysis user postings may be a component of the *formative or summative evaluation* process, and may elicit richer data than (quantitative) surveys.

The ease with which information is accessible for analysis and the anonymity of the Web allows researchers to analyze text and narratives on websites, use newsgroups as global focus groups, and conduct interviews and surveys using e-mail, in chat rooms, on websites, and in newsgroups. Evolving branches of qualitative research include the analysis of interactive communication on the Internet (e-mail), studying Internet communities (virtual self-help groups, newsgroups, mailing lists), investigating communication processes between patients and professionals, reviewing the World Wide Web (www) to study consumer preferences, patient concerns, and information needs, and exploring the "epidemiology of health information" ("infodemiology") on the Web [2–4].

As will be expanded below, the Web population is certainly not representative of the general population, restricting its use for quantitative studies. Qualitative studies, on the other hand, do not necessarily require representative samples, since

in qualitative research we are not interested in an average view of a patient population, but want to gain an in-depth understanding of the experience of particular individuals or groups; we should therefore deliberately seek out individuals or groups who fit the bill. [5]

Still, even in qualitative studies, one should not forget that the experiences, views, and opinions gathered through the Internet may differ systematically from those of the general population, so that these methods are often ideally complemented by doing face-to-face focus groups and interviews with traditional sampling methods. Although some studies have suggested that there are no systematic differences (i.e., the themes emerging from an online focus group are the same as the themes emerging from an offline focus group [6]), this certainly depends on the research question. For example, a study on access barriers to an information system may elicit totally new themes in an offline group because the online group is too self-selected.

Broadly, three different research methodologies for qualitative research on the Web may be distinguished:

1. *Passive analysis*, for example, studying information patterns on websites or narratives and/or interactions in newsgroups, mailing lists, chat rooms, without researchers actively involving themselves.
2. *Active analysis* (can also be called participant observation), meaning that the researchers participate in the communication process, often without disclosing their identity as researchers.
3. *Interviews and surveys*—see below.

These methods have different ethical implications [2], as will be expanded in the following section.

Some examples of (mostly qualitative) research on the Internet are given in Table 5.1.

Ethical Issues

The ethical issues involved in online research (passive analysis, active analysis, and survey research) should not be ignored [2,31–36]. These include informed consent as a basic ethical tenet of scientific research on human populations [37], protection of privacy, and avoiding psychological harm (e.g., by intruding in virtual communities).

In qualitative research on the Web, informed consent is required (1) when data are collected from research participants through any form of communication, interaction, or intervention; or (2) when behavior of research participants occurs in a private context where an individual can reasonably expect that no observation or reporting is taking place. Informed consent is not required

when researchers do research in public places or use publicly available information about individuals (e.g., naturalistic observations in public places, analysis of public records, or archival research). [38]

The question therefore arises whether researchers "passively" analyzing newsgroup postings enter a "public place" (in which case obtaining informed consent would not be necessary) or whether the space they invade is perceived as private (in which case obtaining informed consent is necessary). In the context of research, the expectation of the individual (whether he or she can reasonably expect that no observation is taking place) is crucial. Different Internet venues have different levels of perceived privacy (in decreasing order of privacy: private e-mails → chat rooms → mailing lists → Usenet newsgroups → websites). The perceived level of privacy is a function of the number of participants, but also depends on other arrangements such as the group norms established by the community to be studied. For example, in the controversial study of Finn, the authors studied a virtual self-support group where the moderator was actively discouraging interested professionals who were not sexual abuse survivors from joining the group, which should have deterred researchers from joining the group for research purposes [17].

While the group moderator can and should be consulted for any research with a specific virtual community, the consent of the moderator is rarely sufficient and cannot replace informed consent from the subjects studied. Therefore, in practice, obtaining informed consent, especially for passive research methods, is difficult, as researchers usually cannot post an announcement to a mailing list or newsgroup saying that it will be monitored and analyzed for the next few months, as this may greatly bias the

TABLE 5.1. Framework for and examples of research on the Internet.

	Passive analysis (naturalistic observation)	Active analysis (observation as active participant)	Interviews and surveys
Objectives examples	Identifying research priorities; needs assessments; studying narratives; identifying and studying the "epidemiology" of health beliefs, topics, motives, information and emotional needs etc.; studying gaps between evidence and peoples' experiences	Studying communication processes, e.g., patient–professional interaction, communication processes in virtual self-help groups	Identifying concerns, opinions; generating hypotheses; formative evaluation
Example method	Content analysis of Internet information	Action research; participant observation; ethnography (e.g., participating in a mailing list and studying reactions)	Web-based questionnaires, e-mail questionnaires
IRB/ethical committee approval	Not always necessary, but may be advisable if reporting involves vulnerable online communities	Usually necessary	Usually necessary
Examples of studies on websites	Reviews of Internet information [7]; ethnography on websites [8]; observing usage patterns (log-file analysis) [9]; analyzing search terms.	n/a	Web-based forms: gathering clinical epidemiological data [10]; survey among peers [11]; health status assessment [12]; quality of life research [13]
Examples of studies on newsgroups/ mailing lists	Analyzing messages on newsgroups [14–17] or mailing lists [18,19]	Asking questions on a newsgroup and analyzing feedback [20,21]	Posting questionnaires on a newsgroup [22]
Examples of studies on chat rooms	Using case stories from a chat room and other venues [23]	No study published yet	Online focus groups [6]
Examples of studies on e-mail interaction	Analyzing unsolicited e-mails to identify motives and information needs [24] or improving information systems [25]	Posing as a patient and sending a fictitious case to physicians [21,26–29]	E-mail surveys [30]

results. Subjects who know that they are being monitored may behave differently than under normal circumstances (*Hawthorne effect*). Apart from this threat to validity of the research, postings of researchers may in extreme cases disrupt or even destroy a virtual community.

A much better alternative would be to analyze the communication retrospectively and write individual e-mails to all participants whose comments are to be analyzed or quoted, asking for permission to use them; this technique has been used, for example, by Sharf [39].

Informed consent may also play a role when researchers report aggregate data on usage patterns, such as a log-file analysis (reporting data on what websites have been accessed by a population). Crucial here seems to be an appropriate privacy statement to be brought to the awareness of all users, saying that these data may be analyzed and reported in aggregate [33]. For survey research, researchers may obtain informed consent by declaring the purpose of the study, disclosing which institutions are behind the study, and explaining how privacy will be assured, with whom data will be shared, and how data will be reported before participants complete the questionnaire.

When reporting results, it is obvious that the total anonymity of research participants needs to be maintained. Researchers must keep in mind that, by the very process of quoting the exact words of a newsgroup participant, the confidentiality of the participant may already be broken. This is because powerful search engines such as AltaVista or DejaNews can retrieve the original message, including the e-mail address of the sender if a direct quote is entered into the query. Therefore, it is essential to ask newsgroup participants whether they agree to be quoted, pointing out the risk that they may be identifiable.

Problems can also potentially arise from just citing the name of the community (e.g., of a newsgroup), which may damage the community studied. For example, King [35] quotes the complaint of a group participant that he feels uncomfortable being observed and retreats from a group with the remark that "When I joined this, I thought it would be a support group, not a fishbowl for a bunch of guinea pigs. I certainly don't feel at this point that it is a safe environment, as a support group is supposed to be, and I will not open myself up to be dissected by students or scientists."

Internet Surveys

Taxonomy of Internet Surveys

Interviews versus Questionnaires

In general, surveys may be conducted by means of interactive (one-to-one, in the case of individual interviews, or one-to-many, in the case of focus groups) interviews or by questionnaires designed for self-completion. Both methods can be used on the Internet: electronic interviews can be conducted via e-mail or in chat-rooms [6]; survey questionnaires can be administered either by e-mail (e.g., using mailing lists), posted in newsgroups or discussion forums, or on the Web using HTML forms.

Email versus Web Questionnaires

Surveys distributed by e-mail or posted in discussion forums are usually simple plain text (ASCII) versions and usually instruct participants to e-mail the completed questionnaire back to the researcher, who then needs to enter the responses into a database. In contrast, Web-based surveys allow for survey elements such as radio buttons, checkboxes, drop-down lists, and text fields, and store the responses directly in a database, where they are immediately accessible for real-time analysis.

Web-based surveys have the advantage (or disadvantage, depending on the context and objective) that the respondent can stay anonymous (as opposed to e-mail-based surveys, where the e-mail address of the responder is revealed).

If e-mails are used to administer (and reply to) questionnaires, they are usually sent to a selected group with a known number of participants, so that the response rate can be calculated. Server-side software used to administer mailing lists (e.g., listserv or majordomo) often have commands that allow users of mailing lists to view the list of subscribers or at least determine their number (e.g., WHO for majordomo), so that the researcher can determine the denominator when sending an e-mail to a mailing list. However, the list owner can also disable this command, meaning that the number of subscribers of a mailing list may also be unknown.

Surveys posted on a discussion forum such as a Usenet newsgroup are even more problematic since it is usually impossible to determine who and how many people read the questionnaire. Thus, a response rate (which serves as indicator of how representative the responses are) cannot be calculated. In the continuum between highly controlled survey administration for rigorous research on one hand and uncontrolled surveys for explorative purposes, this method is more on the right hand of this spectrum (see Figure 5.1). However, there are "tricks" allowing the researcher to determine how many people have read a posting on a Web-based forum. If the forum allows HTML postings, the researcher can include an IMG-tag in the body of the message that loads a 1×1 pixel invisible image from a remote server, to which the researcher has access. A simple log-file analysis may then determine how often the image has been served, as an approximation for how often the message has been opened.

Invitation-Only versus Open Web Surveys

If HTML forms are used, they can be either "invitation-only surveys" or "open surveys." In invitation-only surveys, researchers usually publish the survey on a password-protected area of a website and invite only a defined

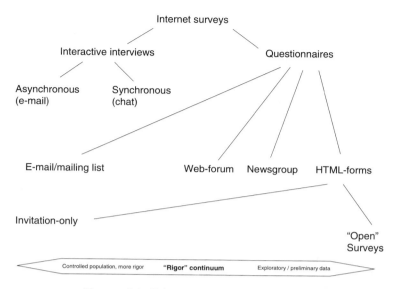

FIGURE 5.1. Taxonomy of Internet surveys.

group of people to participate, for example, by sending the invitation to participate with a password to a select group. In "open (public) surveys," a survey is simply published on a website and is open to the public (e.g., anybody who visits the site can fill in the survey). These two methods are fundamentally different, and the latter ("open" survey) is often regarded as an "unscientific" poll, because the sample usually will be highly self-selected, the response rate is often unknown, and it is not clear who filled in the questionnaire. On the other hand, open surveys may also generate interesting data (even if they are not necessarily generalizable), in particular if qualitative analysis and/or hypothesis generation is the aim, or if the objective is to study trends over time. Also, as outlined below, while more difficult, it is not impossible to calculate response rates for open surveys (if cookies are used), and multiple completions by the same individual usually can be detected using log-files and cookies.

Survey Tools

A number of commercial "survey construction kits" exist, for example, www.surveywriter.com, SurveyShare.com, www.websurveyor.com, www.quask.com, or www.researchexec.com, to name a few. These products allow researchers to set up a Web questionnaire within minutes. Often, however, these "turnkey" solutions have some limitations in respect to the more sophisticated features such as setting cookies to prevent or identify multiple entries from the same person, or creating more complex multipage surveys with multiple branching options.

Internet Surveys in Health Research

Communication scientists, sociologists, and psychologists were among the first to use the Internet for survey research, while its use for *health* research is still emerging [40–46]. Soetikno [13] used the Internet for quality-of-life research. Eysenbach [10] reported the collection of clinical data from atopy patients. Bethell and collegues explored the use of online consumer surveys as a methodology for assessing the quality of the U.S. healthcare system [47]. Hilsden et al. report a Web-based survey among 263 patients with inflammatory bowel disease [48], Potts and Wyatt surveyed general practitioners on the Web [49], and Schleyer used the Web to conduct a survey among 314 dentists [11,50]. A recent systematic review identified 17 Internet-based surveys of health professionals [51].

In addition to gathering data, the Internet may also be used in the course of developing the questionnaire itself, as it allows rapid prototyping and iterative testing of instruments, for example, to quickly evaluate the effect of framing the questions differently [52].

Several studies have checked the validity of Web-based surveys by comparing the results of studies conducted on the Web with identical studies in the real world. Some seem to suggest that data obtained through the Web are comparable to classical methods [6,40,41,53–55], but issues of limited external validity (questionable generalizability mainly due to selection bias, discussed in detail below) remain important concerns [56], and the researcher should carefully select his or her research question and interpret the results within the limits of the methodology. The benefits and problems of Web-based surveys and some draft guidelines for when they may be appropriate have been summarized by Wyatt [57].

Selection Bias

Selection bias is a systematic error in a research project that occurs because of the nonrepresentative way participants were selected or assigned. Selection bias is a major factor limiting the generalizability ("external validity") of results of Internet surveys. Selection bias in Internet surveys occurs for two reasons: (1) due to the nonrepresentativeness of the Internet population and (2) due to the self-selection of participants (i.e., nonrepresentativeness of respondents, also called the *volunteer effect*) [58].

Selection Bias Due to Internet Demography

While it has been argued that the Internet community is "becoming more representative of society as a whole" [59], in reality the Internet community is far from representative of the world's population, or even the population in any given country, and it is unlikely that this fact is going to change in the near future. Household or individual income are important determinants of the presence of personal computers and the extent of Internet access in homes [60]. In higher-income groups, costs of computer equipment and Internet access are less of a barrier than for low-income groups. High income is also associated with better education, which leads to early uptake of information technology. Thus, it is the socially disadvantaged groups who are likely to be underrepresented on the Web. There is also a gender inequality on the Web, with men being overrepresented, but with women being more interested in health issues and generally more likely to complete online surveys.

Another factor to be taken into account is the age distribution—the population above the age of 50 is, while catching up, still underrepresented on the Web.

Considering whether the topic chosen for the survey is suitable for the Internet population is a first and probably the most important step to minimize bias and to increase external validity of the results, but also to make the survey a success in terms of response rates [57]. For example, an online survey targeting elderly homeless alcoholics is unsuitable for an Internet survey and the results are likely to be heavily skewed by hoax responses.

If the demographics of survey respondents are known, results can be weighted and adjusted to extrapolate how the results would look if a representative sample had completed the questionnaire, although whether these methods are sufficient and lead to meaningful data is controversial [56].

Self-Selection Bias

Self-selection bias ("volunteer effect") comes from the fact that people are more likely to respond to questionnaires if they see items that interest them, for example, because they are affected by the items asked or because they are attracted by the incentives offered for participating. As people who respond almost certainly have different characteristics than those who do not, the results are likely to be biased. This kind of selection bias is more serious than the bias arising from the nonrepresentativeness of the population, because the researcher deals with myriad unknown factors and has few chances to adjust his or her results. Such a bias may be exacerbated by providing nonneutral incentives (e.g., typical "male" incentives such as computer equipment as the prize for a lottery). As women are generally more interested in health topics and display more active information-seeking behavior [61], health questionnaires are often more likely to be filled in by females, which may lead to a different self-selection bias effect for men and women.

Response Rate

In surveys, the potential for self-selection bias can be estimated by measuring the response rate, expressed as the number of people who answered the questionnaire divided by those who have viewed the questionnaire (not to be confused with the participation rate, which can be expressed as the number of website visitors who clicked on the link to the questionnaire divided by the total number of website visitors). A simple way to determine the response rate is to divide the number of unique responses to the questionnaire by the number of accesses to the questionnaire page, counted, for example, by a log-file analysis or with cookies (see below).

A recent systematic review identified 17 Internet-based surveys of health professionals [51] with response rates ranging from 9% to 94%. Sending follow-up reminders resulted in a substantial increase in response rates.

Response rates for online surveys are typically much lower than for traditional surveys. "Open" surveys (i.e., questionnaires on websites offered to anyone) often have a response rate of less than 1%. If the response rates are so low, how can external validity be ascertained? Response *representativeness* is more important than response rate, and if the response rate or participation rate is extremely low, attempts to confirm response representativeness should be undertaken, for example, by

- Comparing the demographics of responders to demographics of non-responders (if known); if the sample is representative, the likelihood for representative responses increases.
- Comparing the answers/survey results of responders to those of non-responders (e.g., nonresponders could be called if their telephone numbers are known).
- Inserting questions into the questionnaire that allow comparison with historical data (or data obtained from offline surveys) so that these results can be compared.

Further Techniques and Tips for Web-Based Surveys

Maximizing Response Rate

The number of contacts, personalized contacts, and precontacts (contacting the participants before the actual survey) are the factors most associated with higher response rates in Web surveys [62]. Offering incentives, such as presents or entering participants into a lottery, increases participation rates but also the danger of introducing selection bias. This is less of a problem with monetary incentives. However, perhaps the best incentives (and the easiest to deliver via the Internet) are to promise the survey results (either after human analysis or an ad hoc real-time analysis of the database), or to give some personalized answer (e.g., a score) to the respondent.

People are increasingly hesitant to fill in online questionnaires and are wary about market research or even bogus surveys that are just designed to collect their e-mail addresses and personal interests. Thus, one should clearly disclose who is behind the study and a university or research institute logo may help to distinguish the survey from market research or dubious advertisements coming in the disguise of a survey.

For certain "sensitive" topics (e.g., AIDS), respondents should have the option of filling in the questionnaire anonymously. However, anonymity also increases the risk of hoax answers.

Several studies have shown that postal surveys are superior to e-mail surveys with regard to response rate, but online surveys are much cheaper [30,63]. Schleyer [11] estimated that the cost of their Web-based survey was 38% less than that of an equivalent mail survey and presented a general formula for calculating breakeven points between electronic and hardcopy surveys. Jones gave the figures of 92p per reply for postal surveys, 35p for e-mail, and 41p for the WWW [30].

Cookies

Cookies can be used as unique identifiers assigned to every questionnaire viewer. As mentioned above, cookies can be used to count unique visitors to a questionnaire Web form. The use of cookies is also strongly recommended to filter out multiple responses by the same person in an open survey. People have a habit of double-clicking the "submit" button, which might lead to a double-storing of the same information. Such multiple entries can be prevented or detected by using cookies. The unique participant identifier, read out of the cookie, can then be stored in the database together with each response, so that during analysis multiple responses by the same participant can be easily identified.

The drawback of using cookies is that some people are very suspicious about sites using cookies, and will not accept cookies. Despite (or because of) these concerns, researchers should:

- State up front that cookies will be sent (and the reasons for this).
- Set the cookie to expire on the day that data collection ceases.
- Cover the issue in a published privacy policy.

Measuring Response Time

The response time can be used to exclude respondents who fill in the questionnaire too quickly, as an indication of a possible hoax response where respondents usually don't read the questions. The total time needed to complete a questionnaire can be easily measured by dynamically plugging the time and date a form was created (called-up) into a "HIDDEN" field in the form (see HTML reference books), as well as recording the time and date the questionnaire is submitted. The time needed to fill in the questionnaire can be calculated by subtracting the call-up time from the submit time. Though different transmission times through the network may not allow comparisons exact to the second [57], one may get a good grasp of how long, on average, the completion of a questionnaire takes.

Avoiding Missing Data

A great advantage of computer-administered surveys is that the software can automatically reject incomplete questionnaires and point out missing or contradictory items. To what degree the researcher wants to point out missing or erroneous data immediately (before submission) depends on the research question. In general, one may choose between client-side checking of the responses with JavaScript before they are submitted and stored in the database, or server-side checking (using any server-side script language such as Perl, ASP, etc.), allowing submission and recording of the incomplete results, before any errors are pointed out to the user. The latter method is more suitable if the Web is used to pilot-test questionnaires.

Randomizing Items

Script-languages such as ASP (Active Server Pages) may be used to build up dynamic questionnaires (as opposed to static HTML forms), which look different for certain user groups or which randomize certain aspects of the questionnaire, for example, the order of the items. This can be useful to exclude any possible systematic influences of the order of the items on responses.

Additional Readings

The methodology of Web surveys has become a research topic in itself, with sources such as the "Web Survey Methodology Portal" (http://www.websm. org) offering references and links to conferences and discussion boards. The *Journal of Official Statistics* (www.jos.nu) has announced a Special Issue on methodological aspects of Web surveys for December 2004. Another good introduction is the Rand report, "Conducting Research Surveys via E-mail and the Web," published in 2001 (hence slightly outdated), which can be downloaded from http://www.rand.org/publications/MR/MR1480/ [64].

References

[1] G. Eysenbach and C. Kohler, What is the prevalence of health-related searches on the World Wide Web? Qualitative and quantitative analysis of search engine queries on the Internet, in: *Procendings AMIA Annual Fall Symposium* (2003), pp. 225–229.

[2] G. Eysenbach and J.E. Till, Ethical issues in qualitative research on internet communities, BMJ 323(7321) (2001) 1103–1105.

[3] G. Eysenbach, J. Powell, O. Kuss, and E.R. Sa, Empirical studies assessing the quality of health information for consumers on the World Wide Web: A systematic review, JAMA 287(20) (2002) 2691–2700.

[4] G. Eysenbach, Infodemiology: The epidemiology of (mis)information. American Journal of Medicine 113(9) (2002) 763–765.

[5] T. Greenhalgh and R. Taylor, Papers that go beyond numbers (qualitative research), BMJ 315(7110) (1997) 740–743.

[6] C.M. Kramish, A. Meier, C. Carr, Z. Enga, A.S. James, J. Reedy, et al., Health behavior changes after colon cancer: A comparison of findings from face-to-face and on-line focus groups, Family Community Health 24(3) (2001) 88–103.

[7] K. Davison, The quality of dietary information on the World Wide Web, J Can Dietetic Assoc 57(4) (1996) 137–141.

[8] K.M. Smyres, Virtual corporeality: Adolescent girls and their bodies in cyberspace, *Cybersociology* (6) (1999).

[9] W.P. Eveland and S. Dunwoody, Users and navigation patterns of a science World Wide Web site for the public, Public Understanding of Science 7(4) (1998) 285–311.

[10] G. Eysenbach and T.L. Diepgen, Epidemiological data can be gathered with World Wide Web [letter], BMJ 316(7124) (1998) 72.

[11] T.K. Schleyer and J.L. Forrest, Methods for the design and administration of web-based surveys, Journal American Medical Informatics Association 7(4) (2000) 416–425.

[12] D.S. Bell and C.E.J. Kahn, Health status assessment via the World Wide Web, in: *Proceedings of the AMIA Annual Fall Symposium* (1996), pp. 338–342.

[13] R.M. Soetikno, R. Mrad, V. Pao, and L.A. Lenert, Quality-of-life research on the Internet: Feasibility and potential biases in patients with ulcerative colitis, J Am Med Inform Assoc 4(6) (1997) 426–435.

[14] N.S. Desai, E.J. Dole, S.T. Yeatman, and W.G. Troutman, Evaluation of drug information in an Internet newsgroup, J Am Pharm Assoc (Wash) NS37(4) (1997) 391–394.

[15] A.J. Winzelberg, The analysis of an electronic support group for individuals with eating disorders, Comput Human Behav 13 (1997) 393–407.

[16] P. Klemm, K. Reppert, and L. Visich, A nontraditional cancer support group: The Internet, Comput Nurs 16(1) (1998) 31–36.

[17] J. Finn, An exploration of helping processes in an online self-help group focusing on issues of disability, Health Soc Work 24(3) (1999) 220–231.

[18] J.D. Culver, F. Gerr, and H. Frumkin, Medical information on the Internet: A study of an electronic bulletin board, J Gen Intern Med 12(8) (1997) 466–470.

[19] M.H. White and S.M. Dorman, Online support for caregivers: Analysis of an Internet Alzheimer mailgroup, Comput Nurs 18(4) (2000) 168–176.

[20] J.A. Seaboldt and R. Kuiper, Comparison of information obtained from a Usenet newsgroup and from drug information centers, Am J Health Syst Pharm 54(15) (1997) 1732–1735.

[21] H. Sandvik, Health information and interaction on the Internet: A survey of female urinary incontinence, BMJ 319(7201) (1999) 29–32.

[22] S.A. King, Analysis of electronic support groups for recovering addicts, Interpersonal Computing and Technology 2(3) (1994) 47–56.

[23] M.D. Feldman, Munchausen by Internet: Detecting factitious illness and crisis on the Internet, Southern Medical Journal 93(7) (2000) 669–672.

[24] G. Eysenbach and T.L. Diepgen, Patients looking for information on the Internet and seeking teleadvice: Motivation, expectations, and misconceptions as expressed in e-mails sent to physicians, Arch Dermatol 135(2) (1999) 151–156.

[25] D.M. D'Alessandro, F. Qian, M.P. D'Alessandro, S.F. Ostrem, T.A. Choi, W.E. Erkonen, et al., Performing continuous quality improvement for a digital

health sciences library through an electronic mail analysis, Bull Med libr Assoc 86(4) (1998) 594–601.

[26] G. Eysenbach and T.L. Diepgen, Responses to unsolicited patient e-mail requests for medical advice on the World Wide Web, JAMA 280(15) (1998) 1333–1335.

[27] G. Eysenbach and T.L. Diepgen, Evaluation of cyberdocs, Lancet 352(9139) (1998) 1526.

[28] J. Oyston, Anesthesiologists' responses to an email request for advice from an unknown patient, J Med Internet Res 2(3) (2000) e16.

[29] A. Sing, J.R. Salzman, H. Sing, and D. Sing, Evaluation of health information provided on the Internet by airlines with destinations in tropical and sub-tropical countries, Commun Dis Public Health 3(3) (2000) 195–197.

[30] R. Jones and N. Pitt, Health surveys in the workplace: Comparison of postal, email and World Wide Web methods, Occup Med (Lond) 49(8) (1999) 556–558.

[31] J.C. Polzer, Using the Internet to conduct qualitative health research: Method-ological and ethical issues, University of Toronto (1998).

[32] H. Cho and R. LaRose, Privacy issues in Internet surveys, Social Science Com-puter Review 17(4) (1999) 421–434.

[33] J. Thomas, The ethics of Carniegie Mellon's "Cyber-Porn" study, http://sun.soci.niu.edu/~jthomas/ethics.cmu (1995), 12-1-2001.

[34] J.E. Till, Research ethics: Internet-based research, Part 1: On-line survey research, http://members.tripod.com/~ca916/index-3.html (1997), 9-1-0001.

[35] S.A. King, Researching Internet communities: Proposed ethical guidelines for the reporting of results, The Information Society 12(2) (1996) 119–128.

[36] H. Karlinsky, Internet survey research and consent, MD Comput 15(5) (1998) 285.

[37] World Medical Association, Declaration of Helsinki: Ethical principles for medical research involving human subjects (last amended Oct, 2000), http://www.wma.net/e/policy/17-c_e.html (2000), 20-1-2001.

[38] American Sociological Association, American Sociological Association's Code of Ethics, http://www.asanet.org/members/ecoderev.html (1997), 12-1-2001.

[39] B.F. Sharf, Communicating breast cancer on-line: Support and empowerment on the Internet, Women Health 26(1) (1997) 65–84.

[40] T. Buchanan and J.L. Smith, Using the Internet for psychological research: Per-sonality testing on the World Wide Web, Br J Psychol 90 (Pt. 1) (1999) 125–144.

[41] T. Buchanan and J.L. Smith, Research on the Internet: Validation of a World Wide Web–mediated personality scale, Behav Res Methods Instrum Comput 31(4) (1999) 565–571.

[42] W.C. Schmidt, World Wide Web survey research: Benefits, potential problems, and solutions, Behav Res Methods Instrum Comput 29(2) (1997) 274–279.

[43] L.N. Pealer and R.M. Weiler, Web-based health survey research: A primer, Am J Health Beh 24(1) (2000) 69–72.

[44] Y. Zhang, Using the Internet for survey research: A case study, JASIS 51(1) (2000) 57–68.

[45] J. Lazar and J. Preece, Designing and implementing Web-based surveys, Journal of Computer Information Systems 39(4) (1999) 63–67.

[46] B.K. Kaye and T.J. Johnson, Research methodology: Taming the cyber frontier—techniques for improving online surveys, Social Science Computer Review 17(3) (1999) 323–337.

[47] C. Bethell, J. Fiorillo, D. Lansky, M. Hendryx, and J. Knickman, Online consumer surveys as a methodology for assessing the quality of the U.S. health care system, J Med Internet Res 6(1) (2004) E2.

[48] R.J. Hilsden, J.B. Meddings, and M.J. Verhoef, Complementary and alternative medicine use by patients with inflammatory bowel disease: An Internet survey, Canadian Journal of Gastroenterology 13(4) (1999) 327–332.

[49] H.W. Potts and J.C. Wyatt, Survey of doctors' experience of patients using the Internet, J Med Internet Res 4(1) (2002) E5.

[50] T.K. Schleyer, J.L. Forrest, R. Kenney, D.S. Dodell, and N.A. Dovgy, Is the Internet useful for clinical practice? Journal of the American Dental Association 130(10) (1999) 1501–1511.

[51] D. Braithwaite, J. Emery, S. de Lusignan, and S. Sutton, Using the Internet to conduct surveys of health professionals: A valid alternative? Family Practice 20(5) (2003) 545–551.

[52] M.A. Suchard, S. Adamson, and S. Kennedy, Netpoints: Piloting patient attitudinal surveys on the Web, BMJ 315(7107) (1997) 529.

[53] A.T. Nathanson and S.E. Reinert, Windsurfing injuries: Results of a paper-and Internet-based survey, Wilderness and Environmental Medicalicine 10(4) (1999) 218–225.

[54] C. Senior, M.L. Phillips, J. Barnes, and A.S. David, An investigation into the perception of dominance from schematic faces: A study using the World Wide Web, Behav Res Methods Instrum Comput 31(2) (1999) 341–346.

[55] J.H. Krantz, J. Ballard, and J. Scher, Comparing the results of laboratory and World Wide Web samples on the determinants of female attractiveness, Behav Res Methods Instrum Comput 29(2) (1997) 264–269.

[56] W. Bandilla, M. Bosnjak, and P. Altdorfer, Survey administration effects? A comparison of Web-based and traditional written self-administered surveys using the SSP environment module, Social Science Computer Review 21(2) (2003) 235–243.

[57] J.C. Wyatt, When to use Web-based surveys (comment) (editorial), Journal of the American Medical Information Association 7(4) (2000) 426–429.

[58] C.P. Friedman and J.C. Wyatt, *Evaluation Methods in Medical Informatics* (Springer-Verlag, New York, 1997).

[59] J.D. Houston and D.C. Fiore, Online medical surveys: Using the Internet as a research tool, MD Comput 15(2) (1998) 116–120.

[60] Organization for Economic Co-Operation and Development (OECD), Understanding the Digital Divide (2001).

[61] S. Fox and L. Rainee, The online health care revolution: How the Web helps Americans take better care of themselves, 26-11-2000 (The Pew Internet and American Life Project, Washington, DC).

[62] C. Cook, F. Heath, and R.L. Thompson, A meta-analysis of response rates in Web- or Internet-based surveys, Educational and Psychological Measurement 60(6) (2000) 821–836.

[63] B.E. Mavis and J.J. Brocato, Postal surveys versus electronic mail surveys: The Tortoise and the Hare revisited, Eval Health Prof 21(3) (1998) 395–408.

[64] M. Schonlau, R.D. Fricker, and M.N. Elliott, Conducting research surveys via e-mail and the Web, Rand (2001).

6
Cognitive Approaches to the Evaluation of Healthcare Information Systems

ANDRE W. KUSHNIRUK and VIMLA L. PATEL

Introduction

This chapter provides an overview of cognitive approaches to the evaluation of healthcare information systems. Cognitive approaches in health informatics focus on understanding the processes involved in the decision making and reasoning of healthcare workers as they interact with information systems to carry out a range of tasks. In the first part of the chapter the motivation and theoretical background to cognitive evaluation are provided. The importance of developing effective methods for understanding how systems impact on cognitive processes is discussed as well as the need for developing new approaches to system evaluation borrowing from advances in cognitive science and the study of human–computer interaction. In particular, methods emerging from the areas of usability engineering and cognitive task analysis have important implications for the improved assessment of cognition involved in complex medical tasks and the impact of information systems. Methodologies are described for considering evaluation throughout the system design and development life cycle. The chapter then illustrates how research in cognitive science can be used to drive the development of new conceptual frameworks for evaluation of healthcare information systems. Specific examples from our research will be provided, ranging from application of cognitive approaches for the laboratory analysis of user interactions with complex information systems such as electronic medical records, to the cognitive evaluation of Web-based information resources.

A wide variety of approaches have been taken in the evaluation of healthcare information systems. Many of these evaluations have focused on assessing outcomes associated with deployment and use of systems in clinical environments. These studies have typically involved measurement of dependent variables such as cost of health care, quality of care, and other outcomes [1]. Although such summative evaluation of completed healthcare information systems is necessary to ensure their effectiveness, in recent years an increasing emphasis has appeared on the in-depth study of the effects of such systems on the complex reasoning, decision making, and cognitive processes involved in health care [2–4]. Closely related to this trend is the assessment and evaluation of the impact of emerging healthcare systems on tasks and workflow in health care. The objective of many of these evaluations has been not only assessing the healthcare outcomes of completed systems, but also, as important, assessing the effects of information systems on the *process* of healthcare delivery. From a *practical* perspective, the objective of such process-oriented evaluations of systems under development is to provide iterative input into the improved design and programming of the systems *before* they are deployed. Closely related to some of the evaluation methods used for providing input to designers of healthcare systems are evaluations targeted even earlier in the systems development life cycle that are aimed at assessing the *information needs* of healthcare workers as a basis for design and development of health information systems. Indeed, as argued by Cysneiros and Kushniruk, improved methods for assessing and reasoning about system requirements in design of health information systems may be the key to delivery of improved healthcare information systems [5]. As a consequence, in this chapter we consider evaluation of healthcare information systems from a cognitive, process-centered perspective, along the entire systems development life cycle, from initial requirements gathering and assessment of user information needs, to the evaluation of completed software components and products.

Assessing Unintended Effects of Information Technology

The introduction of information technologies in health care can profoundly affect the way healthcare workers carry out tasks and provide health care. In addition, it has been shown that the introduction of health information systems can have significant *unintended* or *unexpected* effects not just on workflow but also on the decision making and reasoning of healthcare workers [3]. Evaluation approaches that employ an outcomes-based perspective, where variables of interest are identified prior to subjects interacting with systems (e.g., cost of health care, mortality rates, etc.) and then measured after interaction (e.g., a group of healthcare workers interacting with an information system), are unable to assess *unexpected* effects of an information technology that the evaluators have not expected to find. Thus, although traditional approaches to evaluating information systems involving clinical controlled trials and summative evaluation of systems are needed to ensure that systems meet *expectations* of designers, the assessment of effects of systems that are *emergent* (in that they are unexpected) requires a different kind of approach to evaluation focused around assessing the *process* of use of a system in order to discover what the effects of the system are. For example, in a series of studies we conducted of use of a computerized patient record (CPR) system, we found that the particular system under study (which promoted a high level of organization of medical data) resulted in subjects (i.e., physicians) changing the way they normally requested and processed patient information during the doctor–patient interview. Specifically, we found the physicians were strongly guided by the ordering and sequencing of information in the CPR when interviewing patients using the systems, rather than following their own "knowledge base." After experience in using the system we found that the order and organization of information within the CPR greatly affected the physicians' questioning, with experienced users of the system following what we termed "screen-driven" behavior (i.e., asking questions of patients based on the order of information presented on the computer screen) [3]. Furthermore, such unexpected effects of information technology often constitute the type of information that designers of systems find most useful for modifying and improving system design during the process of system development, described in the next section.

The Systems Development Life Cycle

In the software industry a wide range of methodologies have been developed for guiding the design and deployment of information systems [6]. The phases involved in creation and maintenance of information systems is known as the *systems development life cycle* (*SDLC*). The "traditional SDLC" (see Figure 6.1) that emerged in development of early computer applications several decades ago involves the progression through fixed "phases" (a phase consisting of a set of related activities), beginning with

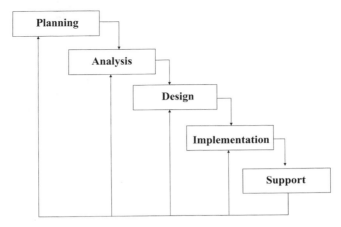

FIGURE 6.1. The classic waterfall system development life cycle.

project planning in Phase 1 and moving to *analysis and requirements gathering* in Phase 2. Once requirements for a project (both technical and user requirements) are obtained, *design* of the system is embarked on in Phase 3. Once design is finalized, in Phase 4 *implementation* (i.e., programming) of the system is undertaken. Finally, in Phase 5, the system is in place and must undergo *support and maintenance* (until it is eventually phased out, replaced, or modified by a new system, leading to a new cycle of development).

Although such an approach to system development has proven to be suitable for many software applications, ranging from applications in industries such as banking to aerospace, it has proven to be a limiting factor in the successful design and deployment of systems in many complex and highly user-centered application domains, in particular health care [2]. The emphasis of the traditional life cycle on fixed and ordered sequence of phases has had a number of drawbacks, including the following: (1) lack of flexibility in moving "back" to previous stages—in particular, if improved knowledge of user requirements would require a costly rethinking of design or implementation decisions once those phases have been passed through (i.e., it is difficult to go back to previous stages), (2) the assumption that user requirements can be adequately defined in the early analysis or requirements gathering phase, and (3) emphasis on waiting until the system is nearly complete (i.e., often during what is known as "beta testing") before conducting intensive end-user testing with a system to be deployed (again making potentially needed rethinking and redesign of major software components difficult and costly). Although such problems are typical in complex domains such as health care when attempting to apply a "traditional" approach to design and development, it should be noted that this traditional approach to software development is commonplace in the healthcare software industry today. In the context of this chapter, of particular interest is the issue of evaluation and testing of systems during the SDLC. Along these lines we will discuss the potential role of cognitive methods in improving the evaluation of systems along the various phases of the SDLC and as an important adjunct to newer approaches to systems development.

In contrast to traditional approaches to software development described earlier, in recent years, a number of software engineering methodologies have been developed that focus on deploying evaluation methods throughout the software life cycle—from the initial analysis of user needs, through the entire design process, as well as the implementation activities. Such approaches to system development are closely related to the concept of *user-centered design*, which emphasizes continued refinement and iteration in the systems development life cycle with a continual focus on evaluation with potential end users of systems at every stage of design and development [7]. As an example, the method known as *rapid prototyping* and other related approaches involve continual and iterative cycles of design and testing of software products and components prior to releasing a system.

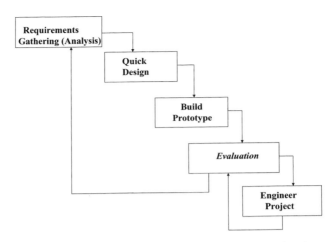

FIGURE 6.2. Rapid prototyping and the role of evaluation.

As can be seen in Figure 6.2, this approach clearly situates *evaluation* of systems as a key aspect of systems development from which decisions to modify or extend design are based. In particular, methods emerging from the fields of usability engineering and cognitive science are of particular value in providing more precise and useful assessments of information systems, particularly from the perspective of potential end users, in providing feedback to designers of systems in cycles of rapid development. This philosophy of system design is consistent with approaches to formative evaluation that have emerged in health informatics and that will form the focus of the discussion of cognitive approaches in this chapter. However, it should be noted that the methods to be described below are also of considerable value in assessing the effects of *completed* information systems on healthcare workers' decision making and reasoning in conducting summative evaluation in health informatics.

The Cognitive Continuum in Health Care, the Role of Expertise, and Cognitive Task Analysis

Prior to discussing specific cognitive methods that can be applied throughout the SDLC (as described above), we will place our work in the context of three important conceptual frameworks emerging from the study of cognitive science: (1) the *cognitive continuum* in reasoning and decision making, (2) the *expertise* continuum, and (3) a methodological framework for analyzing human–computer interactions collectively, known as *cognitive task analysis (CTA)*. According to Hammond, cognitive processes in decision making and reasoning can be located along a *cognitive continuum*, which ranges between *intuition* and *analysis* [8]. Intuitive processing (which is characterized by recognition and quick response) is induced when experienced decision makers are faced with large amounts of information or very short time frames for responding to situations. In contrast, *analysis* is induced by tasks that involve sufficient processing time and presentation of quantitative information. Analytical processes are also associated with information processing by individuals who may lack expertise in a problem solving area, and therefore lack the ability to respond or make decisions based on their prior experiences with similar situations and recognition of similar contexts. In reality, decision making and reasoning may move along the continuum within the same problem solving context. For example, decision makers may apply intuitive (recognitional) processes in solving a part of a problem that they are familiar with or which is routine, and then shift to analytical processing when faced with problem complexity or lack of familiarity with that part of the problem. As demonstrated by Hamm, the concept of the cognitive continuum is of value in helping to explain how decisions are made in complex domains such as health care, which are characterized by complexity of information, shifting constraints, time pressure, and uncertainty of information [9]. As will be seen, knowledge of how healthcare workers move along the cognitive continuum is of considerable relevance in analyzing complex cognitive activity, providing insight into understanding cognitive processes involved in complex tasks, and more specifically, providing guidance in development of frameworks for coding and analyzing qualitative data emerging from cognitive studies. In particular, the knowledge that tasks of differing complexity and nature may dramatically affect the type of processing humans engage in has relevance for designing evaluation studies that take into account not only the expertise of decision makers but also the nature of work tasks, as will be described below.

Closely related to the cognitive continuum in the study of medical cognition is the concept of a continuum of knowledge and expertise that decision makers bring to bear in complex domains such as health care. Expertise in health care can be considered to lie along a continuum, ranging from novices (e.g., medical/nursing students) to intermediates (e.g., medical residents) to experts (e.g., accomplished physicians) [10,11]. Furthermore, the development of expertise in healthcare-related areas is characterized by transitions from novice through to intermediate and expert levels. For example, expert decision making is often characterized by what can be considered along Hammond's cognitive continuum as recognitional processes, where an expert can often quickly arrive at a solution based on analysis of current data in conjunction with his or her knowledge base of similar or related situations. Other characteristics of expert decision making and cognitive processing in general include a greater emphasis on situational analysis of complex problems prior to applying a solution, as exemplified by the research findings of Klein and associates in studying expert decision making in areas ranging from fire fighting to medicine [12].

An important methodological approach to the study of cognition that brings to bear and integrates consideration of both the complexity of decision-making tasks and the prior expertise/knowledge of decision makers is known as *cognitive task analysis* (*CTA*). CTA is a powerful methodological framework for studying and analyzing complex human cognition [13]. In addition, it has been successfully extended to methodological frameworks for studying complex decision-making and reasoning processes of users of computer systems, and as such has definite relevance and relation to methods emerging from usability engineering. The focus of CTA is on the application of scientific and analytical approaches to understanding how people process complex information, reason, and make decisions while undertaking tasks of varying levels of complexity. In contrast to a predominant paradigm in the study of decision making, which has focused on the "decision event" (some hypothesized point in time when the decision maker is supposed to weigh alternatives and arrive at a decision), CTA focuses on understanding the entire process involved in reasoning and decision making, starting with the way a subject first analyses and sizes up a problem or task, and how he or she then proceeds to acquire and process relevant information and finally come up with a decision or course of action.

One approach to CTA typically involves giving subjects (e.g., healthcare workers) specific tasks involving decision making and reasoning, and observing the process of how a decision is made or a problem is solved. This may involve asking subjects to "think aloud" as they process and work through problems in their work domain (that may be presented to them as artificial cases or alternatively as they react to real cases and situations in their work area, as will be described below in the context of situating evaluation along a continuum from experimental to naturalistic approaches). Typically, the entire session is recorded (e.g., audio and video recorded) for further analysis. In addition, CTA may involve comparison of how subjects (e.g., healthcare workers) of varying levels of expertise deal with the same cases (e.g., asking both novices and experts to process medical cases and comparing the differences in their strategies and approaches to problem solving). Currently, there are several research streams from which CTA has emerged, including the study of expertise in the study of problem solving as a basis for design of intelligent tutoring systems [13–15], cognitive engineering [16,17], and the naturalistic study of decision making in domains such as fire fighting and medicine [12].

In our work, we have applied scientific methods from cognitive task analysis (both for setting up studies and for analysis of process data) to the study of how subjects with differing levels of expertise (both in health care and in technology) interact and reason while using computer systems. In this context, the next section presents a discussion of how we have extended and integrated methods from cognitive task analysis with approaches to evaluation collectively known as usability engineering methods.

Usability Engineering Methods and Approaches to Support Cognitive Analysis in Health Informatics

Our work in the evaluation of health information systems has borrowed from research in a number of areas, including cognitive science (as described above), and also from work in the emerging area of usability engineering [18]. Usability engineering has emerged from the integration of evaluation methods used in the study of human–computer interaction (HCI) aimed at providing practical feedback into the design of computer systems and user interfaces. Usability engineering can be distinguished from traditional systems engineering approaches by emphasis on obtaining continual input or feedback from end users, or potential end users of a system, throughout the SDLC. In healthcare settings, a number of researchers have begun to apply methods adapted from usability engineering toward the design and evaluation of clinical information systems. This has included work in developing portable and low-cost methods for analyzing use of healthcare information systems, along with a focus on developing principled qualitative and quantitative methods for analyzing usability data resulting from such study [19]. Since the mid-1990s, a number of groups and laboratories involved in clinical informatics have emerged for testing and designing software applications. For example, Elkin and colleagues describe the use of a usability laboratory for testing a medical vocabulary embedded within the Unified Medical Language System [20]. Kushniruk, Patel, Cimino, and Barrows also describe the use of usability engineering methods for evaluating the design and refinement of a user interface to a CPR system and the analysis of the system's underlying medical vocabulary [21]. Coble and colleagues have described the use of usability engineering in the iterative development of clinical workstations [22]. Others have focused on these methods to deal with the "inspection" of user interfaces [23,24]. Recent work in biomedical informatics has attempted to extend the emerging trend toward usability engineering to include consideration of cognitive issues surrounding design and implementation of clinical information systems, namely cognitive engineering [24,25].

There are a number of specific methods associated with usability engineering, and foremost among these is *usability testing*. Usability testing refers to the evaluation of information systems that involves testing of participants (i.e., subjects) who are *representative* of the target user population, as they perform *representative* tasks using an information technology (e.g., physicians using a CPR system to record patient data) in a particular clinical context. During the evaluation, all user–computer interactions are typically recorded (e.g., video recordings made of all computer screens or user activities and actions). Types of evaluations using this approach can vary from formal, controlled laboratory studies of users, to less formal approaches. Principled methods for the analysis of data from such tests, which may consist of video recordings of end users as they interact with systems, can now be used as tools to aid in the analysis. These techniques generally include the collection of "think aloud" reports, involving the recording of users as they verbalize their thoughts while using a computer. Over the past decade, in the technology industry a range of commercial usability laboratories have appeared for conducting usability testing, ranging from elaborate laboratories with simulated work environments and one-way observation mirrors [26,27], to less elaborate facilities and even portable approaches to usability testing, where the recording equipment is actually taken out to field sites [28]. Many of these techniques borrow from work in the application of cognitive science to the study of human–computer interaction [19,29,30]. The practical role of usability engineering in the development life cycle of clinical information systems has also come under consideration, particularly in the context of use of rapid prototyping methodologies for the design of healthcare information systems [2,22]. Such methods differ from traditional life cycle models, where a system is developed over time using an approach involving fixed stages with limited input from users into redesign. In contrast, rapid prototyping methods typically involve the development of *prototypes* (defined as partially functioning versions of a system), which may be shown to users early in development process in order to assess their usability and functionality. If such assessment indicates that changes are needed, a further cycle of design and testing is initiated. This process continues until the system is deemed to be acceptable to users and shows the desired functionality.

The understanding of how complex information technologies can be successfully integrated into the process of human decision making and practical day-to-day use is critically important in increasing the likelihood of acceptability. Information from usability testing regarding user problems, preferences, suggestions, and work practices can be applied not only toward the end of system development (to ensure that systems are effective, efficient, and sufficiently enjoyable to achieve acceptance), but throughout the development cycle to ensure that the development process leads to effective end products. There are a number of points in the systems development life cycle (SDLC) at which usability testing may be useful in the development of new technologies. As described above, the typical SDLC is characterized by the following phases, which define major activities involved in developing software: (1) project planning, (2) analysis (involving gathering of system requirements), (3) design of the system, (4) implementation (i.e., programming), and (5) system support/maintenance [6]. There are a number of types of usability tests, based on when in the development life cycle they are applied: (1) *exploratory tests* conducted early in the systems development cycle to test preliminary design concepts using prototypes or storyboards; (2) *testing of prototypes* used during requirements gathering; (3) *assessment tests* conducted early or midway through the development cycle to provide iterative feedback into evolving design of prototypes or systems; (4) *validation tests* conducted to ensure that completed software products are acceptable regarding predefined acceptance measures; and (5) *comparison tests* conducted at any stage to compare design alternatives or possible solutions (e.g., initial screen layouts or design metaphors). From this perspective, evaluation in health informatics is seen as being essential throughout the entire life cycle of systems, not just for summative final evaluation.

Cognitive Methods Applied to the Usability Testing of Clinical Information Systems

Given the motivation for applying usability engineering in a clinical setting described earlier, in this section we describe a methodological framework for applying cognitive methods in the evaluation of healthcare information systems. The framework is based on a series of phases employed in performing usability evaluations of healthcare systems and user interfaces extending ideas from both cognitive science and usability testing [19,31,32]. Although there may be some variations in the phases, our evaluation of information systems has typically involved consideration of each of the phases.

Phase 1: Identification of Evaluation Objectives

Possible objectives for conducting evaluations can range considerably, including but not limited to the following examples: (1) assessment of system functionality and usability, (2) input into refinement of emerging prototypes, (3) identifying problems in human–computer interaction, (4) evaluating the effects of a system on decision-making processes, and (5) assessing the impact of a new information technology on clinical practice and workflow. The approach described below can be used to provide practical input into system redesign (e.g., identifying problems with human–computer interaction that need to be rectified).

Phase 2: Sample Selection and Study Design

The second phase involves the identification and selection of a sample of target subjects for the evaluation, resulting in a clearly defined *user profile* that describes the range of skills of target end users of a system. Subjects should be representative of end users of the system under study. For example, if a system is being designed for implementation for use in a particular clinical setting, subjects could consist of personnel who are representative of those who would be expected to actually use the system (e.g., if the system is designed to be used by residents and junior attending staff, it is important to select test subjects that are representative of these groups). Criteria need to be applied for classifying subjects in terms of their prior computer experience. Although there are a number of ways of categorizing users, in our work on usability we have found that considering users along the following dimensions is often useful: (1) expertise of subjects in using computers, (2) the roles of the subjects in the workplace (e.g., physicians, nurses, etc.), and (3) subjects' expertise in the domain of work the information system is targeted for. As evaluation involving cognitive analysis provides a rich source of data, a considerable amount of information may be obtained from a small number of subjects (e.g. 8 to 10 subjects in a group being studied), particularly if subjects selected are representative of target users of the system being assessed.

In addition to describing the tasks that different types of users will be expected to perform using a system, it is also important to describe as much as possible the most critical skills, knowledge, demographic information, and other relevant information about each class of users. Much of our work is an extension of the "expertise approach" [33], which involves comparison of problem solving of subjects with different levels of expertise, to the testing and evaluation of health information systems.

Number of Subjects

Prior studies have shown that carefully conducted usability studies involving as few as 8 to 10 subjects can lead to identification of up to 80% of the surface-level usability problems with an information system [18]. However, more subjects are required in order to conduct inferential statistics (e.g., 15–20 per study group).

Study Design

The study design of our evaluations borrows from approaches in experimental psychology, with a number of options for conducting practical assessments. Study designs may consist of within-group designs where individual subjects may be asked to try out different versions of a prototype system, or one or more subjects may be followed over time as they learn how to use a system. Alternatively, studies may involve between-group designs. Between-group testing might involve, for example, comparison of two different systems, with two groups of different healthcare workers using each system for conducting the same task, such as physicians or nurses looking up patient information in a CPR system. Furthermore, testing may involve use of a CPR system by two groups of subjects of the same medical designation (e.g., attending physicians), one group of which have been identified as being highly computer literate (based on a background questionnaire) and the other group with little experience with computer systems. Within-group studies may focus on longitudinal study of how healthcare workers learn to use and master clinical information systems over time, with testing occurring at specific intervals following initial training in use of a system [3]. Simpler study designs might consist of having a single group (for example, 10 to 15 physician subjects) interacting with a CPR system (with each subject carrying out the same task or set of tasks) in order to assess problems with the design of the user interface.

Phase 3: Selection of Representative Experimental Tasks and Contexts

Studies of use of systems can be situated on a continuum ranging from controlled laboratory studies (e.g., studies involving artificial conditions or tasks) to naturalistic studies of doctor–patient–computer interaction involving use of computer systems in real contexts (e.g., tasks involving subjects being asked to interview a patient while entering data into a computerized patient record system). For laboratory-based evaluations involving controlled experimental conditions, we have sometimes used written medical case descriptions, or vignettes, to be used as stimulus material (e.g., subjects may be asked to develop a diagnosis in response to presentation of a hypothetical or real medical case, while using a CPR). The development of medical cases for use in such studies (often consisting of short written descriptions) may require careful design so that the cases are realistic and representative of real-life clinical situations and elicit high-quality data about user interactions. For example, cases or scenarios can be drawn or modified from the type of cases commonly used for evaluation in medical education, or presented in medical textbooks or journals such as the *New England Journal of Medicine*. They can also be generated from real health data with the assistance of an appropriate medical expert working with the investigators.

Naturalistic studies of actual doctor–patient interactions sacrifice ability to experimentally control the study for an increase in ecological validity (e.g., collection of data on use of a system in a real clinical setting). In naturalistic studies we generally do not present subjects with artificial written cases, but rather monitor the use of systems (using recording methods to be described below) in real clinical contexts (e.g., a physician using a CPR while interviewing a patient). Regardless of the desired level of experimental control, tasks chosen for study should be representative of real uses of the information technology being evaluated.

Phase 4: Selection of Background Questionnaires

A background questionnaire may be given either before or after actual testing of a subject's interaction with a system being evaluated. This questionnaire can be used to obtain historical information about the participants that will help the evaluators to understand their behavior and performance during a test. These can include items to assess level of subjects' typical health practice, or prior experience with computer systems [34]. Some usability tests may include examination of educational systems, where the focus is on assessing how much learning takes place during the process of use of a system (e.g., a Web-based educational resource). This may involve the presentation of questionnaires or multiple-choice test items before and after testing using a system. For example, in conducting an evaluation of physicians using an educational software system on a specific topic (e.g., advances in breast cancer treatment), subjects were given a set of multiple-choice questions to assess their knowledge of that topic both before and after actually recording them interacting with the system, in order to assess the impact of their interactions with systems on their knowledge and learning.

The actual task scenarios to be used during testing also need to be developed during this phase. These may range from simple written descriptions of medical cases, to more elaborate scripts for conducting simulated doctor–patient interviews, where an experimenter plays the part of a patient while the subject interviews or interacts with the "patient" while using a technology such as a CPR system [3].

Phase 5: Selection of the Evaluation Environment

The next step is the selection of the evaluation environment (i.e., where the evaluation will take place). The physical location of the evaluation can vary considerably depending on the degree to which the study is conducted under controlled experimental conditions or in a naturalistic setting. As described in the Introduction to this chapter, a number of fixed laboratories have arisen where commercial organizations conduct testing of developing software products in domains ranging from the aerospace industry to brokerage [27]. During the 1990s there was a trend toward the development of large and expensive fixed commercial usability laboratories, which included simulated environments for testing use of systems (e.g., simulated classrooms or work environments). Such laboratories may consist of testing rooms (containing computer systems with which subjects interact) and adjoining observation rooms with one-way mirrors, for experimenters to watch subjects. However, it has been shown that many of the methods of usability engineering can be applied in a more cost-effective manner, using inexpensive and portable equipment that can be taken to actual work settings. For example, Cimino and colleagues have described the development of a portable usability laboratory for use in clinical settings [35]. For the majority of our studies we have adopted such a portable discount usability engineering approach that involves video recording of subjects in the most convenient setting possible, in some cases right in the hospital or clinic under study [21].

Phase 6: Data Collection—Video Recording and Recording of Thought Processes

Instructions given to subjects may include asking subjects to perform particular tasks using the computer system (e.g., "Please enter data into the computerized patient record system we are testing while 'thinking aloud' or verbalizing your thoughts"). In addition, instructions might involve asking a physician to conduct a doctor–patient interview while using a system, with full video recording of computer screens and concurrent audiotaping of the doctor–patient dialogue [23]. In some studies subjects may also be prompted by experimenters at key points in their interaction with a system to comment on aspects of a system or its design. For example, a study might involve comparison of two screen layouts and for each layout the experimenter might ask the user to comment on the screen's layout. In most of our studies the complete interaction of the subject, starting with the initial instructions to completion of all tasks asked of the user, is video and audio recorded (using equipment such as that detailed below).

Think-Aloud Reports

The collection of "think aloud" reports is one of the most useful techniques emerging from cognitive science. Using this approach, subjects are instructed to "think aloud" (i.e., verbalize their thoughts) as they interact with computer systems (while the computer screens are recorded). There is a principled formal method for analyzing such qualitative data. In our studies of human–computer interaction (HCI), we typically capture the computer screens using video recording (with the computer screen output to a PC–video converter and then input into a VCR) or screen capture software (e.g., the commercially available HyperCam screen recorder software) for detailed analysis of actions, such as mouse clicks and menu selections. The data collected of users' interactions typically include the video recording of all computer screens along with the corresponding audio recording of subjects' verbalizations as they use the system under study [21].

Equipment typically consists of a PC–video converter, for converting the output of computer screens to video (to go into the video-in of a VCR). This allows for recording of all computer screens to video as a user interacts with an information system. In addition, we record all subject verbalizations by using a microphone that inputs into the audio-in of the same VCR. Thus on a single videotape we can record all computer screens and user verbalizations made while a subject performs a task using the computer system under study [31].

A schematic diagram illustrating one approach to collecting video and audio recordings of user interactions with a computer system under study is given in Figure 6.3. In order to obtain video recordings of computer screens, a commercially available PC–video converter is used to convert the VGA computer display output to the video input (i.e., the video-in jack) of a standard VCR. In order to obtain concurrent audio input to the recording of the user–computer interaction we have employed a standard microphone connected to a standard audio mixer (available at most audio stores) or preamplifier, which then outputs into the audio-in jack of the same VCR being used to record computer screens (using a standard RGA cable). This approach allows for recording of user interactions both in the usability laboratory setting as well as in actual clinical settings, since the equipment required is both standard and portable. In a recent paper by Kaufman et al., the use of an inexpensive PC–video converter is described for collect-

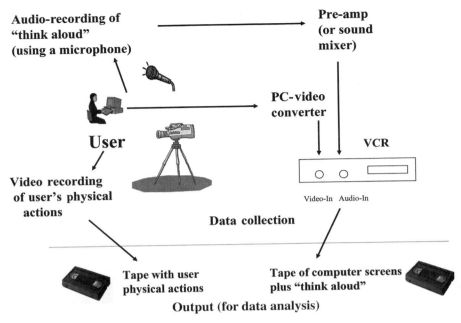

FIGURE 6.3. Video-based usability testing.

ing video data portably [36]. In that study, portable recording equipment was taken to the homes of patient subjects, where complete recordings of subjects' interaction with a diabetes management system were made. The result of this phase includes a complete video recording of user interaction with a computer system along with the audio track containing the verbalizations of subjects interacting with the system.

As indicated in Figure 6.3, video recordings of the actual users themselves (e.g., the faces and gestures of the users as they interact with systems under study) may also be obtained on a separate video recording, although for many of the types of analyses described below, the recordings of computer screens and concurrent audio may be sufficient. If recordings of the actual user are required (e.g., in a study of use of a CPR system where we may want to record how often a physician uses the system as well as physically interacts with other objects such as notes or papers on the desk) in addition to the computer screen recording, this can also be conducted in a cost-effective manner (without requiring the use of an expensive usability laboratory) by using a separate video camera and tripod directed at the user, or users, of the system (see Figure 6.3). In studies requiring unobtrusive observation of user physical interactions with the system, rooms having video cameras placed in unobtrusive locations (e.g., ceiling-mounted cameras) are ideal. In our work in hospital settings, we have on occasion conducted such recordings in rooms that are typically used for other purposes (e.g., rooms outfitted with ceiling-mounted cameras used by medical educators in evaluation of resident and student interviewing skills).

In addition to using standard video recording equipment for recording user interaction with a system, in some studies we have employed a range of software that allows for the recording of screens and audio as movie files directly on the computer being used for testing, removing the need for video cameras and VCRs for recording of the computer screens. For example, the commercially available product HyperCam allows for direct recording of the computer screens, along with audio input to the same computer via a computer microphone. However, due to storage requirements of such approaches (the resulting recordings are stored as large files that may quickly exceed storage allocation on a standard PC), in many studies we continue to employ standard video recording techniques described above, particularly when collecting data in real clinical settings, where the computer equipment and capabilities may be more limited than in the laboratory.

Phase 7: Analysis of the Process Data

The output of Phase 6 may consist of video recordings of computer screens (with an audio overlay of the subject "thinking aloud") and/or a tape of the actual user's interactions with the computer system (e.g., facial expressions, movements, gestures etc.). In many studies, the objective of the evaluation may be to analyze such data to identify problems subjects experience in using a system (e.g., a computerized patient record system or a decision-support system). The transformation of data into recommendations involves qualitative and quantitative analyses of the video-based usability data. The advantages of video recordings as a source data include the fact that videotapes of user–computer interactions provide a record of the "whole event." Furthermore, the same video recordings of user interactions can be examined from a number of theoretical perspectives and analyzed using a range of methodological approaches.

There are a variety of approaches to analyzing data on human–computer interaction from video data, ranging from informal review of the resulting taped data, to formalized and precise methods for analyzing the number and type of errors or user problems. The richness of video data requires principled methods for conducting full analysis and coding. The use of computer tools to aid the analysis of video data has greatly facilitated usability testing [19]. Computer programs are now available that interface between VCR and computer in order to facilitate video coding. A software tool we used extensively in our earlier analyses was called CVideo (Envisionology Inc.)—a program that allowed the verbal transcriptions (e.g., of subjects' "thinking aloud") to be annotated on a MacIntosh computer and linked (time-stamped) to the corresponding video sequence (using a cable that connects the Mac to the VCR while reviewing the tape of a usability testing session). In recent years a number of tools have become commercially available for assisting in the qualitative analysis of audio and video-based data (including MacShapa, Transana, and other related software tools for conducting qualitative analyses that allow for interfacing and indexing of video data). Computer-supported analysis of video data allows researchers to document video frames with textual annotations, notes, and codes on a computer, saving time in analysis, and allows for automatic indexing and retrieval of video frames and sequences. Such analyses also facilitate interrater reliability in coding and allow for coding of user actions and verbalizations.

The procedure for data analysis we employ first involves having the audio portion of the test session ("think aloud" reports) transcribed separately in a word processing file. That file then serves as a computer-based log file for entering annotations and codes that are linked or time-stamped to the corresponding video scenes [21]. However, it should be noted that for the types of analyses described below (involving application of coding schemes), computer-supported coding tools are not a requirement for conducting principled analysis of video data. The coding tool will aid in the annotation of the transcripts by linking the computer word processing file containing the transcripts to the actual video tape sequences. However, this can be also accomplished manually, that is, by watching the videotape and entering into the word processing file containing the audio transcripts the actual corresponding video counter numbers (as will be illustrated below).

Application of a Coding Scheme in Analyzing Video Data

Prior to analyzing video data, a coding scheme should be refined for use in identifying specific occurrences of user problems and aspects of cognitive processes from transcripts of the subjects' thinking aloud and interactions with a computer. Coding categories we have applied in a number of studies include the following: *information content* (e.g., whether the information system provides too much or too little information, etc.), *comprehensiveness of graphics and text* (e.g., whether a computer display is understandable to the user), *problems in navigation* (e.g., whether the user has difficulty in finding desired information or computer screen), and *overall system understandability* (e.g., understandability of icons, required computer operations, and system messages). In addition to these categories, which focus on classical aspects of HCI, one can also extend the analyses to allow for the identification of higher-level cognitive processes. For example, in some studies we code each occurrence of the generation of a diagnostic hypothesis by a subject, or request for information from a patient in the case of studies of doctor–patient interaction involving use of a CPR system.

As an illustration, to assess ease of use of computer systems, a coding system can be used as shown in Figure 6.4. The scheme shows definitions of coding categories, along with examples of coded statements made by test subjects while interacting with a system that fall under each category (an example of a coded transcript will be provided below in our discussion).

1. Examples of Categories Used to Analyze Aspects of Interaction Related Directly to the User Interface:

NAVIGATION
Coded when subject comments on basic navigation, or indicates can't move through program/interface, etc. to find or go somewhere (e.g., "How do I get back to the last screen?").

LAYOUT/SCREEN ORGANIZATION
Coded for if the subject comments on the layout or screen organization (e.g., "I find this page very cluttered").

MEANING OF LABELS
Coded for if the subject comments on the meaning of labels in the interface itself (e.g., "I don't know what this button means here, the one that says "free download" on it").

UNDERSTANDING OF SYSTEM INSTRUCTIONS/ERROR MESSAGES
Coded for if the subject comments on understanding of instructions or errors (e.g., "It says 'fatal error 404' and I don't know what to do now").

CONSISTENCY OF OPERATIONS
Coded for if the subject comments on the consistency of operatons (e.g., "How come there are two different ways to exit on the last two creens?").

OVERALL EASE OF USE
Coded for if the subject comments on the overall ease of use (e.g., "I find this system very hard to use").

RESPONSE TIME
Coded for if the subject mentions response time (e.g., "I seem to be waiting a very long time, and still there is no response from the computer").

VISIBLITY OF SYSTEM STATUS
Coded for if the subject comments on visibility of system status (e.g., "I'm not sure what the system is doing now—it seems to be hanging").

2. Examples of Categories Used to Analyze Aspects of Medical Reasoning/Decision Making Processes:

REQUEST INFORMATION
Coded when subject (e.g., physician) requests information from patient during a doctor–patient interaction (e.g., "How often do you smoke?").

CONSIDER DIAGNOSTIC HYPOTHESIS
Coded when subject considers a diagnostic hypothesis (e.g., "I think this patient has angina").

CHOOSE TREATMENT
Coded when subject chooses a medical treatment (e.g., "At this point I would put him on heparin").

FIGURE 6.4. Excerpts from a coding scheme for analyzing video-based data from cognitive evaluations.

The coding scheme essentially forms a manual for researchers as they watch and annotate the videotapes obtained from experimental sessions. The categories used for coding were developed from examination of categories of interactions from the HCI and cognitive literatures [37,38].

In Figure 6.5, we show the application of coding categories (from Figure 6.4) in analyzing a video log of a user's interaction with a CPR. The

00:00:00 Start of session—user starts up the system.

"I'm just starting up the system; well, what a nice office this is, here we go. This is for patient X. Well I have just tried turning the thing on. OK, here is the first screen, but it looks very poorly laid out."
LAYOUT/SCREEN ORGANIZATION—PROBLEM

00:01:15 User goes to help screen.

"How do I move to the previous screen?"
NAVIGATION—PROBLEM

"I think this patient may have diabetes. So here I go, I'm clicking on this screen about diabetes information."
CONSIDER DIAGNOSTIC HYPOTHESIS—DIABETES

00:01:23 Subject goes to diabetes guideline screen and clicks on help button.

"Now what? It looks like everything has stopped."
LACK OF INDICATION OF SYSTEM STATUS—PROBLEM

FIGURE 6.5. Excerpt of a coded section of a transcript of a user (a physician) interacting with a CPR.

procedure for analysis of the subjects' thinking aloud is based on the method of protocol analysis, as described in detail by Ericsson and Simon [29]. Note that the transcript of the subject's thinking aloud report is marked up with annotations from the coding scheme and that the numbers in the log file (containing the transcript) refer to the corresponding section of the videotape (i.e., the video counter number) where they occurred. Also note that codes that indicate user problems are coded as such (with the additional coding tag "PROBLEM").

We have found that up to 80% of user-interface problems with a particular clinical system can be detected with as few as 8 to 12 transcripts of subjects' interaction with the system under study, which is consistent with the literature emerging from the application of cognitive engineering methods in HCI [18].

Important advances have been made in the development of computer-based tools that aid in the detection and analysis of patterns contained in usability data. In our studies, we have developed a variety of schemes for analyzing video data in a principled manner. These allow coders to identify events of interest, such as user problems, and use of system features (preliminary schemes are typically refined and then verified). Coding schemes can include categories for user/system aspects and problems including categories for human factors issues and cognitive issues. We have developed categories that characterize at a top level the following aspects of human–computer interaction: (1) the *usefulness* of the system being tested in terms of its contents, and (2) the *ease of use* of the system or interface. The first top-level category deals with issues such as whether the system being tested provides useful, up-to-date or valuable information to a user, while the second category characterizes potential problems or issues related to the actual user interface or system design. The coding schemes we have developed are based on and extend categories that have been applied in protocol analysis in the study of medical cognition (see [37] for details). In particular, our coding schemes contain categories used to assess key aspects of medical decision making and reasoning (e.g., choice of treatment) in addition to categories used to code for aspects of usability, allowing us to relate aspects of user interfaces (and their usability) to reasoning and decision-making processes.

Phase 8: Interpretation of Findings

The data collected from usability testing can be compiled and summarized in numerous ways, depending on the goals of the evaluation. The results may summarize any number of aspects of system use, including task accuracy, user preference data, time to completion of task, frequency, and classes of problems encountered. In addition, qualitative analyses of the effects of the technology on healthcare professional reasoning and decision making can be conducted. Results of process evaluations may include a summary of types and frequency of problems that occur when subjects interact with a computer system under evaluation. If the system under study is under development, the information provided from the analysis phase should be communicated to system designers. For further investigations, the findings should be interpreted for what they mean, within the context of the theoretical framework.

Phase 9: Iterative Input into Design

After implementation of changes to a system, based on the recommendations to the programming team (for studies involving formative evaluations), evaluation may be repeated to determine how the changes now affect the system's usability. In this way, evaluation can be integrated in the process of design and development of information systems, iteratively feeding information back into their continual improvement.

Application of Cognitive Approaches to Evaluation: From Medical Informatics to Consumer Informatics— E-health and Beyond

Cognitive approaches to system evaluation can be applied throughout the life cycle of information systems, to answer a range of evaluation questions. In this section of the chapter we describe some of our experiences in applying a cognitive approach to the practical evaluation of a range of types of health information systems. In our initial work along these lines, we have applied the approach to the evaluation of educational software designed for use in continuing medical education. In one study, subjects (physicians involved in a continuing education program) were given the task of exploring a multimedia tutorial in order to improve their knowledge about the treatment of heart disease. After completing a pretest multiple-choice test to assess their prior knowledge in this area, subjects were video recorded as they interacted with the system while asked to think aloud. After completion of the task, subjects were given a follow-up questionnaire (containing the same questions) to assess if the subjects had improved their knowledge of heart disease by interacting with the system. All of the subjects' interactions with the system were video recorded. The audio portions of the sessions were transcribed and the transcripts were coded to identify problems and issues in using the system. The study approach was used both to assess learning that took place while interacting with the system, as well as to identify from the video data specific problems with the interface that needed improving (e.g., use of more meaningful icons, better navigational facilities, etc.).

Following from this initial work in applying a cognitive task analysis approach to assessing an educational program, we began a line of research into assessing the effects of emerging clinical information systems, in particular CPRs, on the decision making and reasoning of healthcare professionals [3,23]. A range of studies were conducted with the objective of evaluating the effects of introduction of a CPR system on physician decision-making and reasoning processes in a diabetes clinic. One component of this research program involved in-depth cognitive analysis of 14 subjects learning how to use and master the system over a six-month period. Subjects were video recorded as they entered information into the system (all computer screens were recorded) and subjects were also asked to think aloud while they interacted with the system. In addition, in another experimental condition, subjects were asked to interview a "simulated" patient (i.e., a research collaborator playing the part of a patient, a technique used in the evaluation of medical trainees' interviewing skills) and their interaction with both the computer system and the patient were video recorded. By both analyzing the data obtained from the experimental condition involving subjects thinking aloud, as well as analyzing the data from recording subjects interacting with simulated patients over time as they learned to use the CPR and became familiar with its capabilities, the effects of use of the system on physicians were assessed. Through analysis of both video and audio data it was found that the layout of the information on the CPR screen had a significant impact on the way the physician subjects interacted with patients and reasoned about patient cases. Specifically, it was found that as the physicians became familiar with the system they became guided by the order and organization of medical findings on the computer screen in requesting information from patients, which ultimately affected reasoning about patient cases, a pattern of interaction with patients we described as being "screen-driven." The implications of such findings of unexpected yet profound effects of CPR systems on physician information processing and reasoning have had important impact in the design of subsequent CPR user interfaces.

In a second line of studies, we applied cognitive approaches to the evaluation of emerging CPR systems at Columbia University [21]. This line of research involved the evaluation of both the user interface and the underlying medical vocabulary of a CPR system. Subjects, consisting of nine physicians, were initially asked to enter information from paper records into the CPR. Full audio transcripts of the subjects' thinking aloud were made, along with video recording of the corresponding computer screens as the subjects transferred information from paper records into the new CPR system. The approach to analysis involved annotation of the audio and video transcripts, using the method described above, to identify the frequency of categories of problems related to both the usability of the interface and the effectiveness of the underlying medical terminology to represent information about the patients' condition. Based on the analysis of the data, it was found that users found use of the system difficult due to design problems ranging from lack of consistency of the user interface (e.g., multiple and confusing ways to carry out procedures such as data entry) to problems in representing medical findings using the system. The frequency of particular usability problems was compiled and presented to the design team and consequently changes were made to the CPR based on the recommendations. Subsequent usability testing with a new set of nine different physicians (who had not used the system before) indicated that the number of problems had decreased from an average of 19 problems per user testing session prior to the suggested changes, to 1.9 problems per user session after the changes were applied. Work such as this has underlined the value and effectiveness of employing cognitive approaches to evaluation in improving the usability of healthcare information systems during the iterative process of system design and implementation.

In another line of research we have been involved in the evaluation of a number of information systems targeted to patient users of health information systems. In a recent study Kaufman and colleagues used a cognitive task analysis approach involving usability testing methods to assess use of a home-based telemedicine system for diabetes [36]. The interactions of 25 subjects, ranging in age and educational background, were recorded in their homes using portable recording equipment. In another related study the usability of an experimental text summarization system was compared to three commercial search engines [39]. This study involved having subjects (consisting of family members of patients in the hospital for cardiac surgery) pose their questions to the different search engines while thinking aloud. Based on this approach we found that although no one search engine was favored by all subjects, there were specific features of each of the systems that users invariably liked. The results have been extended to the design of new approaches to providing information to patient users, based on a reverse-engineering approach (i.e., based on the results of our analyses of search engine use by patients).

In a more recent line of research, we have extended the overall approach to evaluation of information systems described in this paper to the remote evaluation of Web-based information systems, an approach we call "televaluation" of healthcare information systems. Our first work along these lines involved the distance evaluation of a Web-based patient information system, known as PatCIS, which allows patients at home to access their own patient records over the Internet [40]. Data were collected from both in-depth study of individual users interacting with the system as well as statistics on usage of the different components (e.g., advice, review of medical information, and links to educational resources). In one set of studies, we developed an "evaluation server" that intercepts a user's request for information from a Web-based information resource and can automatically query the user for his or her impressions regarding usefulness of the information obtained from the information resource. Thus in this recent line of work we are moving toward automated evaluation of use of Web-based information resources and systems in healthcare and extending the concept of task analysis to include automated probing and tracking of users as they interact with systems remotely.

Our work has shown that cognitively based analyses of information systems can be applied throughout the systems development life cycle, and in a recent work it has been shown that the approach can be extended to the early analysis of systems requirements as a basis for systems design. Along these lines, Cysneiros and Kushniruk have recently described the development of an ontology for classifying and reasoning about cognitive aspects of use of information systems in healthcare and other domains [5]. As the issue of designing improved healthcare systems based on a better understanding of the complexities of the healthcare environment and the varied types of users becomes more widely acknowledged, cognitive approaches will likely increase in importance for evaluating systems (as well as preliminary design ideas) throughout the entire SDLC.

From Laboratory to Naturalistic Evaluations in Health Informatics: A Continuum

Approaches to evaluation of healthcare information systems using cognitive approaches can be located along a continuum of study types ranging from artificial laboratory-based studies at one end of the continuum to naturalistic studies conducted in real work settings at the other end of the continuum (as depicted in Figure 6.6).

At one end of the continuum an attempt is made to conduct studies in controlled artificial conditions. This might, for example, involve use of a

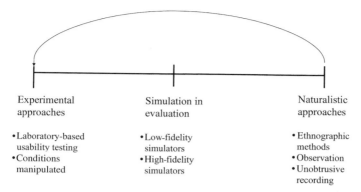

Experimental approaches	Simulation in evaluation	Naturalistic approaches
• Laboratory-based usability testing • Conditions manipulated	• Low-fidelity simulators • High-fidelity simulators	• Ethnographic methods • Observation • Unobtrusive recording

FIGURE 6.6. A continuum of approaches to evaluation of healthcare information systems.

fixed usability laboratory—often consisting of facilities designed for conducting usability testing (with built-in recording devices, ceiling-mounted video cameras, and one-way observation mirrors to view subjects interacting with systems). It should be noted that other approaches to conducting laboratory-type testing of users interacting with information systems also can be carried out using low-cost portable recording equipment. In any case, for this type of study, subjects may be given artificial medical cases as stimulus material (e.g., a written case description) and the procedure often involves subjects thinking aloud or verbalizing their thoughts (which are audio recorded) while carrying out a specific task (e.g., entering the information from the written case description into a CPR that is being evaluated). At this end of the continuum, studies may be designed that exert a higher degree of experimental control with laboratory testing of subjects interacting with the system with only one or a few variables (e.g., display format) manipulated during testing, with the test being conducted under controlled artificial conditions, either in a usability laboratory, or using portable recording equipment (as described in [31]).

Evaluations involving simulation techniques are located halfway along the continuum ranging from controlled to naturalistic approaches to assessment. Such evaluations may allow for a high degree of experimental control while also maintaining a high degree of realism in the tasks presented to subjects during testing. For example, as described above, we have recorded subjects interacting with a CPR system while interviewing a simulated patient, consisting of a research collaborator playing the part of a specific type of patient (borrowing from the concept of a "standardized patient" used for assessing medical residents in medical training). From such studies we have been able to extend our understanding of use of a CPR system from individual physicians interacting with the system to the understanding of how the computer system interacts with the physician in the context of carrying out the task of interviewing a patient in a realistic medical context. A range of other possibilities exist for carrying out evaluations using simulations, including use of high-fidelity computer-controlled mannequins that are now becoming more widely available in medical schools (for providing training to students and residents in areas such as surgery). Such simulators, not unlike their counterparts in areas such as aviation, can be used both for training and also for use in assessment of technology in carrying out work tasks in healthcare.

At the far end of the continuum shown in Figure 6.6 are naturalistic approaches to evaluation. Here user interactions with systems in real-life contexts are monitored with little or no intervention from the evaluators (e.g., recording real use of a CPR system in a doctor's office for entering and retrieving patient data). Also included at this end of the continuum would be studies described above, where use of Web-based information systems is tracked or monitored over time. It has been argued by many that such studies are necessary as results from classical controlled experimental studies may be limited in how well they generalize to real-world situations. In our work we have worked at all points along the continuum, with some of our evaluations beginning with in-depth laboratory study of use of a computer system in healthcare being followed up with collection of data from naturalistic settings. Likewise, study of use of a system using naturalistic approaches (e.g., tracking or logging of real system usage) may lead to specific research questions that may be best answered by applying experimental control and rigor (e.g., following up with laboratory testing of subjects interacting with a system to deal with specific cases using the "think aloud" method).

Cognitive approaches also can be considered in the context of where they can be applied in the systems development life cycle, as depicted in Figure 6.7. From Figure 6.7 it can be seen that approaches to evaluation that are based on ideas and principles from cognitive science and usability

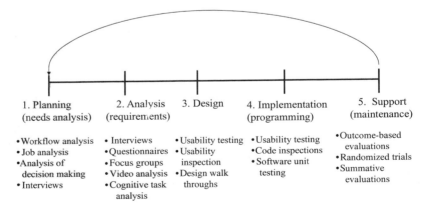

FIGURE 6.7. The systems development life cycle (SDLC) in relation to evaluation methodologies.

engineering can be applied at various points throughout the SDLC. For example, cognitive task analysis and the in-depth recording of subjects interacting with mockups of health information systems can be applied even during early stages of system design. At the other end of the continuum, approaches such as those described in this paper can be applied to assess how completed systems (at the far right of the SDLC in the figure) impact on physician reasoning and decision making in summative evaluation late in the SDLC.

Conclusions and Future Directions

In this chapter we have examined a range of techniques for evaluation of healthcare information systems that borrow from the fields of both cognitive science and usability engineering. The chapter has presented a framework for conducting evaluation at various stages throughout the systems development life cycle (SDLC) in developing healthcare information systems. In this context we consider evaluation to be closely related to system design and implementation within the process of iterative system development. A focus of our work has been on understanding and assessing the impact of new information technologies in healthcare on cognitive processes involved in reasoning, decision making, and using new technology to improve complex work activities. In recent years there has been a move in evaluation of health information systems from a nearly exclusive focus on summative evaluation of completed systems (using methods related to controlled clinical trials) to the formative evaluation of systems being developed in order to lead to their improvement. Furthermore, there has been a newly emerging focus on the analysis of the cognitive *processes* involved using information systems, as such study makes it possible to identify and assess emergent and unexpected effects of these systems on cognitive and work processes.

A challenge for future work will be to integrate data and findings from multiple evaluation approaches (e.g., methods of cognitive task analysis and methods associated with outcome-based evaluations of systems). One area where such synergy will be important is in the evaluation of information systems to ensure patient safety and to lead to design of systems that will reduce error. Recent work in this area has included study of the relationship between cognitive evaluation, using methods such as those described in this chapter, and the analysis of how medical information technology may reduce or introduce error into medical practice. Along these lines, Kushniruk, Triola, Borycki, Stein, and Kannry have demonstrated how coding of usability problems can lead to accurate predictions of actual medical errors resulting from use of medical information systems [41]. Along related lines, Zhang and colleagues have worked on developing taxonomies and frameworks for studying error in medicine based on cognitive analysis [24]. The work we are doing in evaluation is ongoing and constantly being refined as the technology we evaluate changes and advances. Important developments along these lines include work on the automated analysis of qualitative data emerging from cognitive studies [32] and work toward extending many of the approaches described in this chapter to the automated analysis of Web-based information systems from a distance, an approach we have termed "televaluation." As healthcare technology advances, the greatest challenge for evaluation of health information systems will be in understanding the effect of such systems on complex cognitive processes involved in healthcare and in finding ways to apply this understanding in creating systems that facilitate and enhance human information processing.

Additional Readings

V.L. Patel, A.W. Kushniruk, S. Yang, and J.F. Yale, Impact of a computer-based patient record system on data collection, knowledge organization and reasoning, Journal of the American Medical Informatics Association 7(6) (2000) 569–585.

V.L. Patel and D.W. Bates, editors, Special issue of the *Journal of Biomedical Informatics:* Patient safety. Journal of Biomedical Informatics 36(1/2) (2003).

V.L. Patel and D.R. Kaufman, Cognitive science and biomedical informatics, in: E.H. Shortliffe and J.J. Cimino, editors, *Biomedical Informatics: Computer Applications in Health Care and Biomedicine*, 3rd ed. (Springer-Verlag, New York, in press).

A.W. Kushniruk and V.L. Patel, Cognitive and usability engineering approaches to the evaluation of clinical information systems, Journal of Biomedical Informatics 37(1) (2004) 56–76.

A.W. Kushniruk, Analysis of complex decision making processes in health care: Cognitive approaches to health informatics, Journal of Biomedical Informatics 34(5) (2001) 365–376.

A.W. Kushniruk, D.R. Kaufman, V.L. Patel, Y. Levesque, and P. Lottin, Assessment of a computerized patient record system: A cognitive approach to evaluating an emerging medical technology, MD Computing 13(5) (1996) 406–415.

References

[1] C.P. Friedman and J.C. Wyatt, *Evaluation Methods in Medical Informatics* (Springer, New York, 1997).

[2] A.W. Kushniruk, Evaluation in the design of information systems: Applications of approaches from usability engineering, Computers in Biology and Medicine 32(3) (2002) 141–149.

[3] V.L. Patel, A.W. Kushniruk, S. Yang, and J.F. Yale, Impact of a computer-based patient record system on data collection, knowledge organization and reasoning. Journal of the American Medical Informatics Association 7(6) (2000) 569–585.

[4] J. Moehr, Evaluation: Salvation or nemesis of medical informatics? Computers in Biology and Medicine (2002) 113–125.

[5] L. Cysneiros and A.W. Kushniruk, Bringing usability to the early stages of software development, in: *Proceedings of the 11th IEEE International Requirements Engineering Conference* (2003), pp. 359–361.

[6] S. McConnell, *Rapid Development: Taming Wild Software Schedules* (Microsoft Press, Redmond, WA, 1996).

[7] J. Preece, Y. Rogers, and H. Sharp, *Interaction Design: Beyond Human–Computer Interaction* (Wiley, New York, 2002).

[8] K. Hammond, Naturalistic decision making from a Brunswikian viewpoint: Its past, present, future, in: G. Klein, J. Orasanu, R. Calderwood, and C. Zsambok, editors, *Decision Making in Action: Models and Methods* (Ablex, Norwood, NJ, 1993), pp. 205–227.

[9] R. Hamm, Moment-by-moment variation in experts' analytic intuitive cognitive activity, IEEE Transactions on Systems Management Cybernation SMC-18, 5 (1988) 757–776.

[10] V.L. Patel, J.F. Arocha, and D.R. Kaufman, Diagnostic reasoning and medical expertise, in: D.L. Medin, editor, *The Psychology of Learning and Motivation: Advances in Research and Theory* (Academic Press, San Diego, 1994), (31), pp. 187–252.

[11] V.L. Patel and D.R. Kaufman, Cognitive science and biomedical informatics, in: E.H. Shortliffe and J.J. Cimino, editors, *Biomedical Informatics: Computer Applications in Health Care and Biomedicine* 3rd ed. (Springer-Verlag, New York, in press).

[12] G.A. Klein, A recognition-primed decision (RPD) model of rapid decision making, in: G. Klein, J. Orasanu, R. Calderwood, and C. Zsambok, editors, *Decision Making in Action: Models and Methods* (Ablex, Norwood, NJ, 1993), pp. 138–147.

[13] S. Gordon and R. Gill, Cognitive task analysis, in: C. Zsambok and G. Klein, editors, *Naturalistic Decision Making* (Erlbaum, Mahwah, NJ, 1997), pp. 131–140.

[14] R. Glaser, A. Lesgold, S. Lajoie, R. Eastman, L. Greenberg, D. Logan, M. Magone, A. Weiner, R. Wolf, and L. Yengo, Cognitive task analysis to enhance technical skills training and assessment (Report, Learning Research and Development Center) (University of Pittsburgh, 1985).

[15] B. Means and S. Gott, Cognitive task analysis as a basis for tutor development: Articulating abstract knowledge representations, in: J. Psotka, L. Massey, and S. Mutter, editors, *Intelligent Tutoring Systems: Lessons Learned* (Hillsdale, New Jersey, 1988).

[16] J. Rasmussen, A. Pejtersen, and L. Goodstein, *Cognitive Systems Engineering* (Wiley, New York, 1994).

[17] K.J. Vicente, *Cognitive Work Analysis: Toward Safe, Productive and Healthy Computer-Based Work* (Lawrence Erlbaum, New York, 1999).

[18] J. Nielsen, *Usability Engineering* (Academic Press, New York, 1993).

[19] A. Kushniruk and V. Patel, Cognitive computer-based video analysis: Its application in assessing the usability of medical systems, Medinfo (1995) 1566–1569.

[20] P.L. Elkin, D.N. Mohr, M.S. Tuttle, W.G. Cole, G.E. Atkin, K. Keck, T.B. Fisk, B.H. Kaihoi, K.E. Lee, M.C. Higgins, H. Suermondt, N. Olson, P.L. Claus, P.C. Carpenter, and C. Chute, Standardized problem list generation, utilizing the Mayo Cannonical Vocabulary embedded within the Unified Medical Language System, in: *Proceedings of the AMIA Symposium* (1997), pp. 500–504.

[21] A.W. Kushniruk, V.L. Patel, J.J. Cimino, and R.A. Barrows, Cognitive evaluation of the user interface and vocabulary of an outpatient information system, in: *Proceedings of the AMIA Symposium* (1996), pp. 22–26.

[22] J.M. Coble, J. Karat, M. Orland, and M. Kahn, Iterative usability testing: Ensuring a usable clinical workstation, in: *Proceedings of the AMIA Symposium* (1997), pp. 744–748.

[23] A.W. Kushniruk, D.R. Kaufman, V.L. Patel, Y. Levesque, and P. Lottin, Assessment of a computerized patient record system: A cognitive approach to evaluating an emerging medical technology. MD Computing 13(5) (1996) 406–415.

[24] J. Zhang, T.R. Johnson, V.L. Patel, D.L. Paige, and T. Kubose, Using usability heuristics to evaluate patient safety of medical devices, Journal of Biomedical Informatics 36(1–2) (2003) 23–24.

[25] J. Horsky, D.R. Kaufman, M.L. Oppenheim, and V.L. Patel, A framework for analyzing the cognitive complexity of computer-assisted clinical ordering, Journal of Biomedical Informatics 36(1–2) (2003) 4–22.

[26] J. Rubin, *Handbook of Usability Testing: How to Plan, Design and Conduct Effective Tests* (Wiley, New York, 1994).

[27] M.E. Wiklund, *Usability in Practice* (Academic Press, New York, 1994).

[28] A.W. Kushniruk and V.L. Patel, Cognitive evaluation of decision making processes and assessment of information technology in medicine, International Journal of Medical Informatics 51 (1998) 83–90.

[29] K. Ericsson and H. Simon, *Protocol Analysis: Verbal Reports as Data* (Academic Press, Cambridge, MA, 1993).

[30] J.M. Carroll, *Human-Computer Interaction in the New Millennium* (Addison-Wesley, New York, 2002).

[31] A.W. Kushniruk, V.L. Patel, and J.J. Cimino, Usability testing in medical informatics: Cognitive approaches to evaluation of information systems and user interfaces, in: *Proceedings of the AMIA Symposium* (1997), pp. 218–222.

[32] A.W. Kushniruk and V.L. Patel, Cognitive and usability engineering approaches to the evaluation of clinical information systems, Journal of Biomedical Informatics 37(1) (2004) 56–76.

[33] K. Ericsson and J. Smith, *Toward a General Theory of Expertise: Prospects and Limits* (Cambridge University Press, New York, 1991).

[34] A.W. Kushniruk, C. Patel, V.L. Patel, and J.J. Cimino, "Televaluation" of information systems: An integrative approach to design and evaluation of Web-based systems, International Journal of Medical Informatics 61(1) (2001) 45–70.

[35] J.J. Cimino, V.L. Patel, and A.W. Kushniruk, Studying the human-computer-terminology interface, Journal of the American Medical Informatics Association 8(2) (2001) 163–173.

[36] D.R. Kaufman, V.L. Patel, J.L. Starren, P.C. Morin, C. Hilliman, J. Pevzner, R.S. Weinstock, R. Goland, and S. Shea, Usability in the real world: Assessing medical information technologies in patients' homes, Journal of Biomedical Informatics 36(1–2) (2003) 45–60.

[37] A.W. Kushniruk, Analysis of complex decision making processes in healthcare: Cognitive approaches to health informatics, Journal of Biomedical Informatics 34(5) (2001) 365–376.

[38] B. Shneiderman, Designing the User Interface, 4th ed. (Addison-Wesley, New York, 2003).

[39] A.W. Kushniruk, M.Y. Kan, K. McKeown, J. Klavans, D. Jordan, M. LaFlamme, and V.L. Patel, Usability evaluation of an experimental text summarization system and three search engines: Implications for the reengineering of health-care interfaces, in: *Proceedings of the AMIA Symposium* (2002), pp. 420–424.

[40] J.J. Cimino, V.L. Patel, and A.W. Kushniruk, The patient clinical information system (PatCIS): Technical solutions for and experience with giving patients access to their electronic medical records, International Journal of Medical Informatics 68(1–3) (2002) 113–127.

[41] A. Kushniruk, M. Triola, E. Borycki, B. Stein, and J. Kannry, Technology induced error and usability: The relationship between usability problems and prescription errors when using a handheld application. International Journal of Medical Informatics, in press.

7
Work-Sampling: A Statistical Approach to Evaluation of the Effect of Computers on Work Patterns in Health Care

Dean F. Sittig

Introduction

An increasing number of medical informaticians in particular, and health-care institutions in general, are in the process of implementing clinical computing systems. These systems range from small, standalone, PC-based record-keeping systems to mid-sized laboratory/pharmacy management systems, and full-scale hospital information systems. Several institutions are currently working on integrating systems of all sizes into medical center-wide academic information management systems (IAIMS) [1–4]. The need for an accurate assessment of the clinical, administrative, social, and financial effects of such systems has been recognized [5–7]. Sound, statistically valid evaluations of all types of these systems are crucial in determining the future role of computers in health care.

Miller and Sittig [8] identified five reasons for conducting an evaluation of a medical informatics research project, including: (1) to test a prototype, (2) to refine the system, (3) to assure safety, (4) to determine clinical effects, and (5) to develop new evaluation methodologies. This chapter focuses upon yet another reason for conducting a medical informatics research project evaluation: to determine its effect on the work patterns of participants in the healthcare delivery process.

Many different evaluation strategies have been employed in an attempt to determine the optimal assignment of duties and responsibilities to healthcare practitioners of differing skill and training levels. This chapter attempts to review and synthesize information concerning the pluses and minuses of these various work evaluation strategies from a broad spectrum of sources. Following a brief review of several evaluation methodologies, it focuses on the subject of Work-Sampling (WS). While the work-sampling technique has been in use since the mid-1930s [9] and there are citations in the healthcare literature of its use as far back as 1954 [10], there is still no single source that describes in detail the steps and numerous tools available to help an investigator carry out and interpret the results of a work-sampling evaluation.

Review of Work Evaluation Methodologies

There are many questions which can be asked when evaluating the effect of computers on work patterns, including: (1) how and by whom was the system used, (2) how much time was spent using the system, (3) what effect did it have on other work-related activities, (4) how long should it take to use the system, and (5) how can the work patterns, environment, and/or the computer (i.e., the input/output devices, placement and/or numbers of devices, software options and/or data entry flow, etc.) be improved so as to utilize each member of the healthcare, team's knowledge and training to its fullest extent.

Each of these questions requires specific evaluation strategies. The methodologies, described below, each seek to focus on a particular aspect of these questions. The following sections briefly describe particular study designs giving (1) an, overview of pluses and minuses and (2) a review of their findings. Of particular interest is the manner in which many of the investigators combine several evaluation methodologies to obtain a more global view of the effect of their particular computer implementation

Time-Motion Analysis

Time-motion analysis (TM) provides a direct measurement of the amount of time a specific worker spends doing a specific activity. A TM is carried out by a trained observer with a watch, who continuously observes multiple trials of selected activities and records the time spent doing each small part. Often, when looking at the time required to use a computer for a particular task, the total time spent as well as specific timing intervals, can be recorded directly by the computer with little, or no, extra human effort [11]. TM studies are particularly appropriate when one is trying to compare two different work patterns that produce the same result. Such a study might be used to compare the time spent entering a medication order into the computer via lightpen, keyboard, bar-coded chart, or a free-hand pen-based operating system with automatic optical character recognition.

For example, in a TM comparison Minda [12] found that the time required to complete a nursing assessment manually versus a menu-driven computer-based charting system, the computer was 21% faster (558 ± 237 sec vs. 706 ± 223 sec, $p < 0.05$, two-tailed t-test). She also calculated a "productivity index" that measured the number of seconds required to record an observation, and found that the computer system was more than twice as fast (3.5 ± 1.6 vs. 7.6 ± 2.2 sec/observation, $p < 0.05$). To carry out this study, Minda spent 17 days collecting data from 40 nurses on one specific task.

A clear benefit of a TM study is the accurate timing figures obtained. Disadvantages of TMs include: (1) it is labor intensive, that is, usually requiring, a one-to-one observer-to-worker ratio, (2) it is subject to both observer and worker biases (e.g., some workers are always "better" than others), (3) many trials of the same activity must be observed and measured to obtain reliable results, and (4) data-entry source code must be modified to use the computer as the timing mechanism.

Subjective Evaluations

Subjective evaluations usually take the form of questionnaires. Well-designed questionnaires can provide a personal assessment of attitudes and estimates of the time spent in completing a specific task. They may be administered orally, on paper, or even by the computer itself. Obvious advantages of using questionnaires include: (1) easy to administer, (2) easy to interpret, and (3) easy to obtain valuable cognitive information. Unfortunately, such evaluations also carry with them severe limitations, including: (1) giving imprecise measurements of work activities, (2) based on personal biases, and (3) possibly strongly influenced by recent events which may skew the results. Although subjective evaluations of the effect of a new computer system should not be used alone, when used in conjunction with one of the more quantitative methods, they provide important information to the researcher and administrator alike.

For example, Andrews and Gardner [13] combined a computer-based timing analysis with a questionnaire to evaluate the effect of using portable laptop computers for respiratory therapy charting. Their timing study found no significant differences in the amount of time required, or in the "productivity" of the therapists in the study. They did find through a questionnaire administered to six respiratory therapists involved in the pilot implementation that "*all* six therapists preferred (to chart on) ward terminals" rather than laptops. In addition, they found that work patterns varied considerably between the six therapists.

Review of Departmental Records

Departmental records, or statistics, provide a valuable source of information concerning the overall function of a particular department. Unfortunately, such retrospective epidemiologic studies or chart reviews have inherent methodological flaws [14]. In addition, unless they are extremely detailed, they tell little about what actual employees or even groups of employees do on a shift-by-shift basis. For example, if one were interested in the overall change in productivity following implementation of a new computer-based order/entry system in an out-patient pharmacy, one could check the average number of prescriptions filled in the three-month period before implementation and compare that to the average number filled in a three-month period following implementation.

In a review of departmental records conducted in the respiratory therapy department of LDS Hospital in Salt Lake City, Utah, Andrews et al. found that implementation of a computer-based charting system increased productivity (as measured by procedures billed) by 18%, while the number of therapists remained constant [15]. Following presentation of these results, they remind the reader that it is possible that all the computer actually did was "assure that all work done was billed." Their conclusion from this study was that "computer charting did not *decrease* productivity." Perhaps by using a different technique, such as TM or work-sampling, they could have made an even stronger claim for their system.

Personal Record of Activities

Each member of the staff can keep a log of activities performed and the amount of time spent on each activity [10]. Problems arise, however, during periods of intense activity resulting in periods of unaccountable behavior. In addition, if the log is done periodically, a tremendous emphasis is placed on the subject's memory; a known error source.

Description of the Work Sampling Technique

Work sampling, originally developed by Tippett in 1935 [9], consists of a series of instantaneous, randomly spaced observations of the activities being carried out by the group of workers (or possibly machines) under study [16]. WS is a fact-finding tool based on the laws of probability.[1] It can be used to measure the working time and nonworking time of a person (or machine), or to establish a time standard for a specific activity (i.e., to identify the number of minutes required to perform a certain task) [17].

Example

If, for example, one were interested in the percentage of time that the nursing staff on a particular unit spends in interacting with a new bed-side computerized charting system versus the time spent in direct patient care, a work-sampling study could be performed [18]. Such a study is based on the theory that the percentage of randomly made observations in which nurses are using the computers and/or caring for the patient compared to the total number of observation made, represents an estimate of how nurses spend their working day.

---

[1] That is, that a sample taken at random from a large population or group, tends to have the same distribution or percentage of occurrence, as that of the population at large.

TABLE 7.1. Sample work-sampling data collection.

State	Observations (%)
Nurse patient care	18 (50)
Nurse using system	11 (31)
Miscellaneous/other	7 (19)
Total	36 (100)

Table 7.1 shows a simple data collection and analysis form for an example of a WS study. If a nurse is observed using the system, a tally is placed in the OBSERVATIONS column next to "Nurse using system"; if a nurse is caring for the patient, then the mark is placed in the OBSER-VATIONS column next to "Nurse patient care." When enough observations have been made (a formula and sample calculation for determining the appropriate number of observations will be presented in a following section) then the number of OBSERVATIONS are totalled—for each category (across) and then for all categories (down)—and the percentage calculated (e g., $[11/36]*100 = 31\%$). The more observations made, the more certain one can be that the estimates represent the true percentage of time nurses spend interacting with the computer and in direct patient-care activities.

Steps in Designing a Work-Sampling Study

There are many excellent references which describe many of the steps required to design, and tools available to carry out a WS-study [17,19,20]. The following is a synthesis of those descriptions.

Step 1. *Identify research objective.* To choose the appropriate work-study technique and data-collection procedure, one must carefully identify the main hypothesis that one would hope to be able to accept or reject upon completion of the study.

Step 2. *Identify a study site and obtain approval of the manager.* Care must be taken when attempting to identify a particular unit or ward within a hospital to insure that the study site is as "normal," or representative, of the entire range of activities to be studied as possible. The departmental manger will often be able to offer sound advice on the "normal" work activities to be studied and their associated definitions [21].

Step 3. *Identify work categories and carefully define the content of each.* The work-activity categories must be selected and defined so as to leave no doubt in the mind of the observer how each activity that is observed should be categorized (see the appendix) [19]. A key point is that all activities must be able to be accounted for. Therefore, one of the most important categories in every WS study is that of *Other* or *Miscellaneous Activities.*

Step 4. *Create a data entry form.* Once the categories have been adequately described in writing, one should develop an easy-to-use data-entry or observation-recording form. The carefully worded list of categories and their associated definitions should be kept with the data collection forms at all times for easy reference.

Step 5. *Identify and train appropriate observers.* One must identify an appropriate group of WS observers. Key elements in deciding exactly who should collect the data include: (1) do they understand the job being observed, (2) can they do the observations without "getting in the way," (3) do any of the categories require that the observers know "what the subject is thinking," (4) is there someone in the area who can make the observations while also performing their regular job (i.e., a clerk or technician, or perhaps even the manager of the unit). During the training phase, attention must be given to carefully explaining the philosophy behind the description of each work category since many activities are not explicitly described. By walking around the unit and observing the myriad nursing activities for 30 minutes to an hour, one should be able to explain adequately the procedure.

Step 6. *Conduct a pilot study.* Once all the preliminary details have been worked out, one should conduct a pilot study. This study allows one to test the work categories and their definitions, and provides one with a rough estimate of the percentages of time subjects spend in each of the categories. It may be preferable to perform a short TM rather than a short WS-study at this point. A TM pilot will help to insure that all work-related activities are covered by the chosen categories as well as providing a "touchstone" against which the results of the WS-study can be compared.

Step 7. *Design the WS study.* The most important elements of the study to be determined are:

a. *The total number of observations needed* to obtain the desired accuracy. The following formula describes this relationship: $n = p(1 - p)/\sigma^2$, where n = the total number of observations, p = expected percent of time required, by the most important category of the study (from pilot), and σ = standard deviation of percentage.

Example: Determine the number of observations needed to establish that the percentage of time nurses spend charting is 30% ± 2% (estimated from pilot study) with a 95% confidence interval (i.e., we want to be able to state with 95% confidence that nurses spend between 28 and 32% of their time charting); therefore, we set $p = 0.3$, $2\sigma = 2\%$ (or $\sigma = 0.01$), so that $n = 0.3 (1 - 0.3)/(0.01)^2 = 2100$ observations, where n represents an estimate of the actual number of samples needed. There are also published nomograms which provide the WS-study designer with a rough estimate of the value of n [16,19,22].

b. Once the total number of observations is determined, one needs to determine *the frequency for making these observations.* A good rule-of-thumb is to limit the number of randomly made observations to less than eight per hour.
c. Another key element is *whether the observations will be made randomly or at fixed intervals.* This decision is based on whether the underlying work activities are random (lacking any prominent periodic component), such as most healthcare activities, or occur with some regularity or pattern, such as assembly-line work. If the work activities are random, then one can sample (and [23] has shown it to be preferable) at fixed intervals, otherwise the sampling intervals should be randomly selected.
d. Next, *the total length of the study needs to be established.* This decision should be based on some naturally occurring rhythm within the work pattern, for example, a five or seven-day work week, or some other cyclic pattern of activities. It is very important to make sure that equal numbers of subcycles (e.g., day vs. night and/or weekend vs. weekday) are included in the study.

Therefore, to continue with our previous example, if we assume that we need to make 2100 observations over a seven-day period, then we need to make: 2001 observations/7 days = 300 observations/day. If we anticipate that there will be four nurses on duty at all times, then: 300 observations/day × 1 day/1440 min gives 4.8 min/observation, but since there will be four nurses on duty at all times, we can make four observations at each time point. Based on these calculations, observations could be made every 20 minutes around the clock. This would result in 288 observations/day (3 observation periods/h × 24 h/day × 4 nurses) or a grand total of 2016 observations in the entire week (which is within 5% of our original estimate (2100) of the total number of observations needed). If one wanted to be ultraconservation, then one could make observations every 15 minutes resulting in a grand total of 2688 observations (4 observations/h × 24 h/day × 4 nurses × 7 days/week).
e. Finally, *one needs to pick "normal" time* to actually perform the study. For example, one would not want to conduct a study of a cardiovascular surgical ICU during the week that many of the surgeons will be away at their annual meeting.

Step 8. *Establish independent measures of workload.* It is important to establish temporally relevant workload measures in as great a detail as possible. This will help insure that many of the underlying variables which govern the work performed will be accounted for. For example, Bradshaw et al. [21] utilized the daily patient census, a measure of patient acuity (used as an estimate of severity of illness), and the nurse staffing levels in an attempt to explain the differences in the amount of patient care provided by the nurses in the two phases of the study. In another study, Kohout et al. [24] used the total volume of prescriptions filled and the number of full-time equivalents to adjust their results.

Step 9. *Conduct the study.* Apprise all staff members being observed of the study. No matter what precautions one takes, it will only be a short time before everyone is aware of what is going on and they may be quite angry at not being informed beforehand. In addition, a carefully prepared description of the study's goals can relieve staff concerns of losing their jobs, and so on. Keep careful records of all "special events" that occur during the study period. Construct and update control charts at the end of each day [25].

Control charts are an excellent method of monitoring the quality of the data as it is being collected. Briefly, a control chart is a graph of the percentage of time spent in any single work category (although most investigators would use the key category, i.e., the one the null hypothesis is based upon) plotted for every complete shift on day (e.g., see Figure 7.1). One also plots the cumulative percentage of time spent in that particular category. As the study progresses, this cumulative line should begin to approach the final result. Control limits, for the daily percentage estimates, are then calculated using the equation under Step 7, with the terms rearranged to solve σ. Control limits are generally set at ±3 σ.

Continuing with the previous example, assume that we constructed a control chart at the end of the fifth day of the study (i.e., after 1414 total observations were made). Control limits are calculated from the equation of Step 7 and rearranged to solve σ. The numerator contains the

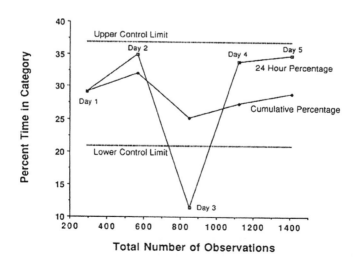

Figure 7.1. Control chart from example work-sampling study. Notice that the data collected on day 3 is not within control limits which indicates a potential problem with the data.

cumulative percentage of time spent in the charting category up to this point in time (28.9%). We use the average number of samples collected for each 24-hour period in the denominator (1414/5 = 282); σ^2 = 0.289(1 − 0.289)/282, or σ = 2.7%. Therefore, we set our upper control limit to be 28.9% + (3 × 2.7%) = 37% (lower limit = 20.8%).

In other words, we would expect that 99% of the time each 24-hour sample should show that the nurses are spending between 20.8 and 37.0% (28.9 ± 8.1%) of their time charting. Therefore, we should carefully interview the observers who collected the data for the third day to see what, if anything, went wrong since the percentage for the third day was only 11.4%. Upon doing this we might find, for instance, that the computer terminals were down for 16 of the 24 hours under study (which accounts for the figure being 2/3 lower than it should have been). For that reason we should eliminate this particular 16-hour period from our final data analysis. It may then be necessary to continue the study for an additional 16 hours to accumulate the data required to obtain our acceptable level of accuracy. This example helps illustrate the benefits gained by constructing and maintaining current control charts as the study progresses. If we had been monitoring this example study more closely we could have quickly eliminated the bad data and increased the frequency of the observations from every 20 minutes to every 15 minutes for the remainder of the study, insuring that we would finish the study on time with enough samples to reach our predetermined confidence levels.

In addition, it is possible to use the same control-chart methodology to quantify the intraobserver reliability. To accomplish this, one would plot each observer's totals along with the overall figures and their associated confidence intervals (i.e., ±3 σ). One would anticipate that, if all observers were equally adept and/or conscientious at classifying the various working activities, all the individual observer's data points would fall within three standard deviations of the final mean. If this is not the case, then one should investigate the outlier observer to ascertain the problem. If indeed there is a methodological problem that cannot be corrected, then this observer's data should not be included in the final analysis.

Step 10. *Analyze and interpret data collected.* Following completion of the study, one should carefully check the control charts and notes made during the study, and interview all observers to determine whether the data collected were truly representative of the work-related activities. Data that are unrepresentative of the normal work routine should he eliminated. Decide whether the data warrant a thorough statistical analysis or whether simple summary statistics (e.g., sum, average, and range of percentages of time spent in each category, with associated confidence intervals) would allow the research question to be answered.

If one decides that a thorough statistical analysis of the pre- versus postimplementation data is necessary, there are many different approaches one might choose, including: (1) comparison of the mean time percentages by Student's t-test [21,26], (2) comparison of mean time percentages with confidence intervals, looking for areas of overlap [27], (3) adjusting data collected both before and after computerization, using an arcsine transformation followed by analysis of variance (ANOVA) [28], and (4) compare pre- and postimplementation activity categories using a chi-square test with Cramer's V statistic to measure the strength of the hypothesized relationships [24].

Step 11. *Create final report with suggestions for realizing benefits.* It is quite possible that study will find that the first implementation of the computer system has not had the desired effect on the healthcare providers work-patterns [21,29]. In that case, however, one should not despair, but proceed with the next phase of benefits realization which may require redefinition of specific jobs, revision of software, increases and/or changes in the locations of the terminals, and so on.

Discussion

While WS studies are relatively easy to carry out and can provide important data to both medical informaticians and healthcare management alike, they are not without limitations. Following a detailed look at the results of several different WS studies, some limitatioin of the WS methodology will be outlined. We conclude with a brief look at the advantages of the work-sampling methodology.

Results form WS Studies

Several WS studies have been conducted in an attempt to "prove" that computer-based nurse charting reduces the amount of time nurses spend charting [6,18,21,29]. By these standards, none of these studies were successful since none was able to document a significant decrease in the amount of time nurses spent charting. On the other hand, they were successful in helping to identify particular programs that needed improvement, preferred terminal placement, and further enhancements to the system to reduce the amount of data that had to be recorded on paper.

By combining the results from other evaluation methodologies (i.e., quality and completeness charting reviews, nursing satisfaction and complaints questionnaire, etc.) with the WS data, managers and developers were able to quantify the effects of the system on the nurses' other work-related activities. Therefore, they were able to determine that the improvements in the documentation of the nurses' patient-care activities more than made up for the slight increase in the time spent charting. In addition, through use of the online charting system, one hospital was able to change the manner in which patients were billed for nursing care [31].

To be more specific, before implementatioin of time on-line charting system, all patients were charged a standard fee for nursing care (included in the room rate), regardless of their need for nursing care. Following implementation, each patient was billed for nursing care based on the actual number of minutes of nursing care they received (derived from the patient-care activities that were charted). This change to variable billing received broad acceptance throughout the hospital and was looked on very favorably by third-party payors, including Medicare. Finally, the nursing department was especially happy with the new system since they became a revenue center rather than a cost center within the hospital. By linking costs to revenue, the nursing department was able to generate productivity measurements which allowed them to look objectively at their organization and to become more efficient and cost-effective without compromising the quality of patient care.

Limitations of Work-Sampling

1. WS is not an economical solution to monitor the job-related activities of one worker or for studying a group of workers spread out over a wide area, because the observer is either idling or walking the majority of the time, rather than observing.

2. WS is not a direct measure of an individual's strengths and weaknesses; it only allows one to draw conclusions about the average behavior of the group. In addition, the percentages of time spent in each work category are only estimates of the true answers and must be treated as such.

3. WS does not provide the researcher with any measure of the quality of the work performed; only of the time spent doing it.

4. If more than one observer is involved, interobserver differences in attention to fundamental details of the WS method may invalidate the study's results. Specifically, one should be careful to insure (1) that each observer makes instantaneous observations at the prearranged times, (2) that the work categories are sufficiently well described to insure that incorrect classifications are not made, (3) that the control charts for each of the observers are relatively consistent, and (4) that enough samples are collected to reach the desired accuracy in the final estimates.

5. Although it is not likely, due to the large number of observations made, workers may be able to change their work-patterns upon sight of the observer. This so-called "Hawthorne effect"[2] has been well-documented.

6. The statistical theory behind the study may be difficult for workers and/or management to comprehend.

---

[2] Named after experiments conducted at the Hawthorne Works of the Western Electric Company from 1927–1932 in which workers productivity increased in response to both positive and negative changes in working conditions. The investigators concluded that the increased attention brought on by the experimental setup motivated the workers to improve their performance regardless of working conditions [17,30].

7. A WS study requires trained observers to make inferences concerning cognitive processes (i.e., what was the worker actually thinking about). Such observers are expensive to train.

Advantages of Work Sampling

1. WS is generally far less expensive to perform than the-motion analyses and provides a quantitative estimate of the amount of time spent in each category rather than a subjective estimate such as the one obtained from a questionnaire.

2. One observer can perform WS studies of different workers and/or different tasks as opposed to a one-to-one (observer/worker) ratio in TM analyses.

3. Observations can be made over an extended time period which decreases time effects of cyclic (i.e., day-to-day, week-to-week, or even seasonal) variations.

4. The chance of obtaining skewed results due to the Hawthorne Effect is reduced in a WS study since no single worker is under direct, continuous observation for extended time periods, and the total number of observations taken makes it extremely difficult for an entire group of workers to manipulate the outcome.

5. The study can be interrupted at any time with a minimal affect on the results.

6. A WS study is not as tedious to perform on the part of the observer as a conventional time-motion analysis [32], because the observer is constantly moving around and looking at different workers. In addition, since the observations are spread out, it is quite possible that the observer can do at least a portion of his or her job.

Conclusions

This chapter has briefly reviewed several work-evaluation techniques and attempted to describe in detail the concepts behind work sampling, a technique based on sampling theory. As described throughout this chapter, work sampling studies are not without problems. Even the most thorough study can be severely compromised by the seemingly endless random occurrences that are the rule rather than the exception in health care. One should not be dissuaded for these reasons, because the potential information gained is critical in determining the future role of computers in health care.

Acknowledgments. A preliminary report of this study appeared in: M.E. Frisse, ed., *Proceedings of the 16th Annual Symposium on Computer Applications in Medical Care*, 1992 in Baltimore MD, USA. This work was supported in part by grants from the National Library of Medicine R29 LM05284 and the Whitaker Foundation.

References

[1] N.W. Matheson and J.A.D. Cooper, Academic information in the health sciences center: Roles for the library and information management, Journal of Medical Education 57 (1982) 1–93.

[2] R.T. West, The National Library of Medicine's IAIMS grant program: Experiences and futures, Journal of American Sco Info Sci 39 (1988) 142–145

[3] W.W. Stead, W.P. Bird, R.M. Califf, et al., IAIMS: Transition from model testing to implementation, MD Computing (1993) (in press).

[4] W.W. Stead, W. Baker, T.R. Harris, T.M. Hodges, and D.F. Sittig, A fast track to IAIMS: The Vanderbilt University strategy, in: M.E. Frisse, editor, *Proceedings 16th Symp Comp Appl Med Care* 16 (1992), pp. 527–531.

[5] R.A. Miller, R. Patril, J.A. Mitchell, et al., Preparing a medical informatics research grant proposal: General principles, Comp Biomed Res 22 (1989) 92–101.

[6] G. Hendrickson and C.T. Kovner, Effects of computers on nursing resource use: Do computers save nurses time? Comp Nurs 8 (1990) 16–22.

[7] R.S. Disk and E.B. Steen, edtiors, *The Computer-based Patient Record* (National Academy Press, Washington, DC, 1991).

[8] P.L. Miller and D.F. Sittig, The evaluation of clinical decision support systems: What is necessary vs. What is interesting, Med Inform 15 (1990) 185–190.

[9] L.H.C. Tippett, Statistical methods in textile research. Uses of the binomial and Poisson distributions: A snap reading method of making time studies of machines and operatives in factory surveys, J Textile Inst Trans 26 (1935) 51–55.

[10] F.G. Abdellah and E. Levine, Work-sampling applied to the study of nursing personnel, Nurs Res 3 (1954) 11–16.

[11] L.E. Garrett, W.E. Hammond, and W.W. Stead, The effects of computerized medical records on provider efficiency and quality of care, Meth Inform Med 25 (1986) 151–157.

[12] S. Minda, *Manual and Computer Recorded Nursing Assessment: A Comparison of Time Required and the Number of Observations Made* (master's thesis), Department of Nursing, Duke University School of Nursing, Durham NC (1990).

[13] R.D. Andrews and R.M. Gardner, Portable computers used for respiratory care charting, Int J Clin Monit Comp 5 (1988) 45–51.

[14] A.R. Feinstein, Scientific standards in epidemiologic studies of the menace of daily life, Science 242 (1988) 1257–1263.

[15] R.D. Andrews, R.M. Gardner, S.M. Metcalf, and D. Simmons, Computer charting: An evaluation of a respiratory care computer system, Resp Care 30 (1985) 695–707.

[16] A. Field, Activity sampling, in: *Method Study* London, (Cassell, 1969), chapter 13.

[17] R.M. Barnes, *Motion and Time Study: Design and Measurement of Work*, 6th ed. (Wiley, New York, 1968), chapter 32.

[18] D.S. Johnson, M. Burkes, D.F. Sittig, D. Hinson, and T.A. Pryor, Evaluation of the effects of computerized nurse charting, in: W.W. Stead, *Proceedings 11th Symp Comp Appl Med Care*, Washington DC (1987), pp. 363–367.

[19] D.W. Karger and F.H. Bayha, *Engineered Work Measurement*, 2nd ed. (Industrial Press, New York, 1966).

[20] N.A. Nickman, R.M. Guerrero, and J.N. Bair, Self-reported work-sampling methods for evaluating pharmaceutical services, Am J Hosp Pharm 47 (1990) 1611–1617.

[21] K.E. Bradshaw, D.F. Sittig, R.M. Gardner, T.A. Pryor, and M. Budd, Computer-based data entry for nurses in the ICU, MD Computing 6 (1989) 274–280.

[22] B.W. Niebel, *Motion and Time Study* (Richard D. Irwin, Homewood, IL, 1967).

[23] H. Davis, A mathematical evaluation of a work sampling technique, Nav Res Log Quart 2 (1955) 111–117.

[24] T.W. Kohout, R.L. Broekemeier, and C.E. Daniels, Work-sampling evaluation of an upgraded outpatient pharmacy computer system, Am J Hosp Pharm 40 (1983) 606–608.

[25] J.A. Larkin, *Work study* (McGraw-Hill, New York, 1969).

[26] X. Wang, *The Design, Development, Implementation, and Evaluation of a Computerized Anesthesia Charting System* (PhD dissertation), Department of Medical Informatics, University of Utah, Salt Lake City (1990).

[27] J.J. Mamlin and D.H. Baker, Combined time-motion and work-sampling study in general medicine clinic, Med Care 11 (1973) 449–456.

[28] K.L. Rascati, C.L. Kimberlin, P.T. Foley, and R.B. Williams, Multidimensional work sampling to evaluate the effects of computerization in an outpatient pharmacy, Am J Hosp Pharm 44 (1987) 2060–2067.

[29] S.H. Tolbert and A.E. Pertuz, Study show how computerization affects nursing activities in ICU, Nursing 51 (1977) 79–84.

[30] E. Mayo, *The Human Problems of an Industrial Civilization* (Viking Press, New York, 1960), pp. 65–67.

[31] M.C. Budd, J. Blaufuss, and S. Harada, Nursing: A revenue center not a cost center, Comp Healthcare (1988) Nov. 24–26.

[32] H.E. Payson, E.C. Gaenslen, and F.L. Stargardter, Time study of an internship on a university medical service, New England Journal of Medicine 264 (1961) 439–443.

Appendix

Definitions of categories used in a work-sampling study designed to measure the impact of computer-based nurse charting on nursing activities (modified from Bradshaw et al., 1989):

Patient care: anything done to the patient by the nurse, e.g. giving medications, turning the patient, starting intravenous medications, i.e., inserting catheter and adjusting drip rate (distinguished from the preparation of the fluid mixture which would be obtaining supplies), fixing bandages, and bathing the patient. Also includes watching the hemodynamic monitors at the central nursing station.

Charting: any activities involving the charting of nursing actions, whether on paper or by computer. Also includes correcting and looking for errors in the chart, as well as looking for the chart itself, and calling-out computer reports.

Oral communication: talking to the patient, or with someone about a patient or other work-related subjects. Talking with physicians, other nurses, technicians, patient's family, laboratories, blood bank, clerks, etc.

Obtaining supplies: going to get anything for a patient within or outside of the unit. Includes obtaining intravenous fluids or medications, preparing medications, getting pillows, bandages, equipment needed for a procedure, or any other supplies needed for patient care.

Planning nursing care: filling out the nursing care plan at a computer terminal (distinguished from time spent performing computer-based chart or data review).

Reporting: time spent giving report at the end of the shift to the next nurse coming on duty. Note: at this time there are approximately twice as many nurses working as there are during the shift; therefore, twice as many observations must be made.

Transferring patients: filling out forms for the transfer of a patient perhaps to the step-down unit or other units within the hospital (distinguished from the actual transport of the patient, for example to surgery or x-ray, which would be considered patient care).

Data review: reviewing data at a computer terminal, e.g., reviewing laboratory test results (distinguished from time spent performing computer-based charting or making nursing-care plans).

Medication scheduling: checking the computer-generated drug schedule against that of the Kardex file.

Non-nursing activities—other: activities unrelated to patient care, such as making personal telephone calls, socializing, taking breaks, etc.

8
Evaluation in Health Informatics: Social Network Analysis

James G. Anderson

Introduction: The Social Network Perspective

Social network analysis comprises a set of research methods that can be used to analyze the relationships among entities such as people, departments, and organizations. The purpose of the analysis is to discover patterns of relationships that affect both individual and organizational attitudes and behavior such as the adoption, discussion, and use of new medical informatics applications. This chapter presents an introduction to the concepts and methods of social network analysis. Several applications to health informatics are described.

Attitudes toward information technology, its adoption and use in healthcare settings are strongly influenced by the pattern of relationships among the individuals who make up the organization [1–5]. Many different occupational groups interact in providing healthcare. These groups include physicians, nurses, administrators, medical technicians, clerical workers, and patients. These groups belong to different professional and organizational groups and different departments. Yet they are interdependent and the provision of healthcare requires cooperation and coordination [6]. Interpersonal interactions among the members of these groups and between groups are essential in sharing information and resources in order to deliver health services. In addition, communication among professionals strongly affects the rate of adoption and diffusion of new information technology [1,2].

Furthermore, electronic medical record systems (EMRs), telemedicine systems and the Internet, where geographically dispersed professionals share a common database or consult and collaborate with one another, create "virtual" departments or organizations whose boundaries are defined by tasks and information flow rather than traditional organizational departments or occupations. Frequently, the introduction of an electronic medical record with its common database alters policies, procedure, work assignments, and interactions among individuals and occupational groups [7].

Traditionally evaluation of information technology has focused on technical aspects of the system and on individual attitudes, work roles, and utilization. However, an understanding of the effects of the introduction of information technology into organizational settings requires an approach that considers patterns of relationships among members of the organization [8,9]. Social network analysis can be used to identify different patterns of relationships within and between occupational groups, departments, and organizations; and to analyze the effects that these patterns have on individual member's attitudes, behavior, and performance [10]. This approach is based on the premise that individuals are influenced by direct and indirect exposure to other person's attitudes and behavior; by access to resources through the network; and by the individual's location in the interpersonal network. For example, studies of the diffusion of innovations have found that individuals who have extensive relations with other professional are more likely to adopt an innovation sooner. In contrast, individuals with fewer relations with other professionals are slower to adopt new approaches [11].

Social Network Analysis

Social network analysis is the study of the pattern of relations among a set of people, departments, organizations, and so on. For example, physicians consult with one another in diagnosing a patient's illness. They interact with nurses, pharmacists, and medical technicians in providing patient care. Physicians, clinics, hospitals, medical laboratories, home care agencies, and insurance companies may all share a common electronic medical record system.

Network analyses may take many forms depending on the purpose of the evaluation. There are four elements of an evaluation design, namely, the units that comprise the network, the type of relations among the units, the properties of the relation, and the level of analysis [12,13].

The units to be studied comprise the nodes of the network. The units or nodes of the network may represent individual; professional or occupational groups, for example, physicians, nurses, technicians; hospital departments; organizations that make up an integrated delivery system; or larger units such as state Medicaid programs.

The type of relation among the units may vary. Frequently, the relation involves communication (i.e., face-to-face, via telephone or the Internet). Other types of relations may involve authority or the exchange of resources or money. Properties of the relations among units also may be of interest. Some of these properties are frequency of interaction, strength of the relation, and whether the relation is reciprocal or multiplex (i.e., involves two or more types of relations).

There are several levels at which the network can be analyzed. One level involves ego networks. Each individual unit or node is involved in a network that comprises all other units with which it has relations and the relations among these units. At another level, a dyad, a pair of units, or a triad, three units, can be investigated. In these networks, relations between or among the units under investigation may be direct or indirect via other units in the network. Most studies involve an analysis of the entire network or system.

Network analysis requires the collection of relational, positional, or spatial data. Usually attributes of individual units are collected as well. Once collected, the relational data are organized into a matrix. Rows and columns represent individuals, departments, or organizations. Within each cell of the matrix, numbers are used to represent the existence or absence of a direct relation or the frequency or strength of the relation. The network also is displayed in graphical form.

Data for a network analysis may be collected by a variety of methods. Members of the organization under study can be provided with a roster of names and asked to indicate the frequency, strength, or importance of their relations with each person. They can be asked to list those with whom they interact. Direct observation by an investigator can also be used to identify relations among individuals.

Information systems also permit the construction of networks involving users. Computers keep track of the number, length, and timing of e-mail messages that are sent among system users [14,15]. Logs are kept of individuals who access electronic patient records. System files of hospital information systems can be used to identify attending and consulting physicians for each patient, and frequency and types of usage of the information system [16].

Network analysis can provide descriptive and inferential information. For example, the strength and direction of relations among units may be of interest. The analysis can be used to identify individual roles in the network such as leaders and isolates. Characteristics of the network as a whole may be important such as density of relations and the cohesiveness of the network. In the next section several applications of social network analysis will be described.

Applications to Health Informatics

Networks and Use of a Hospital Information System

The process by which information technology diffuses in medical settings is poorly understood. The objectives of this study were to identify the structure of the referral and consultation networks that link 24 physicians in a group practice; and to study the effect of the physicians' location in the network on their use of the hospital information system (HIS) [17]. The study site was a large private teaching hospital that had implemented the TDS HC 4000 system. Patient records were accessible by remote terminals throughout the hospital. The system provided communication among hospital services, physicians, nursing services, the medical laboratory, and the hospital pharmacy. Physicians could directly enter medical orders into the HIS and could retrieve patient information.

A questionnaire was used to collect relational data from the 24 physicians. Each physician was asked to indicate which of the other physicians in the group they referred patients to, consulted with, discussed professional matters with, and took on-call coverage for. Self-reported measures of HIS usage were also obtained. A questionnaire was developed to obtain information on physician attitudes toward medical computer applications. Individual attributes measured included the physician's age, speciality, board certification, number of hospital admissions during the past 6 months, involvement in professional activities, and participation in graduate medical education.

Based on the relational data, a number of indices were created for subgroups of physicians and for individual physicians. Densities of relations within subgroups of physicians and between groups were computed. Density measures the proportion of actual relations among group members compared to all possible relations. This measure can range from 0 to 1. Second, a measure of centrality that ranges from 0 to 1 was computed for each group of physicians. This measure describes the degree to which information and resources in the group are dispersed throughout the group or centered on a few individual physicians. A third measure was calculated to describe each physician's role in the network. Physicians were classified as sending, relaying or receiving patients or information based on the ratio of interactions the physician initiated compared to those that were initiated by other physicians. A measure of multiplexity was calculated as the proportion of group members who had more than one type of relation with other physicians in the group. Finally, for each physician, a measure of prestige was calculated ranging from 0, if no one consulted the physician, to 1, if everyone in the group consulted the physician.

The relational data were analyzed by hierarchical clustering and blockmodel analysis [18]. This analysis identified four subgroups of physicians who had similar patterns of referrals, consultations, discussion, and on-call coverage. The results are shown in Figures 8.1 and 8.2.

Figure 8.1 shows the four subgroups of physicians that were identified by the cluster analysis. In Figure 8.2, a circle or a line linking groups indicates that the density of relations among physicians in a group or between groups of physicians is greater than the density of relations in the total network. The results are similar to those of other studies of communication among members of professional groups. Professionals are generally organized around a core of influential individuals who direct and control the flow of information and resources. The results of the current analysis reveal a similar pattern. Physicians in Group 1 control the referral of patients in the network. They consult with and refer patients to physicians in all three of the other subgroups. In a sense, they act as gatekeepers for the group practice.

Figure 8.3 shows the shared attributes and network or relational characteristics of physicians who make up the four subgroups. Physicians in Group

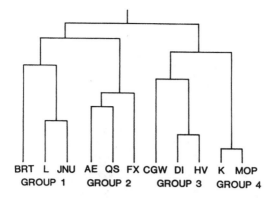

FIGURE 8.1. Clustering of 24 physicians in a group practice. (Reprinted with permission from JG Anderson and SJ Jay. Computers and clinical judgment: the role of physician networks. *Soc Sci Med* 20(10) 1985, 969–979.)

l, who act as gatekeepers, are older and more professionally active than the other physicians. They are central in the referral and consultation networks as evidenced by their scores on the indices of centrality, multiplexity, and role in the network. In general, they initiate 1.5 times as many referrals, consultations and discussions with other physicians as they receive from others. The physicians in Group 1 began using the HIS soon after it was implemented. Also, they are the heaviest users of the system in practice. They directly entered 45% of their own medical orders over a 6-day period.

A Network Intervention

The benefits of direct computer-based physician order entry are significant. However, many attempts to implement such systems have met with limited

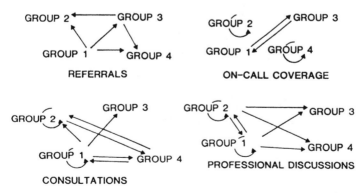

FIGURE 8.2. Professional relations among groups of physicians. (Reprinted with permission from JG Anderson and SJ Jay. Computers and clinical judgment: the role of physician networks. *Soc Sci Med* 20(10) 1985, 969–979.)

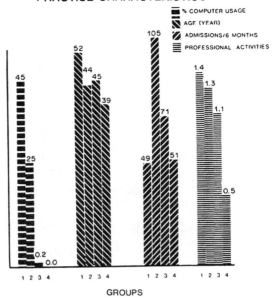

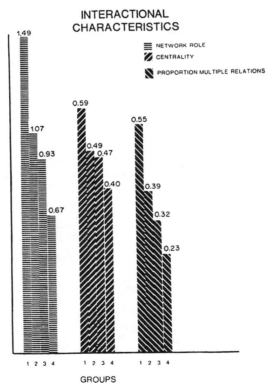

FIGURE 8.3. Characteristics of four groups of physicians. (Reprinted with permission from JG Anderson and SJ Jay. Computers and clinical judgment: the role of physician networks. *Soc Sci Med* 20(10) 1985, 969–979.)

success. The primary objectives of this research was to design, implement, and evaluate an intervention to increase direct order entry into a HIS by physicians' and, secondly, to increase overall physician use of the HIS [16,19]. The study was conducted in the same private teaching hospital described above. The hospital information system permits physicians and other personnel to enter and retrieve patient data at computer terminals through the hospital. Data can be entered with screens that are provided by the vendor of the hospital information system. As an alternative, physicians can create personal and departmental order sets for order entry. These order sets are tailored to the specific procedures that physicians frequently order for their patients. It was hypothesized that if physicians could be encouraged to develop personal order sets, they would use them more frequently for direct order entry and, subsequently, would increase their use of the HIS.

A quasi-experimental design was used. The following hospital services were selected as the experimental group: cardiovascular disease, general surgery, obstetrics and gynecology, and orthopedic surgery. Based on studies of the diffusion of innovations, we initiated an experimental program on these services utilizing physicians identified as educationally influential among their peers. The program was designed to increase the use of the hospital information system through the use of personal and departmental order sets for medical order entry. Physicians on 10 other hospital services were assigned to the control group. Data were collected from 109 and 231 physicians on the experimental and control services, respectively.

Influential physicians were identified on each experimental service by constructing a consultation network such as the one shown in Figure 8.4 for general surgery. Physicians in Group 3 are consulted by physicians in all of the other groups. Consequently, several physicians in this group were recruited to participate in this study to increase the use of personal order sets for direct physician order entry. All of the physicians who were contacted agreed to participate in the study.

At individual meetings with project staff, influential physicians were provided with data that indicated their overall use of the hospital information system as well as their use of personal order sets for order entry. Individual physician profiles were compared to profiles for physicians on their service and to the total hospital medical staff. During the meeting, the project staff discussed with the physician the advantage of using personal order sets to enter medical orders into the hospital information system. Following these meetings, physicians continued their normal practice on their hospital services. A second meeting was held with the educationally influential physicians 6 months later. They were provided with data on order entry times and error rates using the two modes of order entry (i.e., regular hospital information system pathways and personal order sets).

In order to determine whether increased use of personal order sets and overall use of the HIS occurred on the experimental and control services, data were collected before and 6 months and 12 months after the intervention. These data included use of personal and departmental order sets;

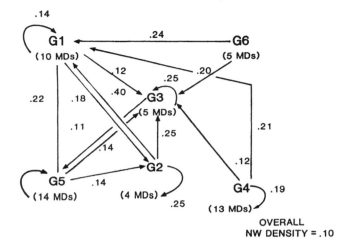

FIGURE 8.4. Groups of physicians with similar consultation patterns on general surgery. (Reprinted with permission from JG Anderson, SJ Jay, H Schweer, M Anderson and D Kassing. Physician communication networks and the adoption and utilization of computer applications in medicine. In: JG Anderson, SJ Jay (eds.), *Use and Impact of Computers in Clinical Medicine* (Springer, New York, 1987), pp. 185–199.)

and frequency of use of the HIS to retrieve patient lists, to access and print laboratory test results, and to access and enter medical orders.

A multivariate analysis of variance with repeated measures was performed on the use of personal order sets by physicians, nurses, and unit secretaries to enter medical orders into the HIS. The mean number of orders entered using personal order sets at three points in time is shown in Figure 8.5. The results of the analysis of variance indicate significant differences between the experimental and control groups ($F1,338 = 15.58, p < 0.000$) and between persons entering the orders ($F1,338 = 10.78, p < 0.000$). Significantly more orders were entered on the experimental services using personal order sets. Also, unit secretaries entered significantly more orders using personal order sets than physicians or nurses. Moreover, the group by time interaction was significant ($F1,338 = 5.80, p < 0.003$). The use of personal order sets for medical order entry on the experimental services increased significantly over the 12 month period.

Significant changes were observed on the experimental services as a result of the network intervention. The use of personal order sets for medical order entry into the HIS significantly increased. In fact, the effect of the educationally influential physicians extended beyond the other physicians on the service. Use of personal order sets for order entry also increased among nurses and unit secretaries on the experimental units.

Computers in the Consulting Room

Computer-based record systems have been rapidly introduced into family practice in the UK. In contrast, only about 1% of physicians in the United

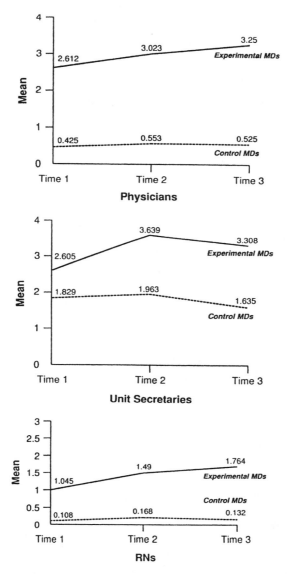

Figure 8.5. Mean number of medical orders entered into the HIS using personal order sets. (Reprinted with permission from JG Anderson, SJ Jay, J Perry, and MM Anderson. Diffusion of computer applications among physicians: a quasi-experimental study. *Clin. Soc. Rev.* 8 (1990) 116–127.)

State uses computer-based patient records [20,21]. This study evaluated clinician reactions to the introduction a computer-based health appraisal system, CompuHx, into the examining rooms at the Department of Preventive Medicine at Kaiser-Permanente, San Diego [22,23]. Initially five of the 22 nurse practitioners and physician assistants who perform examinations began using the system in practice. One user took maternity leave during the study and was excluded from the analysis. The department provides a complete history and physical examination for 50,000 HMO members each year. The CompuHx system is designed to assist practitioners in gathering diagnostic information. A computer database is created during a patient visit containing the patient's history and laboratory results. During the examination, the system assists the practitioner in clarifying items on the patient questionnaire and findings during the physical examination. At the end of the visit, the system produces a summary of the findings.

As part of a social network analysis, examiners were provided with a list of all nurse practitioners and physician assistants, doctors, data processing clerks, chart room clerks, the radiology department, the medical laboratory, and so on. They were asked to indicate the frequency with which they communicated with each person or occupational group while performing their jobs. The frequency of interaction was coded as follows: 0 = never, 1 = once a month, 2 = several times a month, 3 = once a week, 4 = several times a week, 5 = once a day, 6 = several times a day. For the analysis, frequencies of communication of CompuHx users and nonusers with other personnel in the department and with other departments were computed. Also, densities of communication for CompuHx users and nonusers were computed.

Figure 8.6 shows the average frequency of communication for users and nonusers with other examiners and physicians. CompuHx users reported that they communicated several times a week with one another and with the medical director while examining patients. They communicated with other physicians about once a week on average and with nonusers of the system only several times a month. Communication among nonusers of

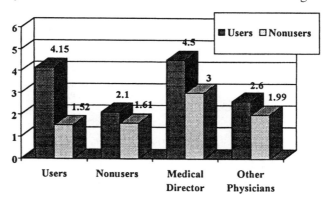

FIGURE 8.6. Frequency of communication with other examiners and physicians. (Score: 0 = no contact to 6 = several times a day.)

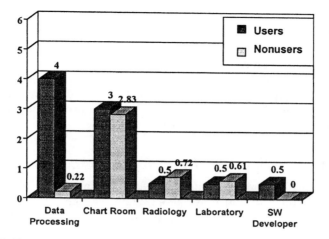

FIGURE 8.7. Frequency of communication with other department staff. (Score: 0 = no contact to 6 = several times a day.)

CompuHx and between nonusers and others in the department was much less frequent.

Figure 8.7 shows the frequency of communication with other department staff. CompuHx users communicated with staff in the data processing department several times a week on average. Nonusers rarely communicated with this department. Communication with the other departments was about the same for both users and nonusers of the system.

Figure 8.8 illustrates the communication patterns for users and nonusers of the CompuHx system. Densities of communication within and between groups are shown. In comparison to nonusers, CompuHx users have higher densities of communication with one another and with nonusers of the system, the medical director, other physicians in the department, and other departments in general.

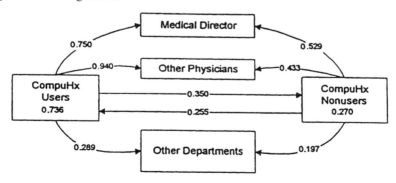

FIGURE 8.8. Network density of CompuHx users and nonusers. (Reprinted with permission from CE Ayding, JG Anderson, PN Rosen, VJ Felitti and HC Weng. Computer in the consulting room: A case study of clinician and patient perspectives. *Healthcare Manag. Sci.* 1 (1988) 61–74.)

The study found that nurse practitioners and physician assistants who used the CompuHx system in their practice communicated more frequently with one another and with other staff who could assist them in performing their professional duties. These communication patterns may have important implications for quality of care and productivity of the department. Other studies indicate that the more co-workers an individual worker communicates with about a new technology, the more productive he or she is likely to be in using the system [24–26].

Computer-Mediated Collaborative Design

The importance of multi-institutional collaboration in medical informatics is increasing. Collaboration allows geographically dispersed institutions and investigators to share resources, to pool expertise, and to standardize tools and methods [27]. Developments in information technology such as the Internet make collaboration at a distance feasible. This study evaluated the InterMed Collaboratory, an Internet-based medical informatics project that involved four institutions [28]. The purpose of the project is to further the development and sharing of software, data sets, procedures, and tools that support the development of new biomedical and clinical applications.

A sociometric analysis was undertaken to measure patterns of interaction among participants in the project [29]. E-mail communication among participants over a 96-week period was analyzed. In Figures 8.9 and 8.10

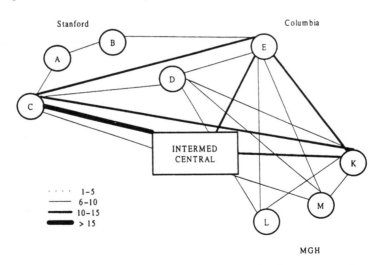

FIGURE 8.9. Sociometric graph of e-mail communication between members of the InterMed group in January and February 1995. (Reprinted with permission from VL Patel, DR Kaufman, VG Allen, EH Shortliffe, JJ Cimino, and RA Greenes. Toward a framework for computer-mediated collaborative design in medical informatics. *Methods Inform. Med.* 38 (1999) 158–176.)

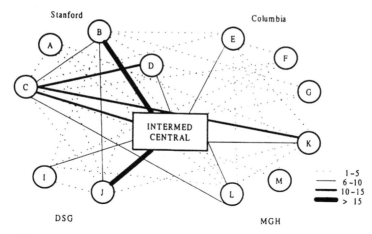

FIGURE 8.10. Sociometric graph of e-mail communication between members of the InterMed group in January and February 1996. (Reprinted with permission from VL Patel, DR Kaufman, VG Allen, EH Shortliffe, JJ Cimino and RA Greenes. Toward a framework for computer-mediated collaborative design in medical informatics. *Methods Inform Med.* 38 (1999) 158–176.)

each node represents a participant from one of four principal sites. InterMed Central is the e-mail distribution list for the entire project.

A comparison of the two networks indicates that participation in the project and communication among participants increased over time. E-mail activity related to guideline development during January and February 1995 was limited. During this period, there were only 45 messages sent between eight participants from three sites. Two individuals, C and E, communicated frequently with the list serve and with individuals at two of the other sites. No members of the DSG group participated during this period.

This reflected a period during which the collaboratory was working on many different activities including creating a common vocabulary and designing clinical guidelines that could be accessed over the Internet. In general, there was a lack of consensus on the goals of the InterMed Collaboratory. Individual roles and tasks were not clearly delineated and areas of focus were unspecified.

Figure 8.10 depicts the communication patterns among participants during April 1996. By this time, the number of participants in the project and the volume of communication had doubled. Eleven active participants generated a total of 107 e-mail messages during this four-week period. Many more of the participants communicated with the list serve at InterMed Central. Individuals B and J appear to have provided leadership on projects underway at this time. Group activities involved intense efforts to complete guideline models and data sets. The distribution of roles and tasks were clearer and more efficient that at the outset of the project.

The results of the analysis of e-mail communication support the findings that the computer-mediated collaboratory design process led to the evolution and refinement of project goals. Over time there was greater differentiation and clarification of individual roles. This led to greater participation from all of the sites involved in the InterMed collaboratory.

Discussion

This chapter demonstrates how social network analysis can be used in evaluating responses to and the impact of the introduction of medical informatics applications into practice settings. The adoption, diffusion and use of information technology in practice settings are influenced by characteristics of the organization's structure and by relationships among individuals and units that make up the organization. The distinguishing characteristic of this approach is that it uses information about relations between individuals and organizational units and their attributes to understand individual and organizational behavior.

From this perspective, the practice setting is conceptualized as a structure of relations among healthcare providers, departments, or organizations. The behavior of providers or units making up the network is explained in terms of the structure of relations in which the behavior occurs. Analyses of these social networks can be used to identify influential individuals or opinion leaders who are critical in the introduction of new information technology. As demonstrated by one application, these influential individuals can be enlisted in planning and implementing new information technology. Evaluation of social networks also helps the investigator to better understand the dynamics of the introduction of new systems or applications into practice settings. In one example, nurse practitioners and physician assistants responded to the introduction of computers into the examining rooms by intensifying their communication with one another and with other practitioners and departments. In a second application, social network analysis indicated that communication patterns among participants in a multi-institutional collaborative project increased significantly over time. The analysis identified individuals who provided leadership on projects.

Summary

Social network analysis can be used to analyze relationships among healthcare providers, departments within healthcare organizations and other organizations. Information obtained using this evaluative methodology can be used to identify influential individuals or opinion leaders who are critical to the successful implementation of medical informatics applications. This methodology can also be used to better understand changes in communication patterns or other interactions over time. Several examples that illustrate this evaluation methodology are presented.

Acknowledgments. I wish to acknowledge the assistance of Marilyn Anderson with the preparation of this chapter.

References

[1] J.G. Anderson and S.J. Jay, Physician utilization of computers: a network analysis of the diffusion process, in: L. Frederiksen, A. Riley, editors, *Computers, People and Productivity* (Haworth Press, New York, 1985), pp. 21–36.

[2] J.G. Anderson, S.J. Jay, H.M. Schweer, and M.M. Anderson, Diffusion and impact of computers in organizational settings: empirical findings from a hospital, in: G. Salvendy, S.O. Sauter, J.J. Hurrell Jr., editors, *Social, Ergonomic and Stress Aspects of Work with Computers* (Elsevier, New York, 1987), pp. 3–10.

[3] J. Kimberly and M. Evanisko, Organizational innovation: The influence of individual, organizational and contextual factors on hospital adoption of technological and administrative innovations, Acad. Manag. J. 24 (1981) 689–713.

[4] R.E. Rice, A. Grant, J. Schmitz, and J. Torobin, Individual and network influences on the adoption and perceived outcomes of electronic messaging, Soc. Networks 12 (1) (1990) 27–55.

[5] J.K. Stross and W.R. Harlan, The dissemination of New Medical Information, J. Am. Med. Assoc. 241 (1979) 2822–2824.

[6] C. Aydin and R.E. Rice, Bringing social worlds together: Information systems as catalysts for interdepartmental interactions, J. Health Soc. Behav. 33 (1992) 168–185.

[7] C.E. Aydin, Occupational adaptation to computerized medical information systems, J. Health Soc. Behav. 30 (1989) 163–179.

[8] J.G. Anderson and C.E. Aydin, Overview: Theoretical perspectives and methodologies for the evaluation of healthcare information systems, in: J.G. Anderson, C.E. Aydin, S.J. Jay, editors, *Evaluating Healthcare Information Systems: Methods and Applications* (Sage Publications, Thousand Oaks, CA), 1994, pp. 5–29.

[9] J.G. Anderson and C.E. Aydin, Evaluating the impact of healthcare information systems, Int. J. Technol. Assess. Healthcare 13 (1997) 380–393.

[10] R.E. Rice and J.G. Anderson, Social networks and healthcare information systems, in: J.G. Anderson, C.E. Aydin, S.J. Jay, editors, *Evaluating Healthcare Information Systems: Methods and Applications* (Sage Publications, Thousand Oaks, CA, 1994), pp. 135–163.

[11] T.W. Valente, *Network Models of the Diffusion of Innovations* (Hampton Press, Cresskill, NJ, 1995).

[12] D. Knoke and J. Kuklinski, *Network Analysis* (Sage, Newbury Park, CA, 1982).

[13] J. Scott, *Social Network Analysis: A Handbook* (Sage, Newbury Park, CA, 1991).

[14] R.E. Rice, Computer-mediated communication and organizational innovation, J. Commun. 37 (4) (1987) 65–94.

[15] R.E. Rice, Computer-mediated communication system network data: Theoretical concerns and empirical examples, Int. J. Man–Machine Stud. 30 (1990) 1–21.

[16] J.G. Anderson, S.J. Jay, H. Schweer, M. Anderson, and D. Kassing, Physician communication networks and the adoption and utilization of computer applications in medicine, in: J.G. Anderson, S.J. Jay, editors, *Use and Impact of Computers in Clinical Medicine* (Springer, New York, 1987), pp. 185–199.

[17] J.G. Anderson and S.J. Jay, Computers and clinical judgment: The role of physician networks, Soc. Sci. Med. 20 (10) (1985) 969–979.

[18] P. Arabie, S.A. Boorman, and P.R. Levitt, Constructing blockmodels: How and why, J. Math. Psychol. 17 (1978) 21.

[19] J.G. Anderson, S.J. Jay, J. Perry, and M.M. Anderson, Diffusion of computer applications among physicians: A quasi-experimental study, Clin. Soc. Rev. 8 (1990) 116–127.

[20] I.N. Purves, Implications for family practice record systems in the USA: Lessons from the United Kingdom, *Proceedings of the American Medical Informatics Association, Spring Congress*, St. Louis, MO (1993), p. 54.

[21] G.L. Solomon and M. Dechter, Are patients pleased with computer use in the examination room? J. Family Practice 41 (3) (1995) 241–244.

[22] J.G. Anderson, H.C. Weng, C.E. Aydin, P.N. Rosen, and V.J. Felitti, Computers in the examining room: Evaluating the social impact on practice patterns, in: J.N.D. Gupta, editors, *Association for Information Systems, Proceedings of the American Conference on Information Systems*, Indianapolis (August 15–17, 1997), Association for Information Systems, Georgia State University, Atlanta, pp. 909–911.

[23] C.E. Aydin, J.G. Anderson, P.N. Rosen, V.J. Felitti, and H.C. Weng, Computers in the consulting room: A case study of clinician and patient perspectives, Healthcare Manag. Sci. 1 (1998) 61–74.

[24] M.J. Papa, Communication network patterns and employee performance with new technology, Commun. Res. 17 (1990) 344–368.

[25] J.G. Baggs, S.A. Ryan, C.E. Phelps, J.F. Richeson, and J.E. Johnson, The association between interdisciplinary collaboration and patient outcomes in a medical intensive care unit, Heart Lung 21 (1) (1992) 18–24.

[26] A.B. Flood, The impact of organizational and managerial factors on the quality of car in healthcare organizations, Med. Care Rev. 51 (4) (1994) 381–428.

[27] R.T. Kouzes, J.D. Myers, and W.A. Wulf, Collaboratories: Doing science on the internet, IEEE Comp. 229 (1996) 40–46.

[28] E.H. Shortliffe, V.L. Patel, J.J. Cimino, G.O. Barnett, and R.A. Greenes, A study of collaboration among medical informatics laboratories, Artif. Intell. Med. 12 (1998) 97–123.

[29] V.L. Patel, D.R. Kaufman, V.G. Allen, E.H. Shortli, J.J. Cimino, and R.A. Greenes, Toward a framework for computer-mediated collaborative design in medical informatics, Methods Inform. Med. 38 (1999) 158–176.

9
Evaluation in Health Informatics: Computer Simulation

James G. Anderson

Introduction: Evaluation in Medical Informatics

The evaluation of complex medical informatics applications involves not only the information system, but also its impact on the organizational environment in which it is implemented. In instances where these applications cannot be evaluated with traditional experimental methods, computer simulation provides a flexible approach to evaluation. The construction of a computer simulation model involves the development of a model that represents important aspects of the system under evaluation. Once validated, the model can be used to study the effects of variation in system inputs, differences in initial conditions and changes in the structure of the system. Three examples are discussed, namely, a wide-area healthcare network, physician order entry into a hospital information system, and the use of an information system designed to prevent medical errors that lead to adverse drug events in hospitals.

Medical informatics applications are complex. They generally involve information technology that is implemented in a complex organizational setting. While technical aspects of these systems and user interfaces can be evaluated prior to implementation, systems that are implemented in practice settings, in most instances, cannot be evaluated with traditional experimental methods [1,2].

Moehr [3] discusses some of the problems encountered in evaluating medical informatics applications. First, the definition of the system is ambiguous. The evaluation usually involves not only the information system but also its impact on the organizational environment in which it is implemented. In fact, Moehr suggests that, in evaluating medical information systems, we are evaluating a dynamic process of adaptation of a new system and its environment rather than a technical system. Second, measurement methods and instruments for data collection and parameter estimation frequently need to be specifically developed for the evaluation. Third, the use of a randomized controlled design for the evaluation requires a level of specificity and objectivity that may vitiate many important objectives of the evaluation. Moreover, conventional evaluation methods frequently inadequately describe the dynamic properties of the system under investigation.

One approach to evaluation that provides flexibility is computer simulation. System simulation is defined ". . . as the technique of solving problems by following changes over time of a dynamic model of a system" [4]. The model that is used in the simulation is an abstraction of the real system that is being evaluated. Models are used to represent the system because they can be manipulated without disrupting the real healthcare setting. Once validated, they yield accurate estimates of the behavior of the real system. In many instances, the medical informatics system under study is too complex to be evaluated with traditional analytical techniques. Using simulation, an investigator can express ideas about the structure of a complex system and its processes in a precise way. Simulation can be used even in situations where the behavior of the system can be observed but the exact processes that generate the observed behavior are not fully understood. A computer model that represents important aspects of the system can be constructed. By running the model, we can simulate the dynamic behavior of the system over time. The effects of variations in system inputs, different initial conditions, and changes in the structure of the system can be observed and compared.

The Modeling Process

Systems Analysis

The development of a computer simulation model begins with the identification of the elements of the system and the functional relationships among the elements. A systems diagram is constructed to depict subsystems and components and relationships among them. The diagram should also show critical inputs and outputs; parameters of the system; any accumulations and exchanges or flows of resources, personnel, and information; and system performance measures. Relationships may be specified analytically, numerically, graphically, or logically. They also may vary over time.

Frequently applications of information technology that are to be evaluated are multifaceted. Subsystems and components are interrelated in complex ways and may be difficult to completely understand. Model development requires the investigator to abstract the important features of the system that generate the underlying processes. This requires familiarity with the system that is being evaluated and its expected performance.

Data Collection

Qualitative and quantitative information are required in order to adequately represent the system. Qualitative research methods are useful in defining the system under investigation. Quantitative data are necessary in order to estimate system parameters such as arrival and service distributions, conversion and processing rates, error rates, and resource levels. Data may be obtained from system logs and files, interviews, expert judgment, questionnaires, work sampling, and so on. Data may be cross-sectional and/or time series.

Model Formulation

In general, there are two types of simulation models, discrete-event and continuous. Swain [5] reviews 46 simulation software packages and provides a directory of vendors. The first two examples described in the next section are discrete-event models. The third example uses a continuous simulation model to describe the drug ordering and delivery system in a hospital.

Discrete-event models are made up of components or elements each of which perform a specific function [6]. The characteristic behavior of each element in the model is designed to be similar to the real behavior of the unit or operation that it represents in the real world. Systems are conceptualized as a network of connected components. Items flow through the network from one component to the next. Each component performs a function before the item can move on to the next component. Arrival rates, processing times and other characteristics of the process being modeled usually are random and follow a probability distribution. Each component has a finite capacity and may require resources to process an item. As a result, items may be held in a queue before being processed. Each input event to the system is processed as a discrete transaction.

For discrete-event models, the primary objective is to study the behavior of the system and to determine its capacity, the average time it takes to process items, to identify rate-limiting components, and to estimate costs. Simulation involves keeping track of where each item is in the process at any given time, moving items from component to component or from a queue to a component, and timing the process that occurs at each component. The results of a simulation are a set of statistics that describe the behavior of the simulated system over a given time period. A simulation run where a number of discrete inputs to the system are processed over time represents a sampling experiment.

Continuous simulation models are used when the system under investigation consists of a continuous flow of information, material, resources, or individuals. The system under investigation is characterized in terms of state variables and control variables [7]. State variables indicate the status of important characteristics of the system at each point in time. These variables include people, other resources, information, and so on. An example of a state variable is the cumulative number of medication orders that have been written on a hospital unit at any time during the simulation. Control variables are rates of change and update the value of state variables in each time period. An example of a control variable is the number of new medication orders written per time period. Components of the system interact with each other and may involve positive and negative feedback processes. Since many of these relationships are nonlinear, the system may exhibit complex, dynamic behavior over time.

The mathematical model that underlies the simulation usually consists of a set of differential or finite difference equations. Numerical solutions of the equations that make up the model allow investigators to construct and test models that cannot be solved analytically [8].

Model Validation

Once an initial model is constructed it should be validated to ensure that it adequately represents the system and underlying processes under investigation. One useful test of the model is to choose a model state variable with a known pattern of variation over some time period. The model is then run to see if it accurately generates the reference behavior. If the simulated behavior and the observed behavior of the system correspond well, it can be concluded that the computer model reasonably represents the system. If not, revisions are made until a valid model is developed [9,10]. The behavior of the model when it is manipulated frequently provides a much better understanding of the system. This process has been termed postulational modeling [11].

Sensitivity analyses also should be performed on the model. Frequently, the behavior of important outcome variables is relatively insensitive to large changes in many of the model's parameters. However, a few model parameters may be sensitive. A change in the value of these parameters may result in major changes in the behavior pattern exhibited by the system. It is not only important to accurately estimate these parameters but they may represent important means to change the performance of the overall system.

Advantages of Simulation

Simulation provides a powerful methodology that can be used to evaluate medical informatics applications. Modifications to the system or process improvements can be tested. Once a model is created, investigators can experiment with it by making changes and observing the effects of these changes on the system's behavior. Also, once the model is validated, it can be used to predict the system's future behavior. In this way, the investigator can realize many of the benefits of system experimentation without disrupting the practice setting in which the system is implemented. Moreover, the modeling process frequently raises important additional questions about the system and its behavior.

Applications

A Wide-Area Healthcare Network

A number of health informatics network projects utilize existing telephone networks. The University of Nebraska Medical Center provides an electronic mail service and access to databases for rural physicians [12]. Another project that was developed in conjunction with the University of Virginia Medical Center supports the exchange of electronic insurance claims data [13]. In Europe, the Advanced Informatics in Medicine (AIM) program is designed to support a wide range of health informatics applications [14].

This research project was undertaken to evaluate the behavior and cost of a wide-area healthcare network [15]. The system was a prototype message store and forward telephone system. Simulation studies were performed on two network topologies, namely, star and mesh. A discrete-event simulation model was constructed to represent a telecommunication network that would link general practitioners, specialists, municipal and regional hospitals, and private medical laboratories in the Canadian province of Saskatchewan. The model was used to simulate the distribution of laboratory test results by private, provincial, and hospital laboratories.

Two different network topologies, star and mesh, were analyzed. The networks consisted of eight subnetworks, one in each region of the province. Figures 9.1 and 9.2 depict the two types of networks. Each subnetwork has a hub or gateway that stores and forwards messages to the nodes. In the star network, a message sent from a node in a subnetwork to another node is stored at the hub until its destination node picks it up. If the destination node is in another subnetwork, the message must pass through another hub before it is delivered to a node. In the mesh network topology unlike the star topology, messages can be transmitted directly between two nodes in the same subnetwork without first passing through the hub. Messages transmitted from and to nodes in different subnetworks must pass through both hubs as previously described.

The simulation software used to model the two networks was written for an IBM compatible PC in Visual C++. Model parameters were based on measurements taken from a prototype network and a survey of two medical clinics. Communication among the gateways and between gateways and their nodes for a period of 24h were simulated. Table 9.1 shows the summary results of the simulation. Only messages containing data were simulated.

The two networks differ in performance when communication among the eight gateways or hubs is compared. Over three times as many connections are originated in the star network as in the mesh network. Gateway utilization of the mesh model is two-thirds of the utilization of the star model. Mean message transmission time in the mesh network, however, is greater. Four times as many messages are transmitted by the gateways to the nodes in the star topology as compared to the mesh topology. This reflects the fact that in the star network, messages between nodes in the same subnetwork need to be transmitted by the gateway.

The end-to-end network performance characteristics of the two topologies also differ. In the star network, only two-thirds as many connections

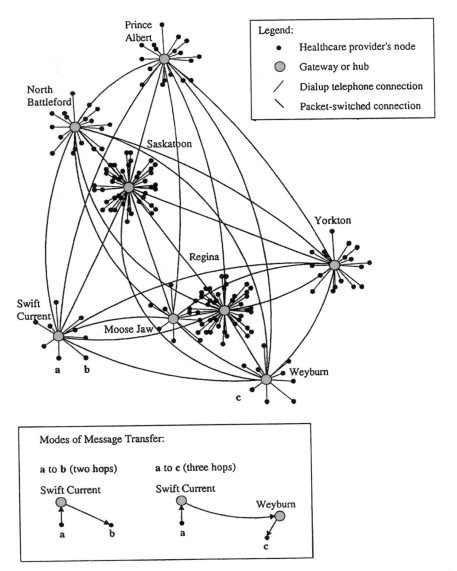

FIGURE 9.1. A schematic of a telecommunication network (star topology). (Reprinted with permission from JG McDaniel, Discrete-event simulation of a wide-area healthcare network. *JAMIA* 2(4) 1995, 220–237.)

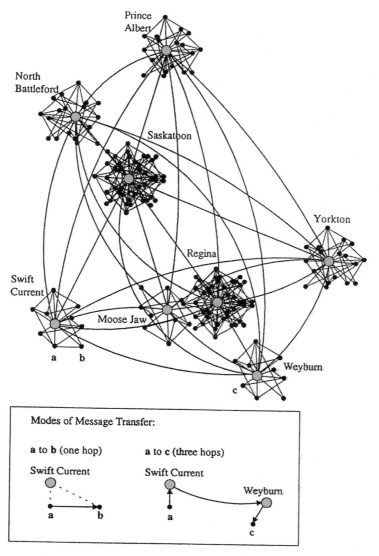

FIGURE 9.2. A schematic of a telecommunication network (mesh topology). (Reprinted with permission from JG McDaniel, Discrete-event simulation of a wide-area healthcare network. *JAMIA* 2(4) 1995, 220–237.)

are originated as compared to the mesh model. This reflects the fact that, in the star topology, nodes within the same subnetwork cannot connect directly to one another. The total connection time is 1.5 times greater in the star network because all messages must pass through subnetwork gateways. The mean message transmission time for the two network topologies is comparable.

TABLE 9.1. Performance statistics for the star and mesh networks.

Statistic	Star	Mesh
Number of connections originated between gateways	10,000	3,000
Percentage gateway port utlization	12	8
Mean data message transmission time(s)	8	10
Number of data messages transmitted by gateways to their respective nodes	80,000	20,000
Number of end-to-end connections between nodes	40,000	40,000
Total connection time at point of origin (h)	300	200
Mean end-to-end message transfer time (h)	1.24	1.23

Table 9.2 summarizes the telecommunication costs for the two network topologies. The estimated total monthly costs for the star network is $58,100 or about 40% of the cost of the mesh topology. This differential is also reflected in the costs per node for the star and mesh network topologies of $37 and $91, respectively. The higher costs of the mesh model are due to the fact that physicians are provided with dedicated telephone access under this network configuration.

The results of the simulation indicate that the telecommunication system in Saskatchewan could be operated for <$100 per node per month. It is estimated that the cost of the star network is about 40% of the cost of the mesh network. A typical message would cost between $0.03 and $0.08. Adding hospital discharge summaries and consultation reports to the messages transmitted by the system would double the data volume and increase the telecommunication costs by 60%. The simulation indicates that this would increase the mean end-to-end transfer time by less than 50%.

Physician Order Entry

There is evidence that direct order entry by physicians into computer-based medical information systems can improve the quality of care and reduce costs. Major advantages of physician order entry include process improvement, clinical decision support, reduction of errors, and improved communication within the healthcare setting [16]. Achieving physician order entry is difficult, however. Both social and logistical barriers to implementation exist [17].

The objective of this study was to develop a computer simulation model to represent the process through which medical orders are entered into a

TABLE 9.2. Telecommunication costs for the star and mesh networks.

Costs	Star	Mesh
Total monthly costs	$58,100	$145,100
Costs per node	$37	$91

hospital information system (HIS) [18]. The model was used to estimate the effects of increasing the percentage of medical orders that physicians enter directly into the HIS.

The study was performed in a large private teaching hospital. The hospital had implemented the TDS HC 4000 hospital information system. During hospitalization, all patient data are entered into the system creating an electronic medical record. Nursing units are equipped with between three to seven computer terminals linked to the HIS. Physicians, nurses, unit secretaries, and other authorized personnel can enter and retrieve patient information using these terminals.

In order to study use of the HIS, data were collected from two sources. Four weeks of patient data were extracted from the information system files. Also, a time and motion study was performed on order entry into the HIS. INSIGHT, a general-purpose discrete-event simulation language, was used to construct a simulation model of the order entry process. The model is shown in Figure 9.3.

At Stage A, a set of medical orders is created for entry into the HIS. Order entry arrival times are generated by a probability distribution. Attributes are assigned to the orders at Stage B. At Stage C, the physician can directly enter orders at a computer terminal, or orders can be written or verbally communicated. If the physician does not enter his or her orders into the HIS at Stage D, orders are entered by a unit secretary. Next, the orders are printed and filed on the nursing unit as well as in the appropriate ancillary services at Stage E. An RN on the nursing unit verifies the orders at Stage F by comparing the written or verbal orders to printed orders. If errors are detected, they are corrected and reentered in the HIS. Otherwise the patient's chart containing the medical orders is stored in the chart rack and the orders are executed at Stage G.

The model was first used to simulate the initial conditions on a hospital unit. Resources included 6 physicians, 3 physician assistants, 2 RNs, 2 unit secretaries, 7 computer terminals, and 2 printers. A total of 227 sets of orders were simulated over a 16-hours period. The initial simulation assumed that 89% of orders were written and that physicians only entered eight percent of the orders. It was also assumed that unit secretaries, physicians, and physician assistants used personal order sets to enter 29%, 50%, and 13% of the medical orders, respectively. Personal order sets are medical orders that are designed for a specific physician or group of physicians and stored on the HIS for use in entering orders. The alternative is to use generic order entry screens provided by the vendor. A second simulation assumed the same resources were available on a hospital unit. However, it was assumed that use of personal order sets for order entry by unit secretaries, physicians, and physician assistants increased to 50%, 75%, and 50%, respectively. Table 9.3 shows the results of the two simulations.

Under the initial conditions, it took 36.9 min on average to process a set of medical orders. Most of this time, 33.6 min, was due to the unavailability

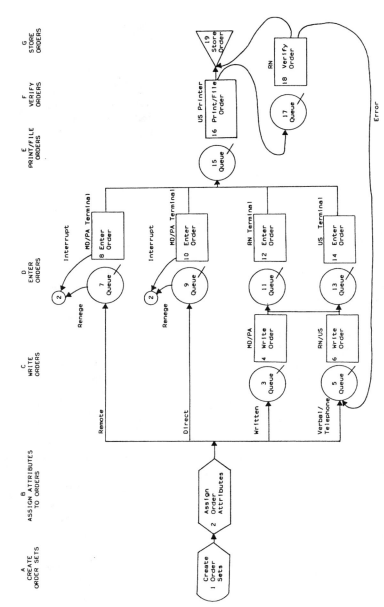

Figure 9.3. Computer simulation model of physician order entry into a hospital information system. (Reprinted with permission from JG Anderson, SJ Jay, SJ Clevenger, DR Kassing, J Perry and M Anderson, Physician utilization of a hospital information system: a computer simulation model. In: *Proceedings of the 12th Annual Symposium on Computer Applications in Medical Care* (1988), pp. 858–861.)

TABLE 9.3. Results of the computer simulation experiments.

Outcome variables	Initial conditions	Experimental conditions
Average time to implement order sets	36.9 min	33.2 min
Average order entry time		
MD	4.6 min	2.9 min
PA	2.6 min	1.6 min
US	1.8 min	1.4 min
Waiting time		
Order entry	12.4 min	9.9 min
Filing orders	3.9 min	3.3 min
Verification	17.3 min	17.3 min
Total	33.6 min	30.5 min
% Time involved with HIS		
MD	4.1%	3.5%
PA	0.5%	0.4%
US	21.9%	17.7%
RN	3.0%	3.0%
Terminal	9.8%	6.9%
Error rates (per 1000 orders)	40.9	33.0

of personnel or a computer terminal. Unit secretaries spent 21.9% of their time processing medical orders. The overall error rate in processing medical orders was estimated to be 40.9 errors per 1000 orders.

When personal order sets are utilized to a greater extent and physicians enter more of their own orders into the HIS, the average time to process orders is only reduced to 33.2 min on average. One reason for this small decrease in processing time is that the waiting time required for RNs to verify the orders remains the same, 17.3 min on average. This step in the process appears to be critical in reducing the time it takes to process medical orders. A significant effect of direct physician order entry and the use of personal order sets is a decrease in the number of errors made in processing medical orders. The model estimates almost a 20% decrease in errors.

This study demonstrates how computer simulation can be used to evaluate a critical process such as order entry into a hospital information system. The model can be used to identify critical steps in the process, such as the lack of sufficient personnel to verify medical orders. Simulation can also be used to explore the effects of changes in the process such as increasing direct physician order entry and the use of personal order sets. In the present example, the simulation suggests that implementation of these changes in the process would significantly reduce errors in order entry.

Prevention of Adverse Drug Events

It is estimated that adverse drug events (ADEs) occur in hospitals at the rate of 6.5 events per 100 hospital admissions [19,20]. The estimated extra length of hospital stay resulting from ADEs is 1.74 days which adds an additional $2012 to the cost of hospitalization on average [21]. The increasing availability of electronic medical record systems makes it possible to detect errors and to prevent ADEs. This study developed a computer simulation model to estimate the effects of various medical informatics applications designed to detect and prevent medical errors that result in ADEs [22].

The study was performed in the private teaching hospital described earlier. Ninety-one percent of medication orders were written by physicians and entered into the hospital information system by unit secretaries. In order to collect data on medication order errors, hospital pharmacists verified every medication order written on two medical-surgical units during the day and evening shifts for a 12-week period. A total of 6966 orders were reviewed for this study. Errors that were detected were classified by the stage of the order and by its severity. In general, physicians made 14% of the errors in writing prescriptions; 83% of the errors were made during transcription and entry into the HIS. The other 3% of errors were made in dispensing and administering medications on the units. Twenty-six percent of the errors could have resulted in serious toxic reactions or inadequate treatment resulting in ADEs if not detected.

A computer simulation model was constructed to model the drug ordering and delivery system using STELLA, a continuous simulation software package [7]. The model is shown in Figure 9.4. The simulation assumes that, on average, 4060 medication orders are written on 14 hospital medical-surgical units each week. Ambulatory clinics and the emergency room were excluded from the simulation. In the baseline simulation, the majority of orders are entered into the HIS by unit secretaries. Medications are dispensed in the central pharmacy and delivered to the nursing units where they are administered by RNs.

The model is used to simulate interventions that have been demonstrated in previous studies to decrease medication error rates. In the first intervention, the computer-based information system provides dosing information and parameters about drugs at the time orders are written. It is assumed that 50% of the physicians would use the system to obtain this information. The second intervention assumes that 50% of the medication orders are directly entered into the information system by physicians thus reducing transcription errors. The third and fourth interventions involve the implementation of a unit dosing system in the pharmacy and an automated medication dispensing system, respectively. The final intervention that was simulated assumes that system-wide changes are introduced that include the provision of information concerning each drug at the time orders are entered, direct order entry by physicians, and predictions of potential adverse drug events based on clinical data. Table 9.4 shows the results of the simulations.

The baseline simulation predicted over 8000 medication errors would be made over the course of 12 months. These errors would result in 2115 ADEs and incur 4654 additional days of hospitalization at a cost of over 5.5 million dollars. The model predicts that each of the individual interventions

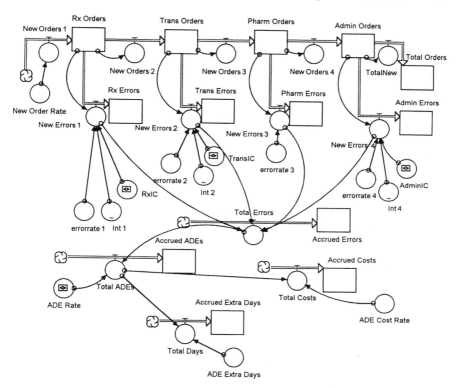

FIGURE 9.4. Computer simulation model of the drug ordering and delivery system of a hospital. (Reprinted with permission from JG Anderson, SJ Jay, M Anderson and TJ Hunt. Evaluating the potential effectiveness of using computerized information systems to prevent adverse drug events, in: *Proceedings of the 1997 AMIA Annual Fall Symposium* (1997), pp. 228–232.)

could reduce medication errors and resulting adverse drug events from 5% to 13%. However, implementation of all three applications could reduce ADEs by over 26%. This would have a substantial effect on excess hospital days and the resulting costs. The model estimates that additional hospital days related to ADEs could be reduced by 1226, saving the hospital $1.4 million in related costs annually.

TABLE 9.4. Estimated medication errors, adverse drug events, and associated extra costs and days of hospitalization.

Run	Orders	Medication errors	ADEs	Hospital days	Cost
Base line	195,392	8,136	2,115	4,654	5,489,752
Intervention 1	195,286	7,714	2,005	4,412	5,205,135
Intervention 2	195,245	7,099	1,845	4,061	4,790,148
Intervention 3	195,288	7,609	1,978	4,352	5,133,856
Intervention 4	195,196	5,993	1,558	3,428	4,044,135

The results of this study demonstrate the importance of viewing interventions designed to detect and prevent adverse drug events from a systems perspective. Errors occur at every stage of the drug ordering and delivery system. This study suggests that system-wide changes in the process are required to significantly reduce ADEs in hospitals. Medical informatics applications that focus solely on a single stage of the process may have a limited impact on the overall medication error and ADE rates.

Discussion

This chapter illustrates how computer simulation can be used to model and evaluate the performance of medical informatics applications. Three examples were discussed in detail. They include the implementation of a telecommunication system, direct physician order entry into a hospital information system, and the use of a hospital information system to detect and prevent medication errors that lead to ADEs. Two of the models used discrete-event simulation, while one used continuous simulation software.

The first example illustrates how simulation can be used before an information system is installed to evaluate the costs and performance of alternative system configurations. The second and third examples indicate how simulation can be used to explore potential improvements to an existing information system that might result in significant cost and error reductions. In all three instances, simulation provides a useful methodology where traditional evaluation methodologies are restricted or costly to employ.

The new generation of simulation software that incorporates graphical interfaces greatly facilitates exploratory studies of complex systems by freeing the investigator from dealing with complex mathematical expressions and programming languages. These computer models, through their use of graphics, provide a powerful means of communicating and exploring model assumptions, structure, and the resulting dynamic behavior of a system. This approach is applicable to a wide variety of medical informatics applications and can be used to better understand their complex dynamic behavior.

Summary

Computer simulation can be used to evaluate complex information systems in situations where traditional methodologies are difficult or too costly to employ. The modeling process is described followed by three examples where computer simulation has been utilized in planning for a wide-area healthcare network and in the use of a hospital information system to reduce costs and errors in order entry.

Acknowledgments. I wish to acknowledge the assistance of Marilyn Anderson with the preparation of this chapter.

References

[1] J.G. Anderson and C.E. Aydin, Overview: Theoretical perspectives and methodologies for the evaluation of healthcare information systems, in: J.G. Anderson, C.E. Aydin, S.J. Jay, editors, *Evaluating Healthcare Information Systems: Methods and Applications* (Sage Publications, Thousand Oaks, CA, 1994), pp. 1–29.

[2] J.G. Anderson and C.E. Aydin, Technology assessment of healthcare information systems, Int. J. Technol. Assessment Health Care 13 (1997) 380–393.

[3] J.R. Moehr, Evaluation: Salvation or nemesis of medical informatics? Comput. Biol. Med. 32 (2002) 113–125.

[4] G. Gordon, *System Simulation* (Prentice-Hall, Englewood Clils, NJ, 1969).

[5] J.J. Swain, Simulation goes mainstream, 1997 simulation software survey, ORMS Today 24 (5) (1997) 35–46.

[6] J. Banks and J.S. Carson, *Discrete-Event System Simulation* (Prentice-Hall, Englewood Cliffs, NJ, 1984).

[7] B. Hannon and M. Ruth, *Dynamic Modeling* (Springer, New York, 1994).

[8] J.L. Hargrove, *Dynamic Modeling in the Health Sciences* (Springer, New York, 1998).

[9] A.M. Law and W.D. Kelton, *Simulation Modeling and Analysis*, 2nd ed. (McGraw Hill, New York, 1991).

[10] N. Oreskes, K. Schrader-Frechette, and K. Belitz, Verification, validation and confirmation of numerical models in the Earth sciences, Science 2163 (1994) 641–646.

[11] M. Katzper, Epistemological bases of postulational modeling, in: J.G. Anderson, M. Katzper, editors, *Health Sciences, Physiological and Pharmacological Simulation Studies* (Society for Computer Simulation, San Diego, CA, 1995), pp. 83–88.

[12] J. Bahensky, University's statewide network links rural doctors, Healthcare Inf. 9 (3) (1992) 10–12.

[13] K. Norman and J.J. Moynihan, The impact of EDI & ANSI standards on administrative cost containment, Healthcare Inf. 9 (11) (1992) 90–96.

[14] J. Villasante, Telematic systems for health in Europe: A look towards the future, Health Inf. Eur. 1 (2) (1993) 10–12.

[15] J.G. McDaniel, Discrete-event simulation of a wide-area healthcare network, J. Am. Med. Inform. Assoc. 2 (4) (1995) 220–237.

[16] D.F. Sittig and W.W. Stead, Computer-based physician order entry: The state of the art, J. Am. Med. Inform. Assoc. 1 (2) (1994) 108–123.

[17] J.G. Anderson, Clearing the way for physicians' use of clinical information systems, Communications of the ACM 40 (8) (1997) 83–90.

[18] J.G. Anderson, S.J. Jay, S.J. Clevenger, D.R. Kassing, J. Perry, and M. Anderson, Physician utilization of a hospital information system: A computer simulation model, in: *Proceedings of the 12th Annual Symposium on Computer Applications in Medical Care* (1988), pp. 858–861.

[19] D.W. Bates, D.J. Cullen, N. Laird, et al., Incidence of adverse drug events and potential adverse drug events, J. Am. Med. Assoc. 274 (1995) 29–34.

[20] L.L. Leape, D.W. Bates, D.J. Cullen, et al., Systems analysis of adverse drug events, J. Am. Med. Assoc. 274 (1995) 35–43.

[21] D.C. Classen, S.L. Pestotnik, R.S. Evans, J.F. Lloyd, and J.P. Burke, Adverse drug events in hospitalized patients: Excess length of stay, extra costs, and attributable mortality, J. Am. Med. Assoc. 277 (1997) 301–306.

[22] J.G. Anderson, S.J. Jay, M. Anderson, and T.J. Hunt, Evaluating the potential effectiveness of using computerized information systems to prevent adverse drug events, in: *Proceedings of the 1997 AMIA Annual Fall Symposium* (1997), pp. 228–232.

Part II
Evaluating Healthcare
Information Systems:
Applications

Chapter 16
Research and Evaluation: Future Directions   334
James G. Anderson and Carolyn E. Aydin

This part includes six applications of various methodologies used to evaluate the impact of healthcare information systems. Chapter 10 provides a study of patient and clinician reactions to a computer-based health appraisal system. Methods used included clinican surveys and interviews, patient surveys, and social network analysis. Findings indicated no difference in patient satisfaction between system users and nonusers. Use of the computer system in the consulting room neither depersonalized nor enhanced patient satisfaction; nurse practitioners and physician assistants were willing to use the system, which they perceived as having benefits for patient care, but were concerned about the increased time required for exams, the effort required to learn the system, and increased monitoring of their performance. Clinicians who used the system showed a higher tolerance for uncertainty and communicated more frequently with each other and others in the department. Implementation was slowed by the need to demonstrate the monetary value of the system.

Chapter 11 provides an evaluation of the implementation of a medical information system at the University of Virginia Medical Center that mandated physician order entry. The implementation process proved to be much more difficult than expected due to cultural and behavioral problems, experienced considerable delays, and cost more than originally estimated. The author describes the problems that occurred and the organizational behavior on which they were based, and analyzes the lessons learned and the challenges that remain. A set of recommendations are provided for those considering similar information technology initiatives in order to reduce the disruptions that may accompany their introduction.

Chapter 12 describes the construction of a computer simulation model representing the medication delivery system in a hospital. The model simulates the four stages of the medication delivery system: prescribing, transcribing, dispensing, and administering drugs. Information technology applications used to reduce medication errors and associated adverse drug events (ADEs) were simulated. The results suggest that an integrated medication delivery system can save up to 1226 days of excess hospitalization and $1.4 million in associated costs annually in a large hospital. The study concludes that clinical information systems are potentially a cost-effective means of preventing ADEs in hospitals and the importance of viewing medication errors from a systems perspective.

Chapter 13 reports the results of a preimplementation study of the internal medicine division of a large physician group practice scheduled to implement an electronic medical record. Data were gathered by participant observation and interviews. The findings indicate that (1) most physicians anticipated enough benefits to use the system; (2) computers must be accessible and easy to log onto, and provide for physician movement and interruptions; (3) physicians were concerned about losing eye contact with patients when using the system; (4) it is unrealistic to expect physicians to enter their long notes; (5) staged implementation, with order entry introduced first, may help physicians to adapt to the system; and (6) training should include protected time for instructional sessions for physicians, simulated patient encounters, and tutors available to answer questions.

Chapter 14 describes a study to determine the amount of time nurses spent on documentation during the implementation of an electronic medical record on an intrapartum unit. A work-sampling study was conducted over a 14-day period. The study found that the total percentage of nursing time spent for documentation was 10.6% on paper and 5.2% on the computer. Despite charting concurrently on both paper and the computer, the amount of time spent on documentation was not excessive and was consistent with previous studies.

Chapter 15 is an evaluation of a respiratory care computer charting system in a hospital. The charting system was evaluated before and after implementation. Four assessments were made: (1) a survey of therapist's attitudes; (2) observation of work patterns; (3) an audit of the content of charts; and (4) analysis of productivity statistics. The study found that computer charting streamlined the process of documentation and allowed more beneficial use of clinical information.

The final chapter provides a brief historical overview of computer applications in health care and outlines current developments. In light of past experience, many of these new systems will result in unforeseen costs, organizational consequences, and possibly failure if developers and administrators neglect to anticipate and evaluate their social impacts. An underlying premise of this book is that the achievement of healthcare reform will require the development of an infrastructure based on computer technology that must be carefully evaluated. This, in turn, will require the application of the methods described in this book.

10
Computers in the Consulting Room: A Case Study of Clinician and Patient Perspectives

CAROLYN E. AYDIN, JAMES G. ANDERSON, PETER N. ROSEN, VINCENT J. FELITTI, and HUI-CHING WENG

Introduction

Few clinicians in the United States use computers during patient encounters and many still worry that computers will depersonalize their interactions with patients. This case study describes patient and clinician reactions to a computer-based health appraisal system. Findings showed no difference in any aspect of patient satisfaction between computer and non-computer groups. Use of a computer in the consulting room neither depersonalized nor enhanced patient satisfaction. Clinicians (in this case, nurse practitioners and physician assistants) were willing to use the system, which they perceived as having benefits for patient care, but were concerned about the increased time required for exams, effort required to learn the system while still interacting appropriately with the patient, increased monitoring of their performance, and other organizational issues. Clinicians who used the system showed a higher tolerance for uncertainty and communicated more frequently with each other and with others throughout the department. Implementation was slowed by the need to demonstrate the monetary value of the system.

The Institute of Medicine of the National Academy of Sciences, in its 1991 report, called for automated medical records [1]. As a result, the U.S. Congress considered mandating automated record systems for all hospitals that receive federal funds [2]. These recommendations are based on a growing body of evidence that properly designed and implemented computerized patient records can be used effectively to change physician behavior and improve patient care [3,4,5].

Spurred by a report by the Royal College of General Practitioners [6], computer systems have been rapidly introduced into consulting rooms in Great Britain. It is estimated that 90% of primary care physicians in that country work in computerized practices and over 50% use computers during consultation [7,8,9,10,11,12]. In contrast, it was recently estimated that fewer than 1% of U.S. physicians use a computer-based patient record [13]. Schoenbaum and Barnett [14] outline a number of reasons for the lack of acceptance of computerized medical records, including the need for clinicians to change long standing habits of data recording and to directly use the computer system while interacting with their patients.

In ambulatory care, recent estimates by industry experts indicate that computer-based patient records are in place at no more than 5% of group practices [15]. While automation is slowly gaining a foothold, roadblocks cited include the need for a leader or active physician champion, the need for reliable information about technology options, getting physicians to invest in information technology, and getting physicians to understand the system and use it appropriately [15,16]. Furthermore, while physicians are willing to embrace applications that make work easier and reject those that make it harder, computer-based patient record systems have had a marginal impact on physician work efficiency [17].

While the technology of computer-based record systems has advanced rapidly, knowledge of the impacts of such systems on physicians and patients during clinical encounters remains sparse. Through 1990, most research on computer use by clinicians has focused on informatics in hospital and specialty medicine. Legler [18] in a comprehensive review could only find 12 reports of the effects of the use of computers during medical consultation upon the physician–patient relationship.

Elson and Connelly [4] provide a more recent review of the impact of computerized patient record and decision support systems on physician behavior and patient outcomes, highlighting the role of these systems in influencing physician compliance with practice guidelines. Clinicians' attitudes and expectations regarding an information system, however, are critical factors in their successful implementation [19]. Anderson et al. [20] found that physicians' attitudes accounted for a significant amount of the variation in use of a hospital information system, even when other variables were controlled. In the UK, where computer use in the consulting rooms is widespread, computer-based patient record systems are perceived by physicians as helpful in improving the structure of medical records, checking prescriptions, providing online medical and regulatory information, and supporting standard protocols determined by the clinician.

Experts in the United States also suggest that when clinicians perceive that a computerized patient information system facilitates their practice, they will learn to use it, even if it requires changes in their practice behavior [16,17]. Bleich et al. [21], for example, reported that over 80% of health-care providers used the computer system at Beth Israel Hospital most of the time to look up laboratory results, in large part because they perceived that the system made their work faster and more accurate. A later study of the use of a computer-based outpatient medical record system at the same hospital found that residents entered almost 50% of their notes directly into the system [22]. The investigators attributed the high level of use of the outpatient system to the overall acceptance and use of the hospital information system. More recently, however, Beth Israel researchers noted that, rather than leading to paperless medical care, computerization had increased the amount of paper produced and managed by the organization. They cited comfort and convenience with paper, legal issues, and difficulty with organizational transitions to online records as reasons for the "paper paradox" [23].

In other settings, research on both physician and nurse acceptance of the HELP system at LDS Hospital suggested that access to patient data and clinical alerts were important factors in acceptance of the system [24]. Aydin and Forsythe [25], in their ethnographic study of a large group practice, reported that physicians said they would be willing to use an electronic medical record in the consulting room, but expressed concerns about learning to use the system and losing eye contact with patients during the consultation. A study conducted at a Veterans Administration General Medical Clinic, however, was unable to measure impacts on physician practice because the study design did not include methods to determine reasons for the unexpected low usage of the system [26].

Research on nurses' use of computers has focused primarily on staff nurses in hospitals. Early studies examined nurses' acceptance of systems such as order entry, measured attitudes toward computerization, including computer anxiety, and also explored whether computer systems would allow nurses more time at the bedside, for example [27,28,29,30,31]. Since computer use is rarely optional for staff nurses in hospital settings, the researchers used their findings to recommend specific teaching and implementation strategies to meet the learning needs of diverse users and enhance computer acceptance and use. More recent studies have continued to measure nurses' attitudes, but have also explored ways in which computer systems can be designed to contribute to and enhance nursing practice [32–34,35,36,37,38,39,40]. Like physicians, nurses have been found to be willing to use computer systems that they perceive can benefit their practice.

Little research to date has addressed the computerization needs of nurses in ambulatory care or of nurse practitioners, that is, advanced practice nurses with masters' degrees who generally see patients in a consulting room and whose information needs and practice patterns more closely resemble those of family practice physicians than of nurses in the hospital setting. Likewise, little research has addressed the needs of physician assistants who practice in ambulatory care. One of the few studies to include the needs of these clinicians was conducted in Kaiser-Permanente's Northwest Region. Chin and McClure [41] and Krall [42] detailed the implementation of an outpatient primary care system used by physician assistants and nurse practitioners as well as family physicians, internists, and pediatricians. Survey findings indicated gradual acceptance of the system over several months, with clinicians spending more time for each patient immediately following system implementation to complete "orders" and "charting" tasks. It took clinicians approximately 30 days to reach the baseline visit rate for their clinic. No direct data was collected on patient satisfaction with the system, although clinicians' survey responses indicted that they felt that patients were more satisfied after system implementation.

The first studies on patient reactions to clinicians using a computer in the consulting room were conducted in the UK, with findings indicating that the overall impact on patients was mixed. Two studies demonstrated no difference in patient satisfaction when physicians used a computer during consultation [43,44]. One study from the early stages of computer use, however, did show increased stress in patients with dyspeptic symptoms when their physicians used a diagnostic computer system. The researchers urged doctors to take care to preserve their human touch [45], a concern still debated in more recent computer literature [46] and also expressed by physicians anticipating system implementation [25]. Also focusing on the patient encounter, Brownbridge et al. [47] found that midwives using a computer were inclined to give less information to patients, especially when they were new to the computer, and used more closed and leading questions. A more recent study conducted in Israel indicated that primary care physicians using computerized medical records during a patient encounter changed their working styles to devote more attention to the computer and longer uninterrupted intervals for data entry than when using the traditional paper record. These physicians changed from a "conversational pattern" in which they alternated frequently between the patient and the record to a "block pattern," first establishing a number of items of information and then entering them into the record [48]. The study did not, however, include patient reactions to the encounter.

Another recent study randomly assigned adult ambulatory care patients to one of three groups where during the encounter the physicians used either a paper-and-pencil charting system, a computerized medical record system with keyboard input, or a computerized medical record system with voice input [49]. Patient reactions were measured with a questionnaire. While there were few differences among the three groups, the voice input group rated explanations of patient problems by physicians significantly higher than the other groups. A similar study was conducted at a family practice office in a metropolitan area [13]. Patients were randomly assigned to a physician who made a written record and a physician who made a computer record during the clinical encounter. There were no significant differences in patient satisfaction between the two groups. Interviews were also conducted with 16 patients seen in the family medicine department at the Medical University of South Carolina where a computerized patient record system has been implemented [50]. Patients perceived that the computerized record provided physicians with ready access to medical information and facilitated the encounter between the physician and patient. The only concern expressed about the computerized record was the confidentiality of patient data.

This chapter extends the literature on clinician use of computers in the consulting room in the United States by examining the impacts of the introduction of CompuHx, a computer-based health record for an interactive health appraisal system, on both clinicians and their patients in a large health maintenance organization. The project focuses on computerization of the health appraisal process in a setting that is likely to become increasingly important as the healthcare delivery system continues to evolve. Furthermore, the study is the first to include both clinician and patient reactions to the same system. First addressing the clinician's perspective, the study was designed to: (1) describe clinician (nurse practitioner and physician assistant) reactions to CompuHx in the consulting room, (2) explore the individual and organizational variables influencing those reactions, and (3) determine whether clinicians who report more stress from uncertainty in patient care have more positive reactions toward a system designed to ensure thoroughness and assist in reaching a diagnosis [51]. Social network analysis was then used to examine the effects of the use of the system on clinician communication patterns. From the patient's perspective, satisfaction of patients whose clinicians use CompuHx was compared to satisfaction of patients whose clinicians do not use the computer during consultations.

The research was designed as a case study of the experience of a single organization [52,53,54,55]. Such case studies rely on analytical rather than statistical generalization [55], that is, they generalize from the experience of the individuals in one organization to broader explanations about why similar change experiences might be expected in other organizations. This is also one of the few systematic studies to include an in-depth examination of the issues and concerns of clinicians and patients alike, using both quantitative and qualitative methodologies [53,56,57]. This multimethod approach can lead to insights beyond those possible with a single approach and help researchers explore some of the reasons for the mixed success of computer projects documented in numerous clinical settings.

The Health Appraisal Setting

The Kaiser-Permanente Medical Care Program provides a detailed complete history and physical examination to 50000 members per year in the San Diego Department of Preventive Medicine. The majority of these patients are the "worried well," patients whose care does not require the traditional, costly, sickness-care portion of the organization [58]. Despite this fact, however, personal interactions with the clinician are an essential part of the health appraisal process for these patients. Interviews with 53 patients indicated that, while about 20% came simply because they wanted (or were required by their employer to have) an annual physical examination, 15% were referred by Primary Care because of specific symptoms or for baseline information, and approximately 60% came with specific symptoms, concerns, or fears to discuss, some of which resulted in a diagnosis or referral to an appropriate physician [59].

A complete medical evaluation is a two stage process with visits two weeks apart. Prior to the first visit, a medical history questionnaire is completed by the patient and mailed in. The first visit consists predominantly of a series of laboratory and other tests (e.g., mammography). During the second visit a nurse practitioner or physician assistant ("examiner") takes the patient history ("yes" answers on the mailed questionnaire define the areas of focus for the history), conducts a complete physical exam, and reviews lab results with the patient. There is a supervisory internist for each six examiners, making it possible to provide a conclusive categorization of each patient as well, ill, or at risk, and make the appropriate referrals [58].

CompuHx in the Consulting Room

CompuHx is designed to record patient information, assist in information gathering for a diagnosis if appropriate, and provide a legible summary of findings. CompuHx enforces thoroughness by (1) addressing all information contained in the original patient questionnaire, (2) ensuring that all information necessary for diagnosis (if applicable) has been obtained, and (3) recording, storing, and reproducing the information in a legible, structured, and easily accessible medium. CompuHx is intended to ensure the performance of the examiners and the quality of patient care.

Two categories of information are initially stored in the data base: patient history (based on the questionnaire completed by the patient prior to the visit) and laboratory values. Stored in the consulting room computer are almost 100 screens, each specific to a question in the medical history. When queried by the examiner, the program displays screens specific to questions answered affirmatively (or left unanswered) on the patient questionnaire. Following the patient history screens is a series of 20 screens to be used in similar fashion during the actual physical examination. At the end of the physical exam, the computer displays a list of all findings and diagnoses. The examiner eliminates findings that have been subsumed, prioritizes the diagnoses, relates a condition to a referral if necessary, and "ties" medications to a condition if prescribed. When complete, all information is sent back to the database and a written summary of the patient history and medical examination is generated along with a "to do" list. A summary letter to the patient discussing the implications of findings was in alpha testing at the time of the study. A new windows version of the program will facilitate products, such as the summary letter, which can be assembled in less than one minute to be sent to patients.

System Implementation

Five of the 22 examiners are CompuHx system users, with four actively using the system at the time of the study. System development and implementation began with one computer installed in one consulting room and was expanded to include one additional computer and examiner within the year, followed by two additional computers and examiners. Since examiners always see their patients in the same consulting room, the number of system users was effectively limited by the number of consulting rooms furnished with computers. The Director of the Department of Preventive Medicine asked for a volunteer to learn the system each time a new computer was to be installed. Once an examiner learned to use the system he or she used it with all patients.

Study Methodology

Examiner Surveys

The study began with a comprehensive survey completed by all 22 nurse practitioners and physician assistants (100% response) in the Department of Preventive Medicine [60]. The survey was distributed with a letter explaining that all responses were confidential and would not be available to anyone in the organization. To ensure confidentiality, completed surveys were mailed directly to an investigator not affiliated with Kaiser-Permanente.

Because research has shown that prior expectations concerning a system are important in understanding later reactions to it (e.g., expectations confirmed, disillusionment, etc.), the survey gathered baseline information from *all* examiners, system users and nonusers alike [61]. Respondents were instructed to answer *either* from their *experience* with the system (users) *or* their *expectations* about what using the system would be like (nonusers). Statistical analyses (*t*-tests) examined differences between responses of users and nonusers.

Independent variables included in the survey were basic demographic information, previous computer experience, personal attitudes about the desirability of computer applications in medical care [20], and reactions to uncertainty in patient care [51]. Dependent variables included expectations or opinions about the accuracy, format, and ease of use of the system [62]; and the impact of CompuHx on numerous aspects of individual job performance and the performance of the department as a whole [63,64,65].

Interviews

Following completion of the surveys, 10–20-min interviews were conducted with 11 of the 22 examiners, including 3 of the 5 system users and 8 nonusers.

The interviewer was not affiliated with Kaiser-Permanente and respondents were assured that their responses were confidential. Interviews were conducted at Health Appraisal on two separate days. The number of interviews was limited by the number of examiners working each day (some work part time) and their ability to make time for the interviews in their schedules (several were seen during their lunch breaks).

Examiners were asked what they knew about the system and how they had acquired the information, their opinions about CompuHx, learning to use the system, impacts on their job, the implementation process, interactions with patients and other clinicians, and other opinions they wished to share. The interview notes were analyzed using established qualitative procedures in which the interviewer codes the major issues or themes mentioned by each examiner [66,67]. Based on these identified themes, the researchers then examined the content of the interviews for explanations of what was going on in the setting.

Social Network Analysis

As part of the survey, examiners were also provided with a list of all nurse practitioners and physician assistants, doctors, and others (e.g., data processing clerks, chart room clerks, health assistants, radiology department, laboratory, etc.) [68]. They were asked to indicate the frequency with which they communicated with each person or occupational group as part of their jobs. The frequency was coded as follows: 0 = never have a contact; 1 = once a month; 2 = several times a month; 3 = once a week; 4 = several times a week; 5 = once a day; 6 = several times a day.

Social network analysis was used to study the pattern of relations among individuals and departments [69]. The following indices were created:

1. The average frequency of communication with other Department of Medicine staff initiated by nurse practitioners (NPs) and physician assistants (PAs) who use CompuHx.
2. The average frequency of communication with other Department of Medicine staff initiated by NPs and PAs who do not use CompuHx.
3. The average frequency of communication of CompuHx users with physicians on the service.
4. The average frequency of communication of nonusers with physicians on the service.
5. The average frequency of communication of CompuHx users with other departments.
6. The average frequency of communication of nonusers with other departments.
7. The density of communications (proportion of the total possible communication ties among and between groups of examiners) among NPs and PAs who use CompuHx.

8. The density of communication of CompuHx users with the other NPs and PAs who do not use the system; the medical director, other physicians in the department; and staff of other departments.

Patient Surveys

During Fall 1994, a convenience sample of 800 Health Appraisal patients were asked by examiners to complete a survey evaluating their experience at the Health Appraisal clinic. A total of 428 patients completed surveys for a response rate of 54%. Respondents included 195 patients whose examiners did *not* use the CompuHx computer program and 233 patients whose examiners used CompuHx during the history and physical exam [70].

Survey design was based on past research indicating that patient satisfaction is related to the affective quality of the clinician's manner, the amount of information conveyed, and the clinician's technical and interpersonal skill [71]. Of particular value to patients are interpersonal skills of the clinician. The scales included on the survey are described below. With the exception of the "global satisfaction with health appraisal scale," all of the scales were adapted for the health appraisal setting from scales with already established reliability and validity. Adaptations were necessary to change terminology (e.g., "examiner" instead of "doctor") and delete items not applicable to the health appraisal setting, for example, items such as "after talking with the doctor, I know just how serious my illness is" were eliminated from the scale [72, p. 396]. Thus, while results are not directly comparable to studies using the source instruments, the research benefited from being able to adapt items and scales with established validity in patient encounters. The reported reliabilities for each scale in the present study (Cronbach's alpha measuring internal consistency) were computed from the survey data.

Global satisfaction with health appraisal: 6-item scale developed for this project measuring different aspects of the patient's experience at Health Appraisal, e.g., "I am satisfied with the physical examination (second half)" (Cronbach's alpha = 0.92).

Cognitive: 6-item scale measuring perceptions of the examiner's explanations and information and the patient's understanding of and confidence in the findings of the exam, e.g., "the examiner is good at explaining the reasons for medical tests," "the examiner answered all of my questions" (Cronbach's alpha = 0.96) [72].

Affective: 7-item scale measuring perceptions of the treatment relationship, the examiner's positive regard for the patient and willingness to listen to his/her concerns, e.g., "the examiner gave me a chance to really say what was on my mind," "I really felt understood by the examiner" (Cronbach's alpha = 0.98) [72].

Behavior: 4-item scale measuring perceptions of the thoroughness of the examination and confidence in the examiner, e.g., "the examiner gave me a thorough examination," "the examiner looked into all the problems I mentioned," (Cronbach's alpha = 0.97) [72].

Acceptance of advice: 5-item scale measuring patient's willingness to accept the examiner's advice, e.g., "I will follow the advice of the examiner completely" (Cronbach's alpha = 0.90) [73].

Computer in exam room: 3-item scale measuring the patient's attitude toward the use of the computer by the examiner—answered by CompuHx group only, e.g., "I think the computer helps the examiner take care of me" (Cronbach's alpha = 0.84) [47].

Responses to the scales, as well as to selected single items (e.g., personal computer use by patients), were analyzed for the total sample and for the CompuHx and non-CompuHx patients separately.

Findings

Examiner Demographic Data

Survey responses indicated that the 22 examiners included 7 nurse practitioners, 14 physician assistants and one examiner who had both credentials. They had a mean of 8.7 years healthcare experience (range = 1–18 years) and had worked in the department a mean of 4.4 years (range = 4 months–14 years). Fourteen (64%) were female and 8 (36%) were male.

Thirteen examiners (59%) had no previous computer experience while 9 (41%) had experience with word processing or other computer applications. Three of the five CompuHx users (60%) had previous computer experience, compared to six of the 17 (35%) nonusers. Four of the five CompuHx users (80%) were male. CompuHx users had volunteered to use the system and the demographic data indicate that male examiners and those with previous computer experience were more likely to volunteer. (In fact, the one woman who had used the system indicated that, while she was willing, she had initially been asked to use the system by the Director. At the time of the study, she had just returned from a leave and was not using the system.) The system had been implemented gradually over a two-year period and examiner experience with the system ranged from 1 month to two years at the time of the study.

Examiner Attitudes Toward CompuHx

Findings showed no significant differences in attitudes toward CompuHx between system users and nonusers. Respondents' ratings of the CompuHx system itself are shown in Table 10.1. The system received higher ratings for content, accuracy and format, but was rated as "easy to use" only "almost half the time." (Cronbach's coefficient alpha, a measure of internal consistency, is shown for scales composed of multiple questions.) The sample sizes are small (users = 5, nonusers = 17), but power analysis for a 5% level two-

TABLE 10.1. Ratings of CompuHx system.

Scoring: 1 = almost never, 3 = almost half the time, 5 = almost always

	Users (n = 5)		Nonusers (n = 17)		Total (n = 22)	
	Mean	SD	Mean	SD	Mean	SD
Content	3.8	0.45	3.7	0.70	3.8	0.64
Accuracy (alpha = 0.90)	3.9	0.22	3.8	0.67	3.8	0.58
Format (alpha = 0.89)	3.8	0.27	3.6	0.88	3.7	0.77
Ease of use (alpha = 0.85)	3.0	0.71	3.3	0.87	3.2	0.82

sided two-group t-test of equal means with these n's indicates 80% power to detect a difference in means of approximately 1.0 (using a standard deviation of 0.7). A 95% confidence interval for the difference in means between the two groups will be approximately ±0.7 (assuming the within group standard deviation is about 0.7). These calculations apply to the items in Tables 10.1 and 10.2 with standard deviations of approximately 0.7. Power analysis for a standard deviation of 1.4 (e.g., some items in Table 10.2 as well as the data in Table 10.4), indicates 80% power to detect a difference in means of approximately 2.0. For the data in Table 10.5, with standard deviations of approximately 2.9, we have 80% power to detect a difference of approximately 4.0. Computations were done using nQuery Advisor based on formulas using the central and noncentral t distribution. (See www.statsol.ie/mtt0u.htm for a validation document and complete references.)

Impacts on Job Performance

Respondents rated potential impacts on job performance (see Table 10.2). Again, there were no significant differences between users and nonusers. Findings showed both groups were uncertain about positive effects on their job performance, but agreed that (1) their performance will be monitored more, (2) top management sees the system as important, (3) external relationships with departments such as primary care (who receive records of health appraisal exams) will improve, and (4) the system is a good teaching tool for new grads. The differences between users and nonusers on the adequacy of training and whether CompuHx would make their jobs more stressful were not statistically significant. Finally, both groups "slightly agreed" that the system would increase the ease and quality of their work and would be worth the time and effort to use it.

Predictors of Attitudes Toward CompuHx

Individual characteristics did not predict attitudes toward CompuHx. t-tests showed no differences between the attitudes of male and female

TABLE 10.2. Impacts on job performance.

	Users (n = 5)		Nonusers (n = 17)		Total (n = 22)	
	Mean	SD	Mean	SD	Mean	SD
Scoring: 1 = strongly disagree, 3 = uncertain, 5 = strongly agree						
Positive effects on job performance (alpha = 0.89)	3.3	0.45	3.1	0.62	3.2	0.58
Performance monitored more	4.0	0.71	3.8	0.75	3.8	0.73
Top management sees system important	3.6	0.55	3.9	0.66	3.9	0.64
Training sufficient/adequate (alpha = 0.63)	3.1	0.74	3.9	0.63	3.7	0.72
Improves external communication/relationships (alpha = 0.85)	3.4	1.24	3.6	0.57	3.6	0.74
Good teaching tool for new grads	3.4	0.89	3.7	1.26	3.6	1.18
Scoring: 1 = negative, 4 = neutral, 7 = positive[a]						
Makes job easier/interesting/fun/pleasant[a] (alpha = 0.89)	3.8	1.79	3.7	1.37	3.7	1.43
Makes job more stressful[a]	3.8	1.79	4.4	1.27	4.2	1.38
Scoring: 1 = strongly disagree, 4 = uncertain, 7 = strongly agree						
Increase overall ease/quality of department work (alpha = 0.89)	4.4	1.24	4.6	1.17	4.5	1.16
System worth the time and effort required to use	4.8	1.30	4.6	1.23	4.6	1.22

[a] Scoring: 1 = more difficult, 7 = easier; 1 = more interesting, 7 = less interesting; 1 = more fun, 7 = less fun; 1 = more pleasant, 7 = less pleasant. Reverse items recoded so that 1 indicates most negative response and 7 indicates most positive response.

TABLE 10.3. Correlation of computer impact on clinician role with selected impacts on job performance ($n = 22$).

	Diminish clinician role
Positive effects on job performance	$r = -0.63$[a]
Makes job easier/interesting/fun/pleasant	$r = -0.75$[a]
Increase overall ease/quality of department's work	$r = -0.61$[a]
System worth the time and effort required to use it	$r = -0.73$[a]

[a] $p < 0.05$ using Bonferroni adjustment for multiple tests.

examiners for survey items and scales (e.g., "system worth the time and effort required to use it", mean for males = 4.63, females = 4.64, t (11.2) = 0.03, $p = 0.98$). There was also no correlation between items such as "system worth the time and effort required to use it" and age ($r = 0.06$, $p = 0.79$), work experience ($r = -0.09$, $p = 0.68$), or prior computer experience ($r = -0.09$, $p = 0.70$).

As would be expected, opinions about the impact of computers in general on the role of the clinician were correlated with attitudes toward CompuHx as a specific system. There were significant correlations between the scale "computers diminish clinician role" (scale includes 5 items: be hard to learn, diminish clinician judgment, be a less efficient use of clinician time, depersonalize practice, and alienate clinicians from their patients, Cronbach's alpha = 0.89) and negative attitudes toward CompuHx. Table 10.3 shows findings for users and nonusers combined, with similar correlations for different aspects of attitudes toward CompuHx. Figure 10.1 illustrates the correlation between the general computer attitude scale and the item "system worth the time and effort required to use it." Responses of users and nonusers are differentiated on the graph. Only two nonusers gave the system negative ratings ("system worth the time and effort required to use it"), both of whom also felt that computers would diminish the clinician's role. Three users and 7 nonusers were uncertain, while 2 users and 8 nonusers gave CompuHx positive ratings.

Uncertainty in Patient Care and CompuHx

Respondents also answered 13 questions designed to measure reactions to uncertainty in patient care (alpha = 0.89). Higher scores indicate greater stress. While Stress from Uncertainty did not correlate with attitudes toward the system, CompuHx users did show less stress from uncertainty in clinical practice (mean 2.37) than did nonusers (mean 3.21), $t = 3.57$, $p < 0.003$. The 95% confidence intervals were (2.02, 2.72) for users and (2.80, 3.62) for nonusers. It is unclear, however, whether those with greater tolerance for uncertainty volunteered to be the first users or whether using the system contributed to their higher tolerance for uncertainty. In other research, both males and physicians in practice longer have shown less stress from uncer-

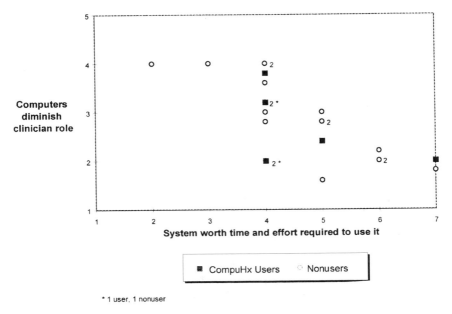

FIGURE 10.1. Relationship between responses to: "Computers diminish clinician role" and "System worth time and effort required to use it."

tainty. There were, however, no significant gender or time differences in the present study, although, understandably, examiners in the preventive medicine setting showed less stress than do physicians in other settings [51,74].

Interview Findings

Of the 11 examiners interviewed, 3 were already using the system and 7 of the 8 nonusers interviewed stated that they were willing to do so. The system was being implemented 1 or 2 examiners at a time and some of the respondents had already volunteered to be included in the future. Coding of the interview findings indicated that respondent attitudes toward the system clustered around four themes: (1) quality control, (2) depersonalization of patient care, (3) time concerns, and (4) the implementation process.

Thoroughness and Quality Control

One of the specific purposes of the system was to enforce thoroughness in history taking and the physical exam. Thoroughness emerged as one of the themes mentioned by respondents as well, although it was mentioned less frequently (by 5 of 11 respondents) than the other three themes. Four respondents (1 user and 3 nonusers) were concerned, however, that the program might not allow enough space for open-ended responses or direct patient quotations.

Depersonalization of Patient Care

Ten of the 11 examiners interviewed brought up the potential for depersonalizing patient care when the examiner's attention is focused on a computer terminal or keyboard and not on the patient. As one respondent noted, this is a "psychological and social visit" for these patients. "They come for the time and attention." While the CompuHx users did not feel that it was a problem, they did mention making a concerted effort (especially when they were first learning the system) to maintain eye contact with patients. One user noted that it was too disruptive to use the computer while conducting the physical exam. Rather, he enters the data into the computer after the patient leaves. A nonuser described mastering the computer system and continuing to meet patients' needs at the same time as an "art" that would have to be learned. Both users and nonusers also thought that patients might be pleased with the thoroughness of the computerized exam, feeling they get more time and attention from the examiner.

Time

Time was a third recurring theme, mentioned by 9 of the 11 examiners interviewed. Both users and nonusers noted that, at the time of study, examinations using CompuHx took more time and had an impact on examiner productivity. The additional time was attributed to the program's thoroughness. Two nonusers, however, also hoped the computer system might help them speed up their history taking.

Implementation Process

The fourth area of concern was the implementation process, mentioned by 8 of the 11 respondents, including the 3 users interviewed. Because implementation was intertwined with continuing system development and modification, all histories completed using CompuHx were reviewed in detail by the Director of Preventive Medicine, who sponsored and guided the development of the system. The Director also reviewed the performance of the examiner using CompuHx, with the process resulting in considerable time required of the examiner to correct or modify the final report for each patient based upon the Director's review. Each examiner learning to use the system actually became something of an apprentice to the Director, altering their working relationship, at least for a time. Several nonusers did not want to use the system until all modifications were complete, not wanting to spend the time editing reports or, as voiced by one respondent, subject themselves to the close scrutiny of the department Director.

Social Network Analysis of Practice Patterns

The survey and interview information was supplemented by analysis of the communication patterns of CompuHx users and nonusers. Only four examiners were classified as users of CompuHx for this analysis since one user stopped using the system when she took maternity leave and was not using the system at the time of the study. Table 10.4 shows the average reported frequency of communications for users and nonusers of CompuHx with other examiners and physicians in the department. System users reported that they communicated several times a week with one another; while they communicated with NPs and PAs who do not use the system only once or twice a month on average. In comparison, examiners who do not use the system with patients reported communicating with users and nonusers of the system with about the same frequency, several times a month on average.

t-tests indicated that differences between users and nonusers in the frequency with which they communicate with physicians in the department were not statistically significant. NPs and PAs who use the system reported communicating with the medical director almost daily. Interview findings indicate that this communication likely resulted from the requirement that he review each history completed using CompuHx, although it is also possible that examiners who already had more frequent communication with the director were also more likely to volunteer to become system users. Nonusers reported communicating with him only about once a week.

Table 10.5 shows the frequency of communication with other department staff. NPs and PAs who use CompuHx communicate with staff in data processing several times a week on average. This difference was expected since data processing prepares data from the patient questionnaire and laboratory tests for examiners. Nonusers rarely communicate with the data processing department. *t*-tests showed no statistically significant differences between users and nonusers in communication with other departments.

Figure 10.2 illustrates the differences in the communication patterns of users and nonusers of the CompuHx system. Densities of communication within and between subgroups are shown. System users have higher densities of communication with one another than do examiners who do not use the system. System users also have more communication with nonusers and

TABLE 10.4. Average frequency of communication for users and nonusers of CompuHx with other examiners and physicians.

Communication with	Users ($n = 5$)	Nonusers ($n = 17$)
CompuHx-users	4.15	1.52[a]
Non-CompuHx-users	2.10	1.61
Medical director	4.50	3.00
Other physicians	2.60	1.99

[a] $p < 0.001$. Scoring: 0 = never have contact, 1 = once a month, 2 = several times a month, 3 = once a week, 4 = several times a week, 5 = once a day, 6 = several times a day.

TABLE 10.5. Average frequency of communication for users and nonusers of CompuHx with other department staff.

Communication with	Users ($n = 5$)	Nonusers ($n = 17$)
Data processing	4.00	0.22[a]
Service representatives	3.25	3.33
Chart room	3.00	2.83
Radiology	0.50	0.72
Laboratory	0.50	0.61
Others	2.02	1.00

[a] $p < 0.01$. Scoring: 0 = never have contact, 1 = once a month, 2 = several times a month, 3 = once a week, 4 = several times a week, 5 = once a day, 6 = several times a day.

with the medical director, medical staff, and other departments than do nonusers of CompuHx.

Patient Demographic Data

Demographic data indicated patient gender to be the only difference between the CompuHx and non-CompuHx groups. There was a significantly larger proportion of males in the CompuHx group (see Table 10.6). Approximately 50% of both male and female patients used computers at home or in the office. Computer users were younger (mean 49.2 years, standard deviation 13.6) than patients who did not use computers (mean 62.5 years, standard deviation 13.4), $t = 9.92$, $p = 0.0001$.

Impacts of CompuHx

There were no significant differences (two-tailed t-tests) in any of the satisfaction scales or items between patients whose examiners used CompuHx and those whose examiners did not (see Table 10.7).

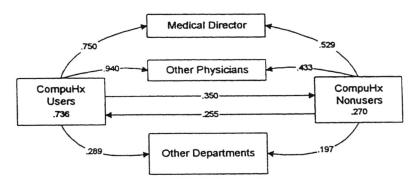

FIGURE 10.2. Network density of CompuHx users and nonusers.

TABLE 10.6. Selected demographic characteristics.

		Total sample (n = 427)	Exams with CompuHx (n = 233)	Exams without CompuHx (n = 194)
Mean age		56.3 yrs	57.5 yrs	54.8 yrs
Gender	Male	52.1%	60.4%	42.3%
	Female	47.9%	39.6%	57.7%
	Chi-square $(1, n = 424) = 13.92, p < 0.001$			
Uses a computer at home or work				
	No	52.1%	54.6%	49.2%
	Yes	47.9%	45.4%	50.8%

In addition, *CompuHx patients* "agreed" with the positive statements in the "Use of Computer in the Exam Room" scale (mean 3.95, standard deviation 0.93). They also "agreed" with the statement, "If given a choice, I would choose an examiner who uses a computer" (mean 3.83, standard deviation 1.15). They "disagreed" with the statement, "The examiner seemed to have trouble using the computer" (mean 1.74, standard deviation 1.26). There were *no* significant differences in patient satisfaction with different examiners for those surveys where examiner codes were available. (Examiners were concerned about being identified and requested removal of examiner codes from the surveys early in the data collection process. Since examiners using CompuHx had begun data collection first, examiner codes were recorded for the first 123 CompuHx patients only and for no non-CompuHx patients.)

TABLE 10.7. Comparison of patient satisfaction with exams conducted with and without CompuHx.

	Total sample		Examinations with CompuHx		Exams without CompuHx	
	Mean (n = 427)	SD	Mean (n = 233)	SD	Mean (n = 194)	SD
Global satisfaction scale	4.43	0.77	4.43	0.73	4.43	0.81
Cognitive scale	4.56	0.77	4.52	0.76	4.60	0.79
Affective scale	4.55	0.79	4.51	0.76	4.60	0.81
Behavior scale	4.54	0.84	4.51	0.82	4.59	0.88
Acceptance of advice scale	4.39	0.75	4.32	0.77	4.47	0.73
Examiner focused on chart or computer (1 item)	3.63	1.39	3.69	1.30	3.57	1.49
Examiner seemed rushed (1 item)	1.81	1.26	1.76	1.17	1.87	1.38

Scoring: 1 = strongly disagree, 3 = neutral, 5 = strongly agree.

The study also included a preliminary exploration of the relationship between a system that enforces thoroughness and aids in gathering information for a diagnosis and the stress clinicians may feel from the uncertainty inherent in patient care. While these cross-sectional data could not address issues of causality, the findings suggest that further research should focus on whether this type of system might contribute to higher tolerance for uncertainty on the part of clinicians.

Role of the System Champion

While computer professionals have pointed out the importance of a leader or champion in system implementation [15], the role of the champion and its implications will differ from setting to setting. In the organization under study, the champion was also the medical director of the organization, and examiner concerns that their performance would be monitored were reflected in both their survey responses and the request to remove examiner codes from the patient surveys. The issue of performance monitoring became particularly salient since the implementation process included a direct evaluation of each CompuHx user's work by the director. His evaluation went beyond system use to examine their overall skills in health appraisal, which he felt also improved as they learned the system. Respondent comments in the interviews indicated that this process was both beneficial and threatening. Comments of several examiners not yet using the system, however, indicated that many practicing health professionals may not welcome becoming students or apprentices again.

Increased Visibility of Clinician Practice

The issue of increased visibility of clinician practice has also begun to emerge in recent ethnographic studies of system implementation. Even in instances when there is no director scrutinizing practice, clinicians are conscious of the increased visibility of their work and may adjust their practice in response. Aydin and Forsythe [25], for example, observed physicians spending time composing longer clinical notes after implementation of a dictation system through which the notes were made available in the electronic medical record. Kaplan [75] focused on imaging systems and clinicians' perceptions of the benefits of making images public by including them in the patient record. In each of these diverse settings, the decisions made by clinicians in their practice are more "public" or visible to others, and consequently also more open to scrutiny.

Clinician Communication Patterns

Communication among clinicians and others can both influence decisions on whether to use a new system, as conversations with colleagues convince individuals that a system might be valuable in their practice; and also help individuals adapt or modify a system to better meet their needs (i.e., the concept of reinvention) [76]. In this study, social network analysis indicated that nurse practitioners and physician assistants who used the system reported that they communicated more frequently with one another as well as with other staff who could assist them in performing their professional duties than did nonusers. This frequent communication can also influence consultation patterns within the organization, with potential benefits for patient care. As expected, users' interactions with the medical director of the department, who was a leader in the development of the system and acted as an important source of information and support for the users, were more frequent than those of nonusers. In addition, NPs and PAs who used the system communicated more frequently throughout Preventive Medicine in carrying out their work. While cross-sectional data does not establish causality, the examiners' own descriptions of their interactions (interview data) support the hypothesis that new communication patterns accompanied the introduction of CompuHx in the organization.

These possible increases in communication may have important implications for the longer term quality and productivity of the department. Research in other healthcare settings has shown that communication and collaboration among caregivers are associated with better patient outcomes [77,78,79,80]. Furthermore, research outside of healthcare indicates that the more co-workers an individual communicates with about a new technology, the more productive he or she is likely to be using the system [81]. The study also illustrates the ways in which communication within social networks becomes an important resource to support system use. In fact, the "heart of the diffusion process is the modeling and imitation . . . of near-peers' experience" [76, p. 304]. New interactions may also arise as individuals learn to use the system and talk to others about it [61]. Managers can facilitate the formation of these networks by designating "superusers" (the user with the highest number of interactions with other users in this setting, for example, was the designated "superuser"), allowing time and encouraging employees to talk to each other about the system.

Patients

Findings showed no difference in patient satisfaction between CompuHx and non-CompuHx groups with *any aspect* of their Health Appraisal experience. The finding that computers in the consulting room did not result in lower affective or cognitive patient satisfaction indicates that clinician use of a computer during consultation did *not depersonalize* the encounter for the patients. The fact that scores on the behavior scale (measuring perceptions of the thoroughness of the exam and confidence in the examiner) also showed no differences, however, indicates that computer use by the clinician *did not enhance* patient satisfaction with their experience either. Furthermore, although CompuHx patients agreed that they would choose an examiner who used a computer, their scores on this item were considerably lower than their highly positive ratings on the other scales. The computer was clearly less important to patients than the other aspects of their relationship with the clinician, with which they were highly satisfied.

Conclusion

In summary, study findings indicate that (1) patients have no problem with the use of a computer in the consulting room; and (2) examiners (NPs and PAs) are willing to use a system that they perceive as having benefits for patient care (e.g., enforcing thoroughness in the exam). For systems to be enthusiastically endorsed and used by clinicians, however, they will need to go beyond the mixed benefits of systems such as CompuHx to include features that clearly make practice easier (e.g., easy retrieval of information clinicians need). Physicians in hospitals, for example, are far more likely to use computers to retrieve laboratory results needed to make clinical decisions than to enter their own orders in the computer, which requires additional work on their part. Also essential is a detailed implementation plan that includes adequate time for training and communication with other users, and addresses issues such as the role of the system champion and any performance monitoring concerns. Implementation may also be hindered by the need to identify the monetary value of the cited benefits in light of the additional time initially required to conduct exams using the system, as well as required capital expenditures. Longitudinal research should examine potential changes in clinician tolerance for uncertainty, as well as the impacts of altered communication and consultation patterns, which have been shown to improve productivity in other settings. The project also highlights the importance of research that focuses not only on system outcomes, but also examines the implementation process and includes the necessary information to evaluate factors influencing clinician usage of the system.

Acknowledgments. This project was supported by a research grant from the Kaiser-Permanente Medical Group. CompuHx was designed by Fuzzy Logic, Inc., La Jolla, CA.

References

[1] R.S. Dick and E.B. Steen, eds., *The Computer-Based Patient Record: An Essential Technology for Healthcare* (National Academy Press, Washington, DC: Institute of Medicine, 1991).

[2] Secretary of Health and Social Services, Medical and Health Insurance Information Reform Act of 1992 (HB 5464, SB 2878), Washington, DC (1992).

[3] J.G. Anderson, Computer-based patient records and changing physicians practice patterns, Topics in Health Information Management 15 (1994) 10–23.

[4] R.B. Elson and D.P. Connelly, Computerized patient records in primary care: Their role in mediating guideline-driven physician behavior change, Archives of Family Medicine 4 (1995) 698–705.

[5] M.E. Johnston, K.B. Langton, R.B. Haynes, and A. Mathieu, Effects of computer-based clinical decision support systems on clinician performance and patient outcome: A critical appraisal of research, Annals of Internal Medicine 120 (1994) 135–142.

[6] Royal College of General Practitioners, Computers in primary care: The report of the computer working party, Occasional Paper 13 (1982).

[7] G. Brownbridge, M. Fitter, and M. Sime, The doctor's use of a computer in the consulting room: An analysis, International Journal of Man–Machine Studies 21 (1984) 65–90.

[8] *Department of Health GP Computing Survey 1991*, London: NHS Management Executive (1991).

[9] G.M. Hayes, Computers in Consultation: The UK experience, in: *Proceedings of the 17th Annual Symposium on Computer Applications in Medical Care* (IEEE Computer Society Press, Washington, DC, 1993), pp. 103–106.

[10] G. Herzmark, G. Brownbridge, M. Fitter, and A. Evans, Consultation use of a computer by general practitioners, Journal of the Royal College of General Practitioners 34 (1984) 649–654.

[11] I.N. Purves, Implications for family practice record systems in the USA: Lessons from the United Kingdom, in: *Proceedings of the American Medical Informatics Association*, Spring Congress, St. Louis, MO (1993), p. 54.

[12] S. Teasdale and M. Bainbridge, Improving information management in family practice: Testing an adult learning model, in: *Proceedings of the 1997 AMIA Annual Fall Symposium*, Nashville, TN (1997), pp. 687–692. (Journal of the American Medical Informatics Association Symposium Supplement.)

[13] G.L. Solomon and M. Dechter, Are patients pleased with computer use in the examination room? The Journal of Family Practice 41(3) (1995) 241–244.

[14] S.C. Schoenbaum and G.O. Barnett, Automated ambulatory medical records systems: An orphan technology, Journal of Technology Assessment in Healthcare 8(4) (1992) 598–609.

[15] J. McCormack, When will smaller medical groups discover computers?, Health Data Management 5(10) (1997) 50–52, 54, 56, 58, 60, 63.

[16] L.L. Berkowitz, Breaking down the barriers: Improving physician buy-in of CPR systems, Healthcare Informatics 14(10) (1997) 73–76.

[17] R.B. Elson, Uniting practice management and the CPR, in: *Healthcare Informatics: Uniting Practice Management and the CPR* (Online, McGraw-Hill, 1997). Available: Http://www.healthcareinformatics.com/issues/1997/09_97/ss_elson.htm.

[18] J.D. Legler, Computers and the physician-patient relationship: What do we know?, in: *Proceedings of the 14th Annual Symposium on Computer Applications in Medical Care* (IEEE Computer Society Press, Washington, DC, November 4–7, 1990), pp. 289–292.

[19] J.E. Bailey, Development of an instrument for the management of computer user attitudes in hospitals, Methods of Information in Medicine 20 (1990) 51–56.

[20] J.G. Anderson, S.J. Jay, H.M. Schweer, and M.M. Anderson, Why doctors don't use computers: Some empirical findings, Journal of the Royal Society of Medicine 79 (1986) 142–144.

[21] H.L. Bleich et al., Clinical computing in a teaching hospital, New England Journal of Medicine 312 (1985) 756–764.

[22] D.M. Rind and C. Safran, Real and imagined barriers to an electronic medical record, in: *Proceedings of the 17th Annual Symposium on Computer Applications in Medical Care* (McGraw Hill, New York, 1993), pp. 74–78.

[23] D.Z. Sands, D.M. Rind, C. Vieira, and C. Safran, Going paperless: Can it be done?, in: *Proceedings of the 1997 AMIA Annual Fall Symposium*, Nashville, TN (1997), p. 887. (Journal of the American Medical Association Symposium Supplement.)

[24] R.M. Gardner and H.P. Lundsgaarde, Evaluation of user acceptance of a clinical expert system, Journal of the American Medical Informatics Association 1 (1994) 428–438.

[25] C.E. Aydin and D.E. Forsythe, Implementing computers in ambulatory care: Implications of physician practice patterns for system design, in: *Proceedings of the 1997 AMIA Fall Symposium*, Nashville, TN (1997), pp. 677–681. (Journal of the American Medical Informatics Association Symposium Supplement.)

[26] B.L. Rotman et al., A randomized controlled trial of a computerbased physician work station in an outpatient setting: Implementation barriers to outcome evaluation, Journal of the American Medical Informatics Association 3 (1996) 340–348.

[27] C.E. Aydin, Occupational adaptation to computerized medical information systems, Journal of Health and Social Behavior 30 (1989) 163–179.

[28] M. Burkes, Identifying and relating nurses' attitudes toward computer use, Computers in Nursing 9 (1991) 190–201.

[29] G. Hendrickson and C.T. Kovner, Effects of computers on nursing resource use, Computers in Nursing 8 (1990) 16–22.

[30] N. Staggers, Using computers in nursing: Documented benefits and needed studies, Computers in Nursing 6 (1988) 164–170.

[31] J.H. Stronge and A. Brodt, Assessment of nurses' attitudes toward computerization, Computers in Nursing 3 (1985) 154–158.

[32] P.Q. Bourie, J. Dresch, and R.H. Chapman, Usability evaluation of an on-line nursing assessment, in: *Proceedings of the 1997 AMIA Fall Symposium*, Nashville, TN (1997), p. 914. (Journal of the American Medical Informatics Association Symposium Supplement.)

[33] P.F. Brennan and M. Anthony, Nursing practice models: Implications for IS design, in: *Proceedings of the 1997 AMIA Fall Symposium*, Nashville, TN (1997), p. 847. (Journal of the American Medical Informatics Association Symposium Supplement.)

[34] S.J. Brown, M.A. Cioffi, P. Schinella, and A. Shaw, Evaluation of the impact of a bedside terminal system in a rapidly changing community hospital, Computers in Nursing 13 (1995) 280–284.

[35] B.A. Happ, The effect of point of care technology on the quality of patient care, in: *Proceedings of the 18th Annual Symposium on Computer Applications in Medical Care*, Washington, DC (1994), pp. 183–187. (Journal of the American Medical Informatics Association Symposium Supplement.)

[36] D.K. Hinson, S.E. Huether, J.A. Blaufuss, M. Neiswanger, A. Tinker, K.J. Meyer and R. Jensen, Measuring the impact of a clinical nursing information system on

one nursing unit, in: *Proceedings of the 18th Annual Symposium on Computer Applications in Medical Care*, Washington, DC (1994), pp. 203–210. (Journal of the American Medical Informatics Association Symposium Supplement.)

[37] M.T. Lush and S.B. Henry, Nurses use of health status data to plan for patient care: Implications for the development of a computerbased outcomes infrastructure, in: *Proceedings of the 1997 Annual Fall Symposium*, Nashville, TN (1997), pp. 136–140. (Journal of the American Medical Informatics Association Symposium Supplement.)

[38] C.A. Murphy, M. Maynard, and G. Morgan, Pretest and post-test attitudes of nursing personnel toward a patient care information system, Computers in Nursing 12 (1994) 239–244.

[39] P.M. Ngin and L.M. Simms, Computer use for work accomplishment: A comparison between nurse managers and staff nurses, Journal of Nursing Administration 26 (1996) 47–55.

[40] R.D. Zielstorff, G. Estey, A. Vickery, G. Hamilton, J.B. Fitzmaurice, and G.O. Barnett, Evaluation of a decision support system for pressure ulcer prevention and management: Preliminary findings, in: *Proceedings of the 1997 Annual Fall Symposium*, Nashville, TN (1997), pp. 248–252. (Journal of the American Medical Informatics Association Symposium Supplement.)

[41] H.L. Chin and P. McClure, Evaluating a comprehensive outpatient clinical information system: A case study and model for system evaluation, in: *Proceedings of the 19th Annual Symposium on Computer Applications in Medical Care*, New Orleans, LA (1995), pp. 717–721. (Journal of the American Medical Informatics Association Symposium Supplement.)

[42] M.A. Krall, Acceptance and performance by clinicians using an ambulatory electronic medical record in an HMO, in: *Proceedings of the 19th Annual Symposium on Computer Applications in Medical Care*, New Orleans, LA (1995), pp. 708–711. (Journal of the American Medical Informatics Association Symposium Supplement.)

[43] G. Brownbridge, G.A. Herzmark, and T.D. Wall, Patient reactions to doctors' computer use in general practice consultations, Social Science and Medicine 20 (1985) 47–52.

[44] J.J. Rethans, P. Hoppener, G. Wolfs, and J. Diederiks, Do personal computers make doctors less personal? British Medical Journal 296 (1988) 1446–1448.

[45] P.J. Cruickshank, Patient stress and the computer in the consulting room, Social Science in Medicine 16 (1982) 1371–1376.

[46] E.H. Shortliffe, Dehumanization of patient care: Are computers the problem or solution? Journal of the American Medical Informatics Association 1 (1994) 75–76.

[47] G. Brownbridge, E.J. Lilford, and S. Tindale-Biscoe, Use of a computer to take booking histories in a hospital antenatal clinical, Medical Care 26 (1988) 474–487.

[48] J. Urkin, S.S. Warshawsky, J.S. Pliskin, N. Cohen, A. Sharon, M. Binstok, and C.Z. Marigolds, How does a computerized medical record (CMR) affect physicians' work style? A video recorded study, in: *Proceedings of the American Medical Informatics Association*, Spring Congress, St. Louis, MO (1993), p. 89.

[49] J.D. Legler and R. Oates, Patients' reactions to physician use of a computerized medical record system during clinical encounters, The Journal of Family Practice 37(3) (1993) 241–244.

[50] S. Ornstein and A. Bearden, Patient perspectives on computer-based medical records, The Journal of Family Practice 38(6) (1994) 606–610.

[51] M.S. Gerrity, R.F. DeVellis, and J.A. Earp, Physicians' reactions to uncertainty in patient care, Medical Care 28 (1990) 724–736.

[52] I. Benbasat, D.K. Goldstein, and M. Mead, The case research strategy in studies of information systems, MIS Quarterly 11(3) (1987) 369–386.

[53] B. Kaplan and D. Duchon, Combining qualitative and quantitative methods in information systems research: A case study, MIS Quarterly 12(4) (1988) 571–586.

[54] J. Van Maanen, ed., *Qualitative Methodology* (Sage Publications, Beverly Hills, CA, 1983).

[55] R.K. Yin, *Case Study Research: Design and Methods* (Sage Publications, Thousand Oaks, CA, 1984).

[56] J.G. Anderson, C.E. Aydin, and S.J. Jay, *Evaluating Health Care Information Systems* (Sage Publications, Thousand Oaks, CA, 1994).

[57] B. Kaplan, Addressing organizational issues in the evaluation of medical systems, Journal of the American Medical Informatics Association 4 (1997) 94–100.

[58] V.J. Felitti, Patient entry into a large, multi-specialty medical group, Kaiser-Permanente Medical Care Program, San Diego, CA (1983), unpublished report.

[59] C.E. Aydin, P.N. Rosen, and V.J. Felitti, Health Appraisal: Why do they really come? Kaiser-Permanente Medical Care Program, San Diego (1993), unpublished manuscript.

[60] C.E. Aydin, P.N. Rosen, and V.J. Felitti, Transforming information use in preventive medicine: Learning to balance technology with the art of caring, in: *Proceedings of the 18th Annual Symposium on Computer Applications in Medical Care*, Washington, DC (1994) pp. 563–567. (Journal of the American Medical Informatics Association Symposium Supplement.)

[61] C.E. Aydin and R.E. Rice, Bringing social worlds together: information systems as catalysts for interdepartmental interactions, Journal of Health and Social Behavior 33 (1992) 168–185.

[62] W.J. Doll and G. Torkzadeh, The measurement of end-user computing satisfaction, MIS Quarterly 12 (1988) 259–274.

[63] C.E. Aydin and R.E. Rice, Social worlds, individual differences, and implementation: Predicting attitudes toward a medical information system, Information and Management 20 (1991) 119–136.

[64] K.H. Kjerulff, M.A. Counte, J.S. Salloway, and B.C. Campbell, Understanding employee reactions to a medical information system, in: *Proceedings of the 5th Annual Symposium on Computer Applications in Medical Care* (IEEE Computer Society Press, Los Angeles, CA, 1981), pp. 802–805.

[65] R.L. Schultz and D.P. Slevin, Implementation and organizational validity: An empirical investigation, in: R.L. Schultz and D.P. Slevin, editors, *Implementing Operations Research/Management Science* (American Elsevier, New York, 1975), pp. 153–182.

[66] R.B. Emerson, R.I. Fretz, and L.L. Shaw, *Writing Ethnographic Fieldnotes* (University of Chicago Press, Chicago, 1995).

[67] M.B. Miles and A.M. Huberman, *Qualitative Data Analysis* (Sage Publications, Newbury Park, CA, 1984).

[68] J.G. Anderson, H.C. Weng, C.E. Aydin, P.N. Rosen, and V.J. Felitti, Computers in the examining room: Evaluating the social impact on practice patterns, in: *Proceedings of the American Conference on Information Systems*, 15–17 August, Indianapolis, IN (Association for Information Systems, 1997), pp. 909–911.

[69] R.E. Rice and J.G. Anderson, Social networks and healthcare information systems: A structural approach to evaluation, in: J.G. Anderson, C.E. Aydin, and S.J. Jay, editors, *Evaluating Healthcare Information Systems: Methods and Applications* (Sage, Thousand Oaks, CA, 1994), pp. 135–163.

[70] C.E. Aydin, P.N. Rosen, S.M. Jewell, and V.J. Felitti, Computers in the examining room: The patient's perspective, in: *Proceedings of the 19th Annual Symposium on Computer Applications in Medical Care*, New Orleans, LA (1995), pp. 824–828. (Journal of the American Medical Informatics Association Symposium Supplement.)

[71] J.R. Lewis, Patient views on quality care in general practice: Literature review, Social Science and Medicine 39(5) (1994) 655–670.

[72] M.H. Wolf, S.M. Putnam, S.A. James, and W.B. Stiles, The medical interview satisfaction scale: Development of a scale to measure patient perceptions of physician behavior, Journal of Behavioral Medicine 1 (1978) 391–401.

[73] J. Kincey, P. Bradshaw, and P. Ley, Patients' satisfaction and reported acceptance of advice in general practice, Journal of the Royal College of General Practitioners 25 (1975) 558–566.

[74] J.G. Anderson, S.J. Trajkovski, R. Campbell, A. Haley, and M.M. Anderson, Determining clinical practice styles from computer-based data, in: *Proceedings Medinfo 92, 7th World Congress on Medical Informatics*, Geneva, Switzerland (September 1992), pp. 6–10.

[75] B. Kaplan, Objectification and negotiation in interpreting clinical images: Implications for computer-based patient records, Artificial Intelligence in Medicine 7 (1995) 439–454.

[76] E.M. Rogers, *Diffusion of Innovations*, 4th ed. (Free Press, New York, 1995).

[77] J.G. Baggs, S.A. Ryan, C.E. Phelps, J.F. Richeson, and J.E. Johnson, The association between interdisciplinary collaboration and patient outcomes in a medical intensive care unit, Heart and Lung 21(1) (1992) 18–24.

[78] A.B. Flood, The impact of organizational and managerial factors on the quality of care in healthcare organizations, Medical Care Review 51(4) (1994) 381–428.

[79] W.A. Knaus, E.A. Draper, D.P. Wagner, and J.E. Zimmerman, An evaluation of outcome from intensive care in major medical centers, Annals of Internal Medicine 104 (1986) 410–418.

[80] S.M. Shortell, J.E. Zimmerman, D.M. Rousseau, R.R. Gillies, D.P. Wagner, E.A. Draper, W.A. Knaus, and J. Duffy, The performance of intensive care units: Does good management make a difference? Medical Care 32(5) (1994) 508–525.

[81] M.J. Papa, Communication network patterns and employee performance with new technology, Communication Research 17 (1990) 344–368.

11A
Introducing Physician Order Entry at a Major Academic Medical Center: Impact on Organizational Culture and Behavior

Thomas A. Massaro

Introduction

In 1988 the University of Virginia Medical Center began implementation of a medical information system based on mandatory physician order entry. The implementation process was much more difficult than expected. The program experienced considerable delays, and cost much more than was originally estimated. Although there were some legitimate questions concerning the user-friendliness of the new technology, these were less significant than the cultural and behavioral problems encountered. The new system challenged basic institutional assumptions; it disturbed traditional patterns of conduct and forced people to modify established practice routines. Real progress toward the integration of the system into the center's operational culture occurred only after a senior management team representing important sectors of the hospital staff and administration began meeting regularly to address the institution-wide issues that had been raised. The chapter describes the problems that occurred and the organizational behaviors on which they were based, analyzes the lessons learned, documents the progress that has been achieved, and outlines the challenges that remain. The center's experience provides insight into the issue of technology-driven organizational transformation in academic medical centers. Recommendations for successful introduction of similar agents of institutional change are presented (Academic Medicine 68 (1993) 20–25).

Increasingly, information technology (IT) is being used to manage the logistical organization that supports healthcare delivery operations. Linking physicians to the IT infrastructure is a major challenge [1]. Physician-order-entry systems establish that linkage by requiring doctors to place orders (for all clinical services including lab tests, x-rays, medications, and nursing interventions) directly into the computer without the assistance of nurses, clerks, or other support personnel. This technology provides an appealing option for many academic medical centers. Under severe cost pressures, they anticipate that having residents online will allow patient care to be delivered more efficiently and will provide one of the operational and strategic innovations that centers need to survive in the present competitive healthcare environment.

There is precedent for this belief. In the retail industry, capturing customer and product information at the "point of sale" has created competitive advantages for numerous firms in different marketplaces [4]. By inference, clinically important information can be generated by the physicians closest to the "point of care" [5]. But, in contradistinction to the retail sector, which can assign relatively inexperienced employees to data-entry positions, the healthcare sector places the most highly trained professional personnel with the greatest opportunity cost in the data-entry role. (Opportunity cost is the value of the activities that must be forgone when one option is chosen over another.) Accordingly, the acceptability of an IT system to physicians is important in any clinical setting but crucial in large teaching hospitals, where balancing education and efficiency is a constant challenge.

This chapter describes what happened when an IT system that mandated order entry by the physician was introduced into the operational environment at one major academic center, outlining some of the behavioral and cultural transformations that occurred, discussing them in the context of technology innovation in the contemporary teaching hospital environment, and drawing several conclusions regarding the management of change in that setting.

Background

The University of Virginia (UVA) Medical Center is a fully accredited 700-bed tertiary referral hospital and is the primary training facility for over 1000 residents and medical students. In 1981, a management consultant firm recommended major IT expansion, including a financial and accounting system and a medical information system (MIS). In recommending the MIS, the consultants projected cost savings of $26.3 million over five years with a payback period of less than two years.

The accounting programs were installed first, with little apparent difficulty and great success. (As an indication of the effectiveness of this effort, accounts receivable were reduced from more than 100 days at the onset to less than 60 days after implementation.)

The MIS installation began in 1985. The basic administrative functions (such as admission, discharge, and transfer) were introduced over the next two years, with no discernable impact on clinical practice. Between 1988 and 1991, clinical functions were added sequentially. The first phase placed dietary and radiology orders on line. Laboratory ordering and results retrieval were provided next. Pharmacy pathways came later, and major ancillaries and nursing procedure orders were introduced in the final phase. In late 1992, over 550 terminals were being deployed in three inpatient locations and in numerous outpatient clinics. More than 3600 nurses, 1200 residents, 800 medical students, and 200 attending physicians had been trained to use the system. Virtually all physician orders were captured, all lab results were obtained, and most radiologists' impressions were retrievable through the MIS.

Although these numbers indicate a significant commitment on the part of the medical center, implementation was much more difficult than expected. The program was three years behind schedule and cost nearly three times the original estimates. The project provoked a major confrontation between the medical staff and the hospital administration. Real progress toward integration of the MIS into the center's operational culture occurred only after the Computer and Information Sciences Executive Committee (CISEC) was created and began to meet weekly so that its members could address the problems. This senior management team included the chairs of three major clinical departments (medicine, surgery, and pediatrics), the executive director of the medical center, the director of nursing, the chief information officer, and the senior associate vice president of the UVA Health Sciences Center.

Analysis

At least four factors contributed to the widespread organizational stress that accompanied the implementation program: the alteration of established workflow patterns and practices; the strict, literal interpretation of rules by the computer (or conversely, an inability of the IT system to identify intent); the ambiguity of governance policies; and the lack of a clear understanding within the physician community of the long-term strategic value of the MIS initiative. The concerns relating specifically to housestaff and medical students' education are discussed separately in a companion article [6].

Questions regarding the quality and user-friendliness of the center's new technology were raised throughout this process. Some of these concerns were quite appropriate and remain valid today. In retrospect, however, the technology issues almost always were used as surrogates for other agenda items related to the challenging of basic institutional assumptions and beliefs. From the organizational perspective, the details of the technology were probably overshadowed by the cultural and behavioral issues, which will continue to be significant even when improved technology is available. Thus, the UVA experience provides insight into the issue of technology-driven organizational change in academic medical centers and is generalizable to other teaching facilities that may be considering similar initiatives.

Work Dynamics

The MIS altered traditional workflow patterns and changed the way the center's professional groups related to each other. Prior to the MIS, an order was written in the chart on the patent's unit. The charge nurse "signed off" on the request, communicated it to the bedside nurse, and assumed responsibility for the unit clerk's delivery of a "hard copy" to the pharmacy. If the order was clear, the pharmacy staff completed the order. If any part of it was unclear, direct contact with the ordering physician was necessary, usually by paging the physician and obtaining clarification by phone. This process changed once the MIS was established. Now, orders are placed by physicians from anywhere in the hospital. No direct communication with other caregivers is required; the bedside nurse is notified of the order from a computer-generated acknowledgement printout generated at each nursing station. Legibility is no longer an issue, and dosage schedules, generally selected from the screen options are less of a problem.

Early in the implementation process a multidisciplinary review committee of practicing clinicians was established to discuss the effect of the MIS on hospital practices. Although in principle this committee was to develop procedures for the MIS, in practice, it was frequently used to enforce policies that had been previously approved but had not been fully implemented. The residents, who were most affected by these policies, often reacted defensively and directed their anger at the MIS and not at the service that initiated the change. They opposed using the MIS for enforcing or policing any behaviors that had not been part of their practice patterns prior to the implementation of the MIS. The CISEC eventually assumed the responsibility for settling these conflicts very late in the implementation process, but only after they had become a source of significant frustration to the residents and other clinical staff.

The attitudes toward the MIS varied across professional groups in proportion to the levels of positive impact on their daily work activities. A survey instrument was designed to quantify those differences. Almost 1500 clinicians completed the survey in 1991, and the results were highly consistent within each group (see Figure 11A.1). The members of each of the three major professional groups (resident physicians, nurses, and pharmacists) tended to assume that their perceptions of the impact of the MIS were similar to the perceptions of the other groups' members. The physicians believed that many clerical functions had been transferred to them from the nurses. Unit secretaries and other nursing personnel were out of the ordering loop. The assistance they had previously provided was no longer available. As a result, housestaff uniformly had a negative view of the MIS and thought that its impact on others was negative as well. Pharmacists, relieved from the tyranny of illegible, incomplete handwritten orders, saw only positive consequences for themselves and for the others. Nurses and respiratory therapists, who gained some independence from the physicians

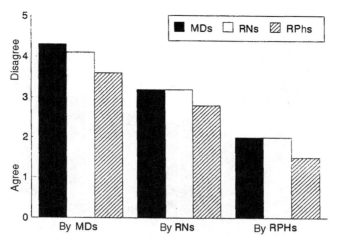

Figure 11A.1. Three professional groups' perceptions in 1991 of how a medical information system (MIS) enhanced their jobs. Nurses, residents, and pharmacists at the University of Virginia Medical Center were asked to rate how much they thought the MIS had enhanced their jobs and the jobs of the other two groups, using a scale of 1 (strongly agree that it had enhanced the job) to 5 (strongly disagree). Differences in responses across groups are significant ($p < .01$ for all cases).

in the ordering process but also assumed additional computer charting requirements, were much more ambivalent about the system. These mixed results are consistent with those reported in previous studies [7–9]. Details of the survey are available elsewhere [10].

Literal Enforcement

Much of what professionals do is based on mutually understood, often unexpressed intent. Protocols and guidelines exist, but rules are not necessarily ends in themselves. Computers are far more rigid. There is no "spirit of the law" subroutine in the MIS systems. Rules are rules; no deviation from a literal interpretation of them is allowed.

As an example, this structural rigidity led to problems with "unsigned verbal orders." Verbal orders had always occurred in certain situations, such as in emergencies or phone communications. Before the MIS, a flag was raised on the patient's chart, indicating that a verbal order had to be cosigned. There were probably instances when these reminders were overlooked, but no one specifically looked for them, and certainly no one had any sense of their volume.

The MIS changed that. Every order placed as a verbal order in the name of a physician by another authorized caregiver (such as a nurse or therapist) was recorded and counted. There was an impression that more verbal

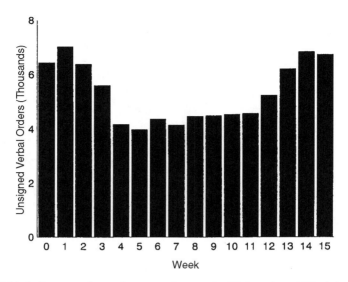

Figure 11A.2. Impact of mandatory review at the University of Virginia Medical Center on the number of unsigned verbal orders during a 15-week period in 1988. Weeks 4–10 represent the trial period. The number of unsigned verbal orders in the trial period was significantly different ($p < .01$) from the number before (in weeks 1 and 2) or after (in weeks 13–15).

orders were being generated, especially in emergency situations, because of the time and effort required to place an order on the MIS. Although it was impossible to confirm whether more were generated, it was certainly easy to see that more were being counted. Figure 11A.2 shows the numbers of unsigned verbal orders recorded by the system before and after a system change (introduced in week 3 as shown in the figure) that required that all unsigned orders be removed before new orders could be entered. The reduction in unsigned orders fell significantly, but did not fall to zero. (The residual orders probably reflect those patient records awaiting dictation and order sign-off after discharge.) Although everyone understood the accountability and potential financial difficulties created by having that number of unsigned orders in the chart, the mandatory signature process proved to be sufficiently unpopular with the residents that a non–computer-based solution to the problem was finally instituted in the twelfth week by the medical staff, and the mandatory requirement was eliminated.

An additional letter-versus-spirit example revolved around "acting interns," that is, fourth-year medical students who often functioned as junior house officers on specific rotations. While supervision was closer than for regular interns, and cosigning of orders was required, acting interns had more latitude in decision making and patient interaction than did third-year students. The MIS made no such distinctions. The fourth-year students do not have an MD degree; therefore they have no ability to enter orders independently or have them cosigned after the fact. This literal interpretation of the rules made the rotations far less attractive to students. A number of creative attempts were made to circumvent this apparent rigidity, but none was successful.

Governance

Alderfer describes an "underbounded system" as an organization where the lines of authority are not well drawn and where the decision-making process is ill-defined [11]. Hanlon applied this concept to teaching hospitals [12]. He suggests that in these large complex organizations there are few firm guidelines regarding the boundaries of administrative and medical control; there is considerable uncertainty about who establishes patient care policies at the institutional level. In such an environment individuals at all levels are unsure about limits or priorities in their roles. This hinders their capacity for systematic planning and contributes to a pattern of short-term focus and crisis management. Also, because patient care activities tend to be highly decentralized, personnel tend to focus on local (unit and department) problems. As a result, it can be difficult to harness the human resources necessary to coordinate and manage a broad institutional initiative. While the management control systems at the UVA center probably do not differ appreciably from those in many other teaching hospitals, they did have many of the characteristics of the underbounded system. This led at least initially to considerable uncertainty in responsibility and authority in dealing with the MIS challenge.

Organizational ambiguity is particularly troublesome when conflicts must be resolved, that is, compromises based on consensus are not easily achieved. In implementing the MIS, the UVA center demonstrated many of the characteristics of an underbounded system; it was virtually impossible to deal with many of the major MIS controversies until the questions of ambiguity in governance practices were addressed.

Broad operational systems such as the MIS tend to cut across functional lines. Integration of cross-functional processes is not easy under the best of circumstances; it is particularly difficult in the traditional department-based functional organization of an academic medical center that has poorly defined governance traditions. In other industries, project management teams are often created to oversee complex cross-functional initiatives, and project managers are generally given the authority to make the necessary decisions. But the delegation of authority to project management is not common in the underbounded academic environment.

At the UVA, the MIS project team was unable to accomplish the project management function. Drawn from within the computing services group, they provided the needed services, but had absolutely no decision-making authority. They clearly owned the problem, but it was far less clear who owned the solution. Eventually the CISEC team assumed ownership of the entire process, but only after the situation had reached crisis level.

One of the continual dilemmas in an underbounded system is determining who speaks for whom. At the UVA, this was especially true for housestaff involvement in MIS decisions. Although residents are nominally employees of the hospital, each relates almost exclusively to the clinical department in which he or she is being trained. The linkages between residents in different departments were very tenuous. In fact, during this process of adjustment to the MIS it became clear that even though there was a central hospital mailbox assigned to each resident, these boxes were checked very infrequently; there was no effective way to communicate directly to the entire community of residents except through their clinical departments. One of the clear and positive tangential results of the MIS has been the establishment of a chief residents' coordinating council, which now meets and exchanges information across residents' teams. This council has provided some elements of continuity and a longer-term horizon to the residents, who originally, and quite appropriately, were oriented to their clinical departments and focused on the short-term aspects of their work.

Short- versus Long-Term Horizons

It is far easiert to deal with short-term difficulties if the long-term benefits are well understood. While the "enabling" benefits of an online physician system (such as decision support, the electronic medical record, automatic capture of quality improvement, and financial performance data) were appreciated by the leadership of the medical center, these benefits were neither perceived nor valued by the attending physician community as a whole. Residents, realistically and appropriately, were concerned with issues of day-to-day survival. Presumably, attending physicians have a greater interest in the long-term future of the institution, but during the implementation they were unprepared or unable to provide incentives or rationalizations for the process or to defend the ultimately beneficial effects of the MIS.

Discussion

In the business world, it is widely appreciated that the introduction of a major new technology can be a destabilizing event [13], but this fact has gone largely unnoticed in medicine, where new technologies are introduced almost daily. Most medical technologies, however, are introduced as part of a natural evolutionary process. They are managed and controlled by a limited number of people who understand them and provide oversight for their use. But the MIS was different in that it required fundamental changes in the ways many individuals worked and, at times, in the ways they perceived themselves.

From an organizational perspective, the projects that tend to be most destabilizing tend to be those that are most "invasive," that is, those that challenge assumptions and routine behaviors. Thus, the invasiveness of a technology relates to how much change in the institution's culture will be demanded by its introduction. The vigor of the response to this invasion can be viewed as a homeostatic reflex to the disturbance introduced by a major cultural challenge. The MIS forced the center's physicians to modify their behaviors in ways they disliked. It was viewed as an administrative initiative, imposed from the "outside" with no real sponsorship in the medical community. All the energies that they normally would direct toward a hostile outside threat were directed at the MIS.

By any criterion, the cost of implementing the MIS, in terms of organizational invasion and resources, was far greater than anticipated. At the same time, the savings have never approached those projected by the original consultants. Pharmacy service has become more efficient, documented ordering errors have been drastically reduced, and the ability to identify reduced, and the ability to identify and capture costs has been enhanced. However, actual personnel reductions, in many ways the raison d'etre for the system at the onset, are not readily identified. Nursing personnel have increased by 30% during this period for a number of reasons, including expansion of services and significant increases in severity of illness, none of which are related to the use of the MIS. Perhaps the personnel growth would have been greater had the MIS not been installed, but the fact remains that five years into the program it is impossible to document even one position that was eliminated as a direct result of the MIS.

Conclusions

The implementation phase of the MIS at the UVA center has concluded with a new equilibrium in place. The organizational accommodations and changes were far greater than expected. In the process of change, we came to understand several things that are relevant to others considering similar initiatives.

First, we learned that information technologies of the scope and invasiveness of an MIS are not culturally neutral. The system was viewed by many as a threat to the values of the organization, and their responses to this cultural assault were predictable. Responses of this magnitude should be anticipated, and they must be managed. The implications of the changes should be explained to those most directly affected, and key personnel should be introduced to the anticipated long-term benefits. Initiatives of this magnitude cannot be managed on a part-time basis using personnel who volunteer time from an already busy schedule. The institution must be prepared to invest resources—both human and financial—that are appropriate to the magnitude of the task, and must be prepared to support those individuals it chooses for this management role. Of course, others have learned similar lessons in many different settings, but we were desensitized to the potential challenge by our success with financial software and our positive experiences with the introduction of clinical technology into the practice environment.

Second, we learned that information technology alone cannot fix problems that it did not create, but that such technology can accentuate existing problems by diverting attention from the root causes and fundamental issues involved. The communication difficulties and governance questions that were identified demanded the attention of the leadership of the institution before the technology could function appropriately. Had these challenges been foreseen and dealt with earlier, the implementation process might have been much less traumatic.

Third, we learned that cross-functional innovation in an institution structured along functional lines requires active and constant support from the top management team. Solomon-like decisions do not come easily at any level, but they appear to be more successful when delivered from individuals in positions well above the fray.

Fourth, we clearly did not generate the operational savings we anticipated. Instead, we adopted an imperfect technology base that has forced us to look at our clinical practices in a different way, and we do things differently because of it. With the experience we have gained, we are better able to understand the technology and ultimately to enhance the care we provide with it.

Finally, we may have gained a strategic and competitive advantage for the future by being forced to deal with issues of institutional change. Although the driving force for this particular crisis was internally generated, numerous other forces demanding change are present for all academic medical centers in the external environment, and our experience may have contributed to our ability to deal more effectively with these others in the future.

Acknowledgment. The author gratefully acknowledges the insight and stimulation derived from numerous conversations with Professor Andrew C. Boynton, Mr. James R. Paul, and Dr. Robert E. Reynolds on the issues of this chapter.

References

[1] W.F. Bria and R.L. Rydell, *The Physician–Computer Connection: A Practical Guide to Physician Involvement in Hospital Information Systems* (American Hospital Publishing, 1992).

[2] J. Schreier, Physicians who use the system help hospital gain advantage, Computers in Healthcare (August 1991) 30–33.

[3] K.K. Kim and J.E. Michelman, An examination of factors for the strategic use of information systems in the healthcare industry, MIS Quarterly 14 (1990) 201–215.

[4] P.G.W. Keen, *Shaping the Future, Business Design though Information Technology* (Harvard Business School Press, Cambridge, MA, 1991).

[5] M.F. Stefanchik, Point-of-care revolution, Computers in Healthcare (April 1991) 19–24.

[6] T.A. Massaro, Introducing physician order entry at a major academic medical center: II. Impact on medical education, Acad. Med. 68 (1992) 25–30.

[7] C.E. Aydin and R.E. Rice, Social worlds, individual differences, and implementation: Predicting attitudes toward a medical information system, Information and Management 20 (1991) 119–136.

[8] B.L. Harris, Becoming deprofessionalized: One aspect of the staff nurse's perspective on computer-mediated nursing care plans, Adv. Nurs. Sci. 13 (1990) 63–74.

[9] C.G. Schroeder and P.G. Pierpaoli, Direct order entry by physicians in a computerized hospital information system, Am. J. Hosp. Pharm. 43 (1986) 355–359.

[10] T.A. Massaro and A. Baglioni, Perceptions of a computer-based hospital information system: Differences across professional groups. Unpublished data.

[11] C.P. Alderfer, Improving organizational communication through long-term intergroup intervention, J. Appl. Behav. Sci. 13 (1977) 193–210.

[12] M.D. Hanlon, D. Nadler, and D. Gladstein, *Attempting Work Reform* (Wiley, New York, 1985), p. 41.

[13] N. Bjorn-Andersen, K. Eason, and D. Robey, *Managing Computer Impact* (Ablex Publishing Corporation, Norwood, NJ, 1986).

11B
Introducing Physician Order Entry at a Major Academic Medical Center: Impact on Medical Education

Thomas A. Massaro

Introduction

The introduction of an information technology (IT) system that mandates order entry by physicians had significant and often unexpected effects on medical education at the University of Virginia Medical Center. The system was deactivated briefly after the introduction of laboratory ordering, and frustration with the pharmacy ordering pathways provoked a major confrontation between the residents and medical center management. With time and experience, however, the housestaff have adjusted to the system and developed facility in using it. Much of the dissatisfaction was derived from the perception that "doctors spend too much time on the computer." In fact, less than 10% of the physicians spent more than an hour each day. However, a small group of residents on call for the busier services were sometimes at the computer for more than four hours each day. Changes in responsibilities, patterns, and priorities of work introduced by the system also contributed significantly to the general dissatisfaction. These issues had not been thoroughly considered in the planning stage, but it was only after accommodation was made to these changes that integration of the technology into routine practice could proceed. The chapter emphasizes the importance of extensive involvement and leadership of attending physicians in the planning and implementation of such a system. It presents a set of recommendations to those considering similar IT initiatives and wishing to reduce the disruptions that may accompany their introduction (Academic Medicine 68 (1993) 25–30).

Considerable attention has been focussed on the application of information technology (IT) to medical education [1–3]. Far less attention, however, has been paid to the influence of IT packages introduced into the patient care environment for administrative purposes, even though these can have broad and sometimes unsuspected influences on teaching activities. Since large IT packages represent major institutional investments and are often custom-configured during the procurement process, it is important that medical educators understand the potential tension that can arise between the requirements of an IT system and a school's educational mission, and participate fully in decisions regarding selection and implementation of these systems.

This chapter describes the introduction into a major teaching hospital of a system mandating order entry by physicians, outlines the difficulties that occurred, discusses the consequences for residents and medical students, and offers a set of organizational recommendations for the successful implementation of such a system in an educational setting.

Background

The University of Virginia (UVA) Medical Center serves as the primary training facility for the 560 medical students and over 500 residents of the UVA Medical School. In 1982, the hospital's executive board (primarily the chairs of the various clinical departments) approved a recommendation to proceed with a medical information system (MIS) featuring mandatory physician order entry. A cost savings of $26.3 million over five years was projected from time-and-motion studies of the activities of nurses and allied care providers. Unfortunately, a corresponding calculation of *additional* physician time was not included in that analysis, but this discrepancy was not appreciated until the selection process was reviewed several years later.

A physicians' advisory board was established to oversee the implementation process in 1984. This group, which included representatives of the housestaff, met regularly under two different chairs and involved a constantly changing membership for several years in the processes of reviewing and approving screen designs, ordering pathways, and operating protocols.

Early in 1988, the first hospital-wide implementation that involved physicians—enabling them to use the computer to give orders for dietary and radiology procedures—was initiated with little difficulty. Later that year, the system was expanded so that orders could be given and results retrieved for laboratory functions also. The initial responses of the housestaff were negative, and these functions were deactivated almost immediately by the center's administration. Computing services personnel worked closely with the housestaff to accommodate their concerns, and the system was reactivated after a three-week downtime.

In July 1989, pharmacy-order communication was implemented, with much stronger opposition from the housestaff. Residents appealed to their chairs and/or program directors, and medical students petitioned the dean for relief from the restrictions imposed on them by the system. In contradistinction to the deactivation of 1988, however, the system remained operational while these problems were discussed. Dissatisfaction peaked in June 1990, when a work action was initiated by a group of the most frus-

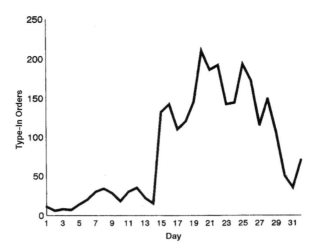

FIGURE 11B.1. Volume of typed-in pharmacy orders (during a residents' 1990 work action at the University of Virginia Medical Center) to avoid placing orders electronically. Type-in orders are far more labor-intensive for the pharmacy staff to fill than are the electronically generated requests.

trated residents. The electronically processed pharmacy-order pathways were bypassed and an optional type-in mode was chosen. (Type-in orders required considerably more processing time in the pharmacy and placed extraordinary demands on the pharmacists, who were throughout very active and enthusiastic supporters of the MIS.) During the peak of the type-in demonstration, 250 orders were generated in the type-in mode, compared with a baseline of no more than 10 to 20 (see Figure IIB.1).

Later that month, in a confrontational open meeting called to discuss the type-in action, many physicians reiterated their displeasure with the system and demanded it be shut down. Senior members of the medical administration stressed the system's strategic importance and reaffirmed their decision to keep it operational. At the time, it was unclear whether additional work actions would be attempted. As it turned out, this public demonstration of frustration and anger, with the countering statement of resolve by management, was the apogee of the resistance to the system. After this meeting, type-ins were discontinued and residents resumed normal ordering procedures. A few days later, the new class of housestaff arrived and were oriented to the system with few difficulties.

In July, a fax-based alternative to physician entry of medication orders was introduced as a pilot on three patient care units [4–6]. Copies of handwritten routine orders were transmitted directly to the pharmacy, where they were entered into the MIS by pharmacy personnel. The fax option initially captured 22% of the orders processed on the pilot floor, but after three months of operation the proportion was down to 2–3%.

Perhaps the most effective innovation during this time was the introduction of departmental and personal order sets (POSs), which allow groups of frequently associated orders to be bundled together for speed and efficiency. Department order sets are developed and utilized by the appropriate service and are maintained by computing services. Personal order sets allow each physician to generate customized groupings of his or her own personal orders on an ad hoc basis.

The academic year 1990–91 passed with no major incidents and by July 1991 the attitude toward the MIS had changed appreciably. New residents were oriented with the help of experienced senior residents and immediately accepted the MIS as part of the practice environment. They quickly developed POSs and acquired facility in using the system to do so. By June 1992, 273 residents had generated 2684 POSs, and a resident-led oversight committee reviewed the POS files and reduced the total to 545 with no problem from their peers [7].

Analysis

From the beginning, almost without exception, the residents complained that they spent too much time "on the computer." In fact, usage data generated during the most difficult period indicated that fewer than 10% of the physicians spent more than 60 minutes during a 24-hour day. It was clear, however, that a small number of residents spent much longer intervals at the terminals. It was equally clear that "excessive" time is much more a function of rotation and/or rotation design than anything else. On those rotations where the junior residents were responsible for entering the majority of orders, terminal times were very high. Figures IIB.2 and IIB.3 show characteristics of usage patterns and breakdowns of efforts. The major impact of the system was clearly on first-year residents. The repeating patterns of long periods of time spent at computer terminals corresponded almost perfectly with the interns' call schedules on specific rotations and services.

The usage pattern of two general surgery interns (Figure IIB.4) is a dramatic but not isolated demonstration of that high-usage phenomenon. Unfortunately, this pattern continues to the present for most of the residents. Figure IIB.4 gives the terminal time data for the new residents' turnover period in June 1991. The number of residents spending over two hours on the MIS increased significantly after June 23, the first day of service for new housestaff.

Medical students were also affected. They received MIS training and passwords, but their pharmacy and laboratory orders were "suspended," to be activated only by the intervention of a licensed physician. While this was not in principle different from pre-MIS procedure, in practice it had several significant ramifications that, in the eyes of the students, reduced the teaching they received on the floors.

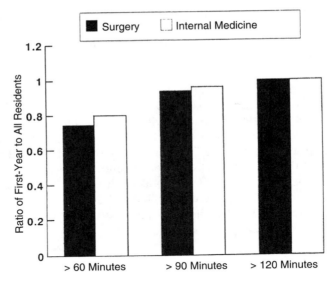

FIGURE 11B.2. Characteristic amount of use of a medical information service by residents in two specialties at the University of Virginia Medical Center, expressed as ratios of first-year residents' use to all residents' use for three lengths of time. The first-year students use the system much more than do the other residents.

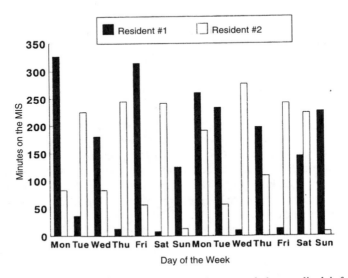

FIGURE 11B.3. Influence of call schedule on the use of the medical information system by residents at the University of Virginia Medical Center in 1990. The figure indicates how two general surgery residents used the system on an every-other-night call rotation over a two-week period.

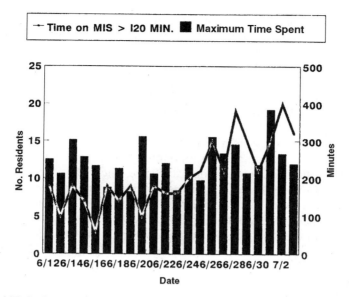

FIGURE 11B.4. Graph showing how use of the University of Virginia Medical Center's medical information system increases as new residents enter service. The bars represent maximum time the residents use the system each day. The graph line indicates the number of residents who are using the system for more than two hours.

A common complaint was that the suspend mode of the MIS system took them out of the ordering loop. Before the MIS system was used, medical students prepared the treatment plans and wrote the orders, which were then cosigned by the resident following a discussion of the plan. With the MIS, it was far less efficient for the resident to go over the suspended orders proposed by the student (which were at various levels in different pathways throughout the system) than it had been to go over handwritten orders on a single sheet. A simple modification could become a time-consuming operation. Thus, the ability of the medical student to help (i.e., save time for) the resident was compromised. In the end, the resident had less time available. As a result, some of the opportunities for teaching, provided on a quid-pro-quo basis for the time saved by the student, were lost.

Another important relationship that was disrupted by the MIS was that between the attending physician and the residents and/or students on the physician's service, Clinical training is in large part based on role-modeling and example-giving, journeyman to apprentice. The MIS turned that upside down. With a few exceptions, attending physicians generally do not place orders themselves and, therefore, do not routinely become adept at doing so. As a result, they could offer no guidance to their trainees. Thus, the residents were faced with a substantive practice problem in which they had more experience than their mentors. The frustration of faculty unable to offer appropriate guidance to trainees was directed at the MIS and to the administrators who had implemented it. This led to a further isolation of the MIS operation. The MIS became even more the administrators' system—"their" problem—and "they" had to fix it.

Technically, the MIS operation functions well; 99.99% of all physician-initiated transactions are processed in much less than one second. The system is off-line for approximately 20 minutes per day between 3:00 AM and 4:00 AM to allow for data to be downloaded to storage. Unscheduled downtime for 1990 and 1991 was less than 12 hours per year, which is really quite impressive for a system of that size.

But physicians entering large amounts of data in the form of orders expect more than data-processing excellence. They want the system to be simple and effortless. In the jargon, they want user-friendliness, that is, easy and flexible conformability to individual practice patterns and styles. Over 95% of our medical students had familiarity with personal computers and expected similar ease of use from the mainframe-based MIS system. One of the perceptions that hindered the early acceptance of the MIS was that there were much friendlier systems "out there" and that "they" had purchased the "wrong one." Only after several attending physicians became knowledgeable about the industry—long after the problems with pharmacy-order entry erupted—and reported that, at least at that time, there was no commercially available system that offered substantially greater flexibility and friendliness did this issue subside.

In reality, the modeling of physician behaviors is not straightforward. Osheroff and colleagues have reported on inquiries of internal medicine residents on rounds [8], but there are major differences in information needs and uses across specialties and levels of training. The first and perhaps second generation of MISs have been developed primarily for administrative functionality without significant involvement of physicians. Perhaps one of the most significant benefits of the MIS to UVA is that we now have several hundred physicians prepared to enter into a dialogue about how physician-friendly IT should be configured.

Discussion

The issue of time is real for the residents, especially for those few individuals on the high-volume services. By almost any criteria, the times recorded in Figures IIB.2, IIB.3, and IIB.4 are excessive. And they are probably an underestimation of the time an on-call resident spends, since they are based on a 24-hour calendar day and not the morning-to-morning schedule of the typical call rotation.

Absolute comparisons, however, are difficult. Unfortunately, there are no good data to indicate how much time a busy resident on a traditional non-computerized service spends writing orders in a chart or phoning the lab for a blood gas result. There is certainly no cataloging of the time lost searching for misplaced records or having to take the elevator from the operating room to the intensive care unit to write admission orders. As pressures build to reduce the time demands on housestaff, an understanding of the time costs of various components of their workload would be very useful information. It would also make possible comparisons of before-and-after changes as "invasive" technologies are introduced.

Although, in principle, there were potential practice options that could have relieved the major impact on the few vulnerable interns (e.g., redistribute assignments, modify coverage, and similar measures), these alternatives were never realistically considered. Organizations tend to resist change and to confine the change to as limited an area as possible. The universal consensus was to attempt to find IT answers to IT questions. Departmental and personal order sets were successful because they were seen as computer-based solutions to computer-generated problems. Restructuring residents' work assignments would have meant adopting a non-IT response to an IT challenge. That went too far in extending the potential option-set into areas that were outside the acceptable range, that is, that were not directly related to the computer system.

In our setting, the MIS required physicians to behave differently. The MIS was viewed as an administrative initiative, imposed from the "outside," with no real sponsorship in the medical community. All the energies that they normally would direct at a hostile outside threat were directed at rected at the MIS.

The MIS-imposed changes were perceived by the physicians as a loss. They responded in ways consistent with Elisabeth Kübler-Ross's stages of grieving and accommodation to misfortune [9]. Their initial reaction prior to and during the initial phase of implementation was one of almost complete denial: "This isn't going to happen to us." Although the process of order entry had been described to the physician community, neither the attending physicians nor the resident staff acknowledged the changes that the MIS required. Their anger was unmistakable—a clear and protracted phase: "How could you do this to us?" The anger ultimately led to bargaining, as "both sides" began to understand the other's predicament and to maneuver for position and control. As the irreversibility of the implementation became clearer (i.e., after the June 1990 confrontation), the residents became disenchanted and depressed. Some of that lingers, but overall this appears to have been a necessary prodrome to the ultimate accommodation and acceptance that have occurred recently. Although today's MIS is technically very similar to that first implemented three years earlier, it has been integrated into the practice environment of the hospital and is no longer a source of great controversy for the medical community. The change, accompanied by a sense of loss to those most involved, has been accommodated and a new equilibrium has been established.

Clearly, one of the major dissatisfiers with the time spent was that it represented effort in "non–physician-related" activities, especially regarding the order-entry functions. (Technically, these systems are known as order-entry and results-retrieval systems.) But physicians understand the need for data in making clinical decisions. As a result, the retrieval process was less of an issue. Most of the debate centered on the ordering component, but there are no physician role models for "point-of-care" order entry. Residents were forced to absorb duties previously performed by clerical staff, and they resented it. The order of priorities, the pecking order, had been changed. Physicians and physicians-in-training no longer had the positions of primacy in the healthcare information process. With time, the harshness of these initial interpretations appears to have softened. The general outlines of the restructuring are now accepted and have become the basis for the current operating procedures on the various units.

Conclusions and Recommendations

In retrospect, the lack of broad and committed attending physician involvement and direction prior to implementation was the biggest single source of problems for the housestaff. Although both residents and attending physicians were involved in the advisory committee, this group functioned like any other hospital advisory committee, supporting a general overview and providing a forum for discussion of procedural issues. But no one in the group really understood the magnitude of the behavioral changes that would be required or the time that would be demanded of the few unfortunate residents on the high-volume services. It was unreasonable to expect the housestaff to anticipate the problems for themselves or to have the institutional acumen to coordinate the necessary compromises and solutions. Residents are relative short-termers in the hospital setting; their input and insight are valuable, but should be used to supplement, not supplant, involvement for long-term faculty. Thus, our first recommendation is to develop a group of clinically respected internal advocates within the attending physician population who know the system and are aware of the associated requirements.

It is not obvious how that level of involvement could have been generated at UVA. The clinical chairs who formally approved the package were told that it would require physicians to interact closely with the computer at the time of the procurement decision, but they had no idea of the scope of this interaction. Most of them had spent time with the consultants prior to the procurement phase and had discussed the future opportunities that computers offered to medicine in general and their specialties in particular. They had received no return visit describing the practical limitations of the available options under consideration. The second recommendation, therefore, is to undersell the proposed system, keep under control everyone's expectations of it, and solicit support for the short-term implementation effort and long-term success of the endeavor.

Had our chairs understood the effort involved, they might have committed the faculty time necessary to develop the skills required and, had the faculty time been so committed, we might have looked more closely at the practice behaviors we were about to instigate. Ideally, this might have prevented some of the excesses seen in the time required for implementation. Even if these practice behaviors had not been modified in advance, we would have at the least understood the precomputer situation better. As a result, we would have been able to more effectively distinguish the problems residing in preexisting conditions from those stemming from the new system. Accordingly, we recommend studying the practice environment carefully, modifying and streamlining problematic operations before automation wherever possible. These early strategies provide important baseline information for evaluation later and also protect the IT team from the "slay-the-messenger syndrome," which is bound to occur in these circumstances. As a corollary, the implementation team should be prepared to stay the course once an operational decision has been carefully considered and made. Although the first impressions of an implementation may be negative, learning-curve advantages may overcome the initial problems and allow the benefits to become relatively more visible.

Finally, in the early stages we did not anticipate problems; we were often surprised by them and had no ready response or alternative prepared. Under these circumstances it is prudent to consider "What if . . . ?", to analyze the potential difficulties, to consider all possible options, and to understand the implications of each decision that may be required. This anticipatory anxiety is both appropriate and perhaps prophylactic in dealing with many of the significant organizational conflicts that are certain to accompany an undertaking as complicated and as invasive as the introduction of an MIS into the patient care environment of an academic medical center.

Acknowledgment. The author thanks James Perkins, Agnes Frankfurter, Reid Adams, Sharon Boyer, and Leah Wachsman for their insight and suggestions during this study.

References

[1] R.B. Haynes, M. Ramsden, K.A. McKibbon, C.J. Walker, and N.C. Ryan, A review of medical education and medical informatics, *Acad. Med.* 64 (1989) 207–212.
[2] J.W. Murphy, N.W. James, P.A. Williams, and R.S. Hillman, A residency-based information system, *Ann. Intern. Med.* 112 (1990) 961–963.
[3] P.A. Jennett et al., Preparing doctors for tomorrow: Information management as a theme in undergraduate medical education, *Med. Educ.* 25 (1991) 135–139.
[4] J.C. McAllister, Pharmacy fax, *Am. J. Hosp. Pharm.* 46 (1989) 255–256.

[5] B.J. Ellinoy, Fax fiction, *Am. J. Hosp. Pharm.* 46 (1989) 1549–1550.
[6] D.W. Joubert, The case for fax machines, *Am. J. Hosp. Pharm.* 46 (1989) 2461–2462.
[7] M. Nadkarni, W.T. Stevenson, J.O. Perkins, and T.A. Massaro, "Enhancement of personal order set use by residents in a university hospital environment," presented at *MISPA, 8th International Conference*, San Francisco, C (October 1992).
[8] J.A. Osheroff et al., Physicians' information needs: Analysis of questions posed during clinical teaching, *Ann. Intern. Med.* 114 (1991) 567–581.
[9] E. Kübler-Ross, *On Death and Dying* (Macmillan, New York, 1979).

12
Evaluating the Capability of Information Technology to Prevent Adverse Drug Events: A Computer Simulation Approach

JAMES G. ANDERSON, STEPHEN J. JAY, MARILYN M. ANDERSON, and THADDEUS J. HUNT

Introduction

The annual cost of morbidity and mortality due to medication errors in the United States has been estimated at $76.6 billion. Information technology implemented systematically has the potential to significantly reduce medication errors that result in adverse drug events (ADEs). A computer simulation model was developed that can be used to evaluate the effectiveness of information technology applications designed to detect and prevent medication errors that result in adverse drug effects.

A computer simulation model was constructed representing the medication delivery system in a hospital. STELLA, a continuous simulation software package, was used to construct the model. Parameters of the model were estimated from a study of prescription errors on two hospital medical/surgical units and used in the baseline simulation. Five prevention strategies were simulated based on information obtained from the literature.

The model simulates the four stages of the medication delivery system: prescribing, transcribing, dispensing, and administering drugs. We simulated interventions that have been demonstrated in prior studies to decrease error rates. The results suggest that an integrated medication delivery system can save up to 1226 days of excess hospitalization and $1.4 million in associated costs annually in a large hospital. The results of the analyses regarding the effects of the interventions on the additional hospital costs associated with ADEs are somewhat sensitive to the distribution of errors in the hospital, more sensitive to the costs of an ADE, and most sensitive to the proportion of medication errors resulting in ADEs.

The results suggest that clinical information systems are potentially a cost-effective means of preventing ADEs in hospitals and demonstrate the importance of viewing medication errors from a systems perspective. Prevention efforts that focus on a single stage of the process had limited impact on the overall error rate. This study suggests that system-wide changes to the medication delivery system are required to drastically reduce mediation errors that may result in ADEs in a hospital setting.

Based on the Harvard Medical Practice study of 51 hospitals in the state of New York [1,2] and a sample of hospitals in Utah and Colorado [3], the Institute of Medicine (IOM) estimated that between 44,000 and 98,000 deaths occur in the United States each year as a result of medical errors [4]. Although the exact number of deaths due to medical errors is a subject of debate [5,6], meta-analyses of 39 prospective studies performed in the United States between 1966 and 1996 indicated that even when drugs are properly prescribed and administered, adverse drug reactions may rank between the fourth and seventh leading cause of deaths in the United States, exceeding car accidents, suicide, homicide, or AIDS [7].

The Harvard Medical Practice study found that the top cause of adverse events in hospitalized patients was drug complications, which accounted for 19 percent of the adverse events [2]. An ADE is defined as "an injury resulting from medical intervention related to a drug" [8]. A recent study found that the rate of ADEs was 6.5 per 100 hospital admissions. Errors were detected at every stage of the process: ordering (56%), transcription (6%), dispensing (4%), and administration (34%) [8,9]. The severity of the adverse drug events was 1% fatal, 12% life-threatening, 30% serious, and 57% significant. Other studies of hospitals in Utah and Colorado [3], pediatric inpatients [10], and hospital intensive care units [11], have also found high rates of ADEs.

Deaths due to medication errors in the United States may be increasing. One study found a 2.57-fold increase in deaths attributed to medication errors between 1983 and 1993 [12]. One factor that may account for this increase is the shift from inpatient to outpatient care [13]. During this decade, inpatient days fell by 21 percent while outpatient visits increased by 75%.

Studies of hospitalized patients indicate that serious adverse drug events increase the length of hospital stay and costs. One study estimated the additional length of stay associated with an ADE was 2.2 days; the increase in cost associated with an ADE was $3,244 [14]. Based on these costs and incidence rates of ADEs, it was estimated that the annual costs attributed to all ADEs for a 700-bed hospital were $5.6 million. A second study conducted at LDS Hospital in Salt Lake City estimated that the extra length of hospital stay attributable to an ADE was 1.74 days, whereas the extra cost of hospitalization was estimated to be $2,013 per patient [15]. During one year of the study a total of 567 ADEs were detected. The direct hospital costs associated with these ADEs were $1.1 million. Over the four years of the study excess hospital costs due to ADEs were estimated at $4.5 million. The total annual cost of morbidity and mortality due to drug-related errors in the United States has been estimated at $76.6 billion [16].

Most hospitals rely on voluntary reporting, which may result in the detection and reporting of only 5% to 10% of ADEs [17–20]. At the same time, the increasing availability of computerized information systems in hospitals makes it possible to develop and implement automated surveillance systems to detect ADEs [21–23]. Moreover, computerized physician order entry systems reduce medication errors and may reduce adverse drug event rates [24–29].

In healthcare settings efforts to reduce errors traditionally have focused on training rules and sanctions. In contrast, a human factors approach advocates changing the system to reduce the likelihood that an error will occur and to permit the detection and intervention before the error causes harm to a patient [9,30]. From this perspective errors can be viewed as a measure of the quality of the medication delivery system. As such, error rates are a measure of the rate of the system's failures [31].

Two studies of medication errors have used a systems approach. In a study of two hospitals in Boston, medical errors that resulted in adverse drug events or potential ADEs were classified according to proximal cause and underlying system failures [9]. Sixteen causes of system failures were identified, including lack of knowledge of the drug or the patient; transcription errors; faulty drug identification and dose checking; failure to check for allergies; and failure to track medication orders. Half of the 16 types of system failures could have been prevented by providing better, timelier information.

More recently, the Institute for Safe Medication Practices sponsored a nationwide test of hospital pharmacy systems to identify and prevent serious drug-related errors [32]. During the test, actual prescriptions that had caused serious injury or death to patients were entered into the system. Only a small percentage of errors were detected by the existing hospital pharmacy systems. Some of the system problems identified included lack of integration between the physician order entry and pharmacy systems, lack of integration between the laboratory and medication order systems, no clinical order screening capability, and complex order entry systems.

In the present study, we describe a computer simulation model that can be used to estimate the effectiveness of information system applications designed to detect and prevent medication errors that result in ADEs. The model was constructed using a systems approach that identifies components of the medication delivery system that make errors more likely to occur and more difficult to detect and prevent. It predicts the number of errors at each step in the medication delivery system, the number of associated ADEs, the extra number of days of hospitalization, and the excess costs of hospitalization attributable to ADEs.

Simulation was used because the medication delivery system in a hospital is complex and difficult to investigate in its entirety with more traditional methods. By building a computer model representing the system, we can simulate the behavior of the system over time and the effects of changes in the system's structure without disrupting the actual practice setting [33]. Several earlier studies have used simulation to study the causes of medical errors. One study used discrete event simulation to estimate transcription errors in order entry into a hospital information system [34]. Another study used a simulation system based on information processing theory to study errors in chemotherapy administration [35–36].

Methods

Hospital Setting

The study was performed in a large private teaching hospital. The hospital had implemented the TDS HC 4000 hospital information system. During hospitalization, all patient data were entered into the computer system, creating an electronic medical record. Nursing units were equipped with three to seven computer terminals linked to the HIS. Physicians, nurses, unit secretaries, and other authorized personnel entered and retrieved patient information using these terminals.

At the time of this study, 91% of medication orders were written by physicians. All written orders were transcribed and entered into the computerized hospital information system by hospital ward clerks. Physicians entered 9% of their orders directly into the system; ward clerks entered 81% of orders; other clinical personnel, such as physician assistants, entered the remaining 10%. Medication orders were printed out in a centralized pharmacy where the drugs were dispensed and transported to the wards for administration.

Data Collection

The quality assurance records for the previous 12 months in the central pharmacy were used to obtain initial data about the number of medication errors that were detected prior to this study by a voluntary reporting system. To collect baseline data about medication errors, a pharmacy committee designed a report form. A list of types of mediation errors was adapted from previous published studies [37–41]. An experienced registered pharmacist was assigned fulltime to the project to supervise and assist with the data collection on two medial/surgical units. During the day and evening shift for a 12-week period, every medication order written by a physician and entered into the HIS by a unit secretary was verified. A total of 6966 drug orders were reviewed. When an error was detected, the pharmacist completed a form that identified the prescribing physician, unit secretary and/or nurse involved with the order, the nature of the incident, and the action taken to correct the error. When necessary, the physician who wrote the order was contacted. Hospital pharmacists were also available for

TABLE 12.1. Types of errors detected on two hospital units.

Type of error	Four North (%)	Four South (%)
Prescription	13	15
Transcription	85	81
Dispensation	0	2
Administration	2	2
Total	100	100

consultation on the units during the day and evening shifts. They recorded information about all consultations. No chart reviews were performed in this study, nor was it possible to study actual adverse drug events that occurred in the hospital.

Analysis

A classification scheme was developed to classify the types of medication errors and their severity [37–41]. During the previous 12 month period, only 48 medication errors or one error per 1000 drug orders were reported throughout the entire hospital under the voluntary reporting system. During the 12-week study period when all drug orders on the two hospital units were reviewed, pharmacists detected 227 errors. This represented a rate of 32 errors per 1000 orders. Rates of medication errors for the two hospital units are shown in Table 12.1.

On Four North, 85% of the errors were made in transcribing the physicians' orders and entering them into the medical information system. Physicians made errors in writing prescriptions in 13% of cases. The other 2% of errors were made in administering medications.

On the second Unit, Four South, 81% of the errors involved transcription of drug orders by ward clerks. Physicians' prescription errors amounted to 15%, whereas errors in dispensing and administering medications each amounted to 2% of the total errors.

Medication errors were classified by their potential severity (Table 12.2). On both hospital units, over 70% of the errors were classified as problem orders. Orders were classified as problems if they involved duplicate

TABLE 12.2. Severity of medication errors detected on two medical/surgical hospital units.

Severity	Four North (%)	Four South (%)
Problem	76	72
Significant	18	18
Potentially serious	6	6
Potentially fatal	0	4
Total	100	100

therapy without the potential for adverse effects on the patient; lacked specific dose, dosage strength, route, or frequency information that would not have harmed the patient; or an incorrect order was written that was unlikely to be carried out.

Eighteen percent of the errors on both units were potentially significant. Potentially significant errors involved orders that specified a high dose of 1.4 to 4 times the normal dose of a medication that had the potential for an adverse effect; the dose was inadequate to produce the intended therapeutic effects; an illegible order, wrong medication or wrong route was specified that may have resulted in adverse effects or inadequate therapy.

Six percent of the medication errors were potentially serious. These errors might have resulted in serious toxic reactions or inadequate therapy for a serious illness. Medication errors classified as potentially serious included a high dose of a medication 4 to 10 times the normal dose that potentially would have resulted in a serious toxic reaction; a dose ordered for a drug used for a serious illness that was too low for a patient; the wrong medication was ordered with the potential for a serious toxic reaction; an illegible order or duplicate order with the potential for a serious toxic reaction.

The last category of medication errors was potentially fatal and might have resulted in the death of the patient. On Four South, 4% of the errors were classified into this category. Potentially fatal errors included an order for a medication with a low therapeutic index that was greater than ten times the normal dose; a dose of a medication that would potentially result in pharmacologic effects or serum concentrations associated with fatal toxic reactions; a drug that had the potential to produce a life-threatening reaction in the patient; and a dose of a lifesaving drug that was too low for the patient.

The coding of the types of errors and their severity was verified by a second registered pharmacist to ensure reliability. Also, similar results obtained on two separate medical/surgical units provide additional evidence of the reliability of the estimates of error rates used in this study.

The Computer Simulation Model

Simulation

A dynamic computer simulation model was constructed to model hospital medication errors using STELLA, a graphically based, continuous simulation software package [42,43]. Continuous simulation models are used when the system under investigation consists of a continuous flow of information, material, resources, or individuals and the system is dynamic, changing over time [33]. The system under investigation is characterized in terms of state variables and control variables. State variables indicate the status of important characteristics of the system at each point in time. Examples of these variables include people, other resources, and information, such as the cumulative number of medication orders that have been written on a hospital unit at any time during the simulation. Control variables are rates of change and update the value of state variables in each time period. An example of a control variable is the number of new medications orders written per time period.

Components of the system are dynamic, may interact with each other, and may involve positive and negative feedback processes. The current model assumes that error rates at the prescription and transcription stage change nonlinearly over the period of time modeled as more physicians adopt interventions one and two. When relationships are nonlinear, the system may exhibit complex, dynamic behavior over time. The mathematical model that underlies the simulation usually consists of a set of differential or finite difference equations. Numerical solutions of the equations that make up the model allow investigators to construct and test models that cannot be solved analytically.

The model, shown in Figure 12.1, assumes that medication orders are written or directly entered into the hospital information system by physicians. Written orders are transcribed by ward clerks on the medical-surgical units. Once entered medication orders are transmitted directly to a central pharmacy where they are printed. After a check by a pharmacist, medications are dispensed and transported to the nursing unit. Registered nurses administer the medications to the patient.

The simulation begins by generating 4060 medication orders, the average number of medication orders written by physicians each week on 14 hospital medical/surgical units. Based on the analysis of medication orders on the two hospital units, it was assumed that error rates at each stage of the process were variable and distributed normally. Means and standard deviations for error rates are shown in Table 12.3.

For example, at the prescription stage the error rate applied to the new medication orders is generated randomly from a normal distribution with a mean error rate of 4.6 errors per 1000 medication orders and a standard deviation of 2.0. Orders without prescription errors move to the transcription stage, where a random error rate based on a mean of 27.0 transcription errors per 1000 orders and a standard deviation of 10 is applied to the orders. This process is repeated for the dispensing and administration stages. The model assumes that an error that occurs at one stage of the process (e.g., prescription) does not propagate through the system, causing compound errors or multiple errors on the same drug order.

The model assumes that on the average an ADE results in 2.2 additional days of hospitalization. The cost of the additional days of hospitalization was estimated to be $2,595 on average. These estimates were based on the results of two published studies [14–15].

Two estimates were made of the number of ADEs and associated excess days of hospitalization and associated costs. The higher estimate assumed

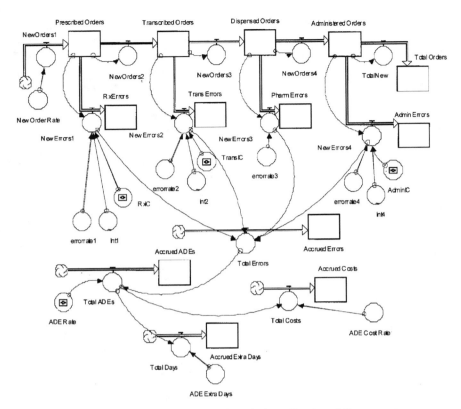

FIGURE 12.1. Systems model of a hospital medication delivery system.

that 26% of the medication errors that could have resulted in serious toxic reactions or inadequate treatment would have resulted in ADEs if not detected and corrected. The low estimate assumed that only the 8% of drug errors that were potentially serious or fatal if undetected would have resulted in ADEs.

The simulation was run for a 52-week period with these baseline parameter estimates. Next, five strategies designed to reduce medication errors and potential ADEs were simulated for the same period of time.

TABLE 12.3. Error rates per 1000 medication orders.

Stage	Mean	SD
Prescription	4.6	2.0
Transcription	27.0	10.0
Dispensing	4.3	2.0
Administration	5.7	2.0

Simulation of Prevention Strategies

First, the actual medication delivery system in the hospital was simulated, using the error rates obtained from the pharmacy study. Next, four simulations were performed with hypothetical changes in the system designed to prevent medication errors. Error rates for these simulations were obtained from the literature. Finally, a fifth simulation was performed assuming changes were made at all four stages of the process in order to prevent medication errors from occurring.

Intervention 1: Provision of Information at the Prescribing Stage

The first intervention involved computerized prescribing. Errors may occur at every stage of the medication process, but our study and others indicated that a significant number of errors are made during ordering. These errors are most likely to result in serious adverse drug events. Efforts to change physician decisionmaking regarding the prescription of drugs, such as dissemination of educational material, lectures, and drug detailing by clinical pharmacists and consultation, have had short-term success [44]. Computerized prescribing systems are potentially more effective.

The first intervention simulated was the implementation of a computer-based system that provides dosing information about drugs at the time orders are written. Such a system decreases the likelihood that an error will occur by facilitating access to information at the time the physician orders medications. Based on the low physician use of the order entry feature of the HIS at this hospital, the model assumes that over the course of one year, 50% of the physicians will gradually adopt the system in ordering medications and that this would result in an overall 20% reduction in prescription errors. It was also assumed that error rates at the other stages of the process would remain the same as in the baseline simulation.

Intervention 2: Physician Computer Order Entry

The second intervention involved computerized physician order entry. Many hospitals in the United States utilize ward clerks, unit secretaries or nurses to enter physician orders into computer-based information systems. At the same time, direct physician order entry into the system can significantly reduce medication errors by reducing transcription errors due to the illegibility of written orders [45].

This study found that ward clerks made over 80% of the errors in transcribing physicians' written orders. Anderson and others [46] demonstrated that by encouraging physicians to develop personal order sets, the percentage of medical orders directly entered into the medical information system could be significantly increased in a teaching hospital. An earlier computer simulation estimated that elimination of the need for transcription of medical orders could reduce errors by as much as 40% [34]. One study at Brigham and Woman's Hospital found that if all medical orders were entered online by physicians, 58% of all adverse events would be identifiable and potentially avoidable [8].

The second intervention involved the implementation of a physician order entry system that permitted physicians to enter their own orders directly into the hospital information system. Because it was assumed that by the end of the first year of implementation only 50% of the drug orders would be directly entered into the information system by physicians, it was assumed that the overall transcription error rate would be reduced by 30%.

Intervention 3: Pharmacy System

The third intervention involved the implementation of a unit dosing system. Pharmacy medication systems such as unit dosing can reduce medication errors. These systems dispense most medications from the pharmacy in a single unit or unit-dose package that is ready to be administered to the patient. One study found that a unit dosing system reduced medication errors by over 80% [47,48]. Based on these studies the third intervention assumed that the implementation of a unit dosing system would reduce dispensing errors on average by 80%. Other rates for prescribing, transcribing, and administering medications were assumed to remain at baseline levels.

Intervention 4: Automated Medication Dispensing Systems

Bar-coding of medications can lead to a reduction in errors at the administration stage. This practice has the potential to eliminate most errors involving drug substitutions. It improves tracking of medications that are administered and when they are given [49]. The fourth intervention involved the implementation of a bar coding system to prevent errors frequently made in administering medications on the hospital units. It was assumed that such a system, once implemented, could reduce administration errors on average by 60%.

TABLE 12.4. Errors by stage of the medication delivery system.

Run	Prescription	Transcription	Dispensation	Administration	Total errors	Total orders
BL	948	5,220	868	1,099	8,136	195,392
1	747	5,063	853	1,050	7,714	195,286
2	1,016	4,050	881	1,151	7,099	195,245
3	924	5,352	247	998	7,523	195,324
4	931	5,457	842	451	7,680	195,268
5	747	4,055	836	354	5,993	195,196

TABLE 12.5. Rates of medication errors and ADEs per 1000 orders by intervention.

Run	Medication errors	ADEs Low estimate	ADEs High estimate
BL	41.6	3.3	10.8
1	39.5	3.4	10.3
2	38.3	2.8	9.4
3	38.5	3.2	10.0
4	39.3	2.9	10.2
5	30.7	2.4	7.9

Intervention 5: Comprehensive Medication Delivery System

Bates has outlined a comprehensive medication delivery system that would include many of the prevention strategies outlined [47,50]. The system would involve the use of a computerized order-entry system that would provide patient and medication information to the physician when medications are being prescribed. Direct order entry into the information system would significantly reduce transcription errors. The information system would transmit medication errors directly to the pharmacy where additional checks would be performed. Medications, as far as possible, would be dispensed at a point-of-care distribution system. When nurses administered a medication, they would scan a bar code to document that the correct medication had been administered. The fifth intervention involved implementation of all four strategies to prevent errors at each stage of the hospital medication process. All four error rates were modified based on the assumptions described above.

Results

The model was used to simulate the medication delivery system on 14 medical-surgical units in a teaching hospital. Tables 12.4 and 12.5 and Figures 12.2 through 12.7 show the results of the baseline run and the five

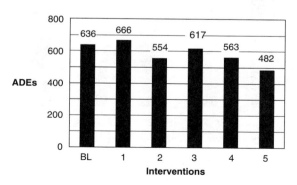

FIGURE 12.2. Estimated ADEs by intervention: low estimate.

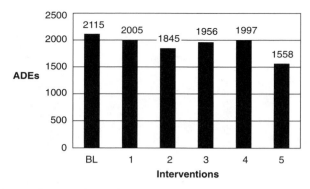

FIGURE 12.3. Estimated ADEs by intervention: high estimate.

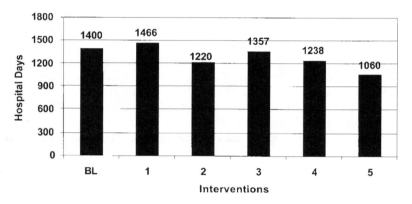

FIGURE 12.4. Estimated additional days of hospitalization by intervention: low estimate.

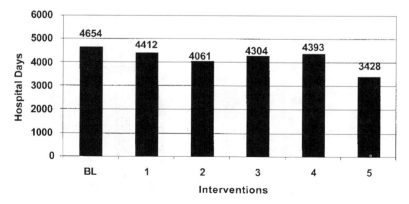

FIGURE 12.5. Estimated additional days of hospitalization by intervention: high estimate.

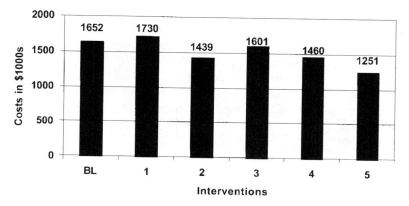

FIGURE 12.6. Estimated additional hospital costs by intervention: low estimate.

runs that simulate potential information system applications designed to prevent medication errors. The baseline simulation generated a total of 195,392 drug orders over a 52-week period. A little over 4% of these orders involved errors. Almost 64% of these errors were made in the transcription stage. The model estimated that medication errors, if undetected, would result in from 1400 to 2115 adverse drug events, a rate that ranges from 3.3 to 10.8 ADEs per 1000 medication orders. The resulting additional days of hospitalization were estimated to cost between $1.6 and $5.5 million per year.

A sensitivity analysis was performed on the baseline parameters. Prescription error rates were varied by ±20% with little effect on the outcomes of the simulation. Changes in the estimates of the total cost of the additional days of hospitalization that resulted from ADEs ranged from 2% to 5%. The model is more sensitive to the estimate of the average cost of the

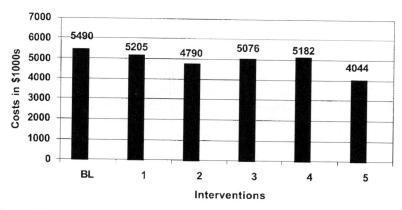

FIGURE 12.7. Estimated additional hospital costs by intervention: high estimate.

additional days of hospitalization due to ADEs. Using the cost estimate from the LDS hospital study, the model estimated that the annual cost of ADEs would be about $4.3 million, which is similar to the estimate of $4 million in our study. When the higher cost estimate from the Harvard study was used, annual costs were estimated to be $6.8 million. Finally the model estimates are most sensitive to the assumption concerning what percentage of errors that result in ADEs. Two percentages were used in this study, 8% and 26%.

The first intervention simulated was the implementation of a clinical information system that provides dosing information, parameters about drugs at the time orders are written, and warnings about excessive doses and drug–drug interactions. Such a system decreases the likelihood that an error will occur by facilitating access to information at the time that the physician orders drugs.

This intervention by itself failed to significantly reduce the overall error rate and ADE rate. While this intervention resulted in about a 21% reduction in prescription errors, total errors were only reduced by about 5%. The model predicts that as many as 2000 ADEs may occur resulting in 4412 excess days of hospitalization costing over $5.2 million annually.

The second intervention involved implementation of a physician order entry system. The simulation estimates that this strategy could reduce medication errors to 38.3 and ADEs to about 9.4 per 1000 medication orders. However, the total number of errors was reduced by only about 4%. Overall excess days of hospitalization could be reduced by as much as 600 days and the associated costs by as much as $213,000 to $700,000 annually.

The third intervention simulated involved the implementation of a unit dosing system in the central hospital pharmacy. These systems reduce medication errors by dispensing medications in a single unit or unit-dose package that is ready for administration to the patient. The model predicts that the implementation of a unit-dose system would reduce medication errors at the administration stage by only about 9%. The overall affect on the error rate and ADE rate is small. The model estimates that at most this intervention would reduce excess hospital days by 350 and annual costs by $413,442.

The fourth prevention strategy simulated involved bar-coding of medications. This intervention could reduce errors when medications are administered and provide more complete documentation of medications that are administered. The model estimates that this prevention strategy would reduce only slightly the overall medication error rate and associated ADEs. Days of hospitalization would be reduced by less than 300 and associated costs by about $300,000 or less annually.

The final run simulates the effects of implementing the comprehensive medication delivery system proposed by Bates [47,50]. The model estimates that errors would be reduced at all stages of the medication delivery system. Medication error rates and associated ADEs could be reduced by over

26%. It is estimated that a comprehensive information system could detect and prevent over 2000 medication errors a year. The final implementation of an information system would have a substantial effect reducing excess hospital days by 1226 and saving the hospital $1.4 million in related costs annually.

Discussion

This study estimated the effectiveness of several computerized information system applications designed to detect and prevent medication errors that result in ADEs. The cost-effectiveness of these systems needs to be documented since current voluntary reporting systems for ADEs detect only a fraction of such events [17–20]. The voluntary reporting system in the hospital that we studied detected only 1 medication error per 1000 drug orders. Our study revealed an error rate of 32 per 1000 medication orders. It was estimated that over 8000 medication errors occur on 14 medical-surgical units each year.

The study that we performed estimated the frequency and types of medication errors in a specific hospital. These rates were used in the model to estimate ADEs, additional days of hospitalization, and associated hospital costs. The distribution of types of errors found in this hospital differed from other published studies in part because of the method we used to detect medication errors and in part because of the use of minimally trained ward clerks to transcribe physicians' written orders.

Based on error rates from our study of medical/surgical units at the teaching hospital and published estimates of the effects of ADEs on length of stay and hospital costs, a computer simulation model was developed. The model estimated that, under the current system, ADEs annually result in from 1400 to 4654 days of extra hospitalization. From $1.6 to $5.5 million in annual excess hospital costs were estimated. The lower estimate of the effects of medication errors assumes that only the 8% of errors that might have led to serious toxic reactions, inadequate treatment, or death of the patient would have resulted in ADEs. The higher estimate assumes that the additional 18% of medication errors that involved omitted drugs, duplicate orders, or incorrect information also could have led to ADEs.

The model indicates that the implementation of a comprehensive medication delivery system designed to detect and prevent ADEs could save up to 1226 days of hospitalization and $1.4 million in hospital costs annually, even if it only prevented 26% of medication errors. These savings reflect only direct hospital costs. They do not include the additional costs of outpatient care, disability, and malpractice awards associated with ADEs. A recent study used the outpatient costs of ADEs to a managed care provider to project that these costs nationwide may be as high as $76.6 billion [16].

This study has several limitations. It was undertaken in only one teaching hospital in the Midwest. Consequently, the results may not be entirely generalizable to other hospitals with different medication delivery systems and information systems. However, the model is general. Therefore, error rates, ADE rates, and cost estimates can be modified to fit other institutions.

Medication error rates were determined by a 12-week study on two medical/surgical units by clinical pharmacists. However, resources were not available to perform chart audits or to investigate the actual adverse drug events that occurred in the hospital during this period. Consequently, we assumed that medication errors classified as potentially serious or fatal, if not detected and corrected, would have resulted in ADEs.

Moreover, we were unable to determine the exact number of additional days of hospitalization that occurred due to ADEs or the actual cost of the additional length of stay to the hospital. Instead we relied on estimates from two major published studies [14,15]. Despite these limitations, estimates of medication error rates, ADE rates, and estimated costs due to excess hospitalization are in line with those reported in other major studies.

The study assumed that serious medication errors would result in ADEs. In reality, some of these medication errors would have been corrected before the medication was administered to the patient. It was also assumed that errors at each stage had an equal chance of resulting in an ADE. This is probably not correct, but the exact proportions of errors at each stage that result in ADEs is not known. Also, the cost estimates in this study underestimate the true costs of ADEs. Only direct costs of hospitalization were estimated. Other costs include outpatient care, disability, legal fees, and malpractice awards resulting from ADEs.

Errors occur at every stage of the medication delivery system. Many result from systems failures and are not detected by the typical hospital self-reporting system. Moreover, this study indicated that systemwide changes to the process are required to significantly reduce medication errors in a hospital setting. Preventive efforts that focus solely on a single stage of the process have limited impact on the overall error rate. Bates and others suggest that clinical information systems that support the medication delivery system should be carefully designed and evaluated to ensure that they identify and prevent medication errors that result in ADEs [50]. Moreover, clinical information systems need to be combined with other prevention strategies to reduce ADEs even more. Our simulation estimated that even a systemwide implementation of information technology would reduce medication errors and associated ADEs by only about 26%. Studies indicate that several other approaches could be used in addition to the ones that we investigated.

One approach would be to significantly improve incident reporting of medical errors [20]. Healthcare providers need to be trained to recognize changes in a patient's medical condition that may indicate an ADE and encouraged to report them promptly. Also, healthcare institutions need to create an environment that encourages the reporting of medication errors and investigation of system, features that contributed to the error [51]. Another promising approach is to more fully incorporate clinical pharmacists into the provision of patient care [52]. At one hospital the participation of pharmacists in patient rounds on ICU units reduced the rate of ADEs from 33.0 to 11.6 per 1000 patient days, almost a two-thirds reduction [53]. This study demonstrates the importance of viewing adverse drug events from a systems perspective.

We conclude that the traditional medical approach to medication error prevention that relies on individual detection and voluntary reporting is reactive and largely ineffectual [54]. If hospitals are to reduce medication errors that lead to ADEs and associated unnecessary costs and days of hospitalization, they will have to recognize the multiplicity of reasons that errors occur at each stage of the medication delivery system. Computerized information systems are an important means of detecting errors in time to take corrective action to prevent ADEs. The results of this study suggest that information systems are potentially a cost-effective means of preventing ADEs in hospitals, especially when coupled with other proven prevention strategies.

Acknowledgments. The authors acknowledge the assistance of Munir Shah, MD, Michael Hamang, RPh, and the pharmacists in the Department of Pharmacy Services at Methodist Hospital of Indiana for their assistance in collecting the data for this study.

References

[1] T.A. Brennan, L.L. Leape, N.M. Laird et al., Incidence of adverse events and negligence in hospitalized patients, New England Journal of Medicine 324 (1991) 370–376.

[2] L.L. Leape, T.A. Brennan, N. Laird et al., The nature of adverse events in hospitalized patients: results of the Harvard medical practice study II, New England Journal of Medicine 324 (1991) 377–384.

[3] E.J. Thomas, D.M. Sudderth, H.R. Burstein et al., Incidence and types of adverse events and negligent care in Utah and Colorado, Medical Care 28 (2000) 261–271.

[4] L.T. Kohn, J.M. Corrigan, and M.S. Donaldson, editors, *To Err is Human: Building a Safer Health System* (National Academy Press, Washington, DC, 1999).

[5] C.J. McDonald, M. Weiner, and S.L. Hui, Deaths due to medical errors are exaggerated in Institute of Medicine report, JAMA 284 (2000) 93–95.

[6] L.L. Leape, Institute of Medicine medical error figures are not exaggerated [comment], JAMA 284 (2000) 95–97.

[7] J. Lazarou, B.H. Pomeranz, and P.N. Corey, Incidence of adverse drug reactions in hospitalized patients: A meta-analysis of prospective studies, JAMA 279 (1998) 1200–1205.

[8] D.W. Bates, D.J. Cullen, N. Laird et al., Incidence of adverse drug events and potential adverse drug events, JAMA 274 (1995) 29–34.

[9] L.L. Leape, D.W. Bates, D.J. Cullen et al., Systems analysis of adverse drug events, JAMA 274 (1995) 35–43.

[10] R. Koushal, D.W. Bates, C. Landrigan et al., Medication errors and adverse drug events in pediatric inpatients, JAMA 285 (2001) 2114–2120.

[11] D.J. Cullen, B.J. Sweitzer, D.W. Bates et al., Preventable adverse drug events in hospitalized patients: A comparative study of intensive care and general care units, Crit Care Med. 25 (1997) 1289–1297.

[12] D.P. Phillips, N. Christenfeld, and L.M. Glynn, Increase in U.S. medication-error deaths between 1983 and 1993, Lancet 351 (1998) 643–644.

[13] B. Honigman, J. Lee, J. Rothschild et al., Using computerized data to identify adverse drug events in outpatients, Journal of the American Medical Informations Association 8 (2001) 254–266.

[14] D.W. Bates, N.S. Spell, D.J. Cullen et al., The costs of adverse drug events in hospitalized patients, JAMA 277 (1997) 307–311.

[15] D.C. Classen, S.L. Pestotnik, R.S. Evans et al., Adverse drug events in hospitalized patients: Excess length of stay, extra costs, and attributable mortality, JAMA 277 (1997) 301–306.

[16] J.A. Johnson and J.L. Bootman, Drug-related morbidity and mortality: a cost of illness model, Arch Intern Med. 155 (1995) 1949–1956.

[17] L.L. Berry, R. Segal, T.P. Sherrin, and K.A. Fudge, Sensitivity and specificity of three methods of detecting adverse drug relations, American Journal of the Hospital Pharmacy 45 (1988) 1534–1539.

[18] A.C. O'Neil, L.A. Petersen, E.F. Cook et al., A comparison of physicians self-reporting with medical record reviews to identify medical adverse events, Annals of Internal Medicine 119 (1993) 370–376.

[19] E.A. Chrischilles, E.T. Seager, and R.B. Wallace, Self-reported adverse drug reactions and related resource use, Annals of Internal Medicine 117 (1992) 634–640.

[20] D.J. Cullen, D.W. Bates, S.D. Small et al., The incident reporting system does not detect adverse drug events: A problem for quality improvement, Journal of Quality Improvement 21 (1995) 541–548.

[21] D.C. Classen, S.L. Pestotnik, R.S. Evans, and J.P. Burke, Computerized surveillance of adverse drug events in hospital patients, JAMA 266 (1991) 2847–2851.

[22] D.W. Bates, A.C. O'Neil, D. Boyle et al., Potential identifiability and preventability of adverse events using information systems, JAMIA 1 (1994) 404–411.

[23] A.K. Jha, G.J. Kuperman, and J.M. Teich et al., Identifying adverse drug effects: Development of a computer-based monitor and comparison with chart review and simulated voluntary report, Journal of the American Medical Information Association 5 (1998) 305–314.

[24] R.S. Evans, S.L. Pestotnik, D.C. Classen et al., Prevention of adverse drug events through computerized surveillance, in: *Proceedings of the Annual Symposium on Computer Applications in Medical Care* (1993), pp. 161–165.

[25] R.S. Evans, S.L. Pestotnik, D.C. Classen et al., A computer-assisted management program for antibiotics and other antiinfective agents, New England Journal of Medicine 338 (1998) 232–238.

[26] D.W. Bates, L.L. Leape, and D.J. Cullen, Effect of computerized physician order entry and a team intervention on prevention of serious medication errors, JAMA 280 (1998) 1311–1316.

[27] D.W. Bates, J.M. Teich, J. Lee et al., The impact of computerized physician order entry on medication error prevention. Journal of the American Medical Informations Association 6 (1999) 313–321.

[28] R.A. Raschke, B. Collihare, T.A. Wundertlich et al., A computer alert system to prevent injury from adverse drug events, JAMA 280(15) (1998) 1317–1320.

[29] Agency for Healthcare Research and Quality, Reducing and preventing adverse drug events to decrease hospital costs, Research in Action, Issue 1. AHRQ Publication Number 01-0020, March 2001. Agency for Healthcare Research and Quality, Rockville, MD, <http://www.ahrq.gov/qual/aderia/aderia.htm>.

[30] N. Moray, Error reduction as a systems problem, in: M.S. Bogner, editor, *Human Errors in Medicine* (Erlbaum, Hillsdale, NJ, 1994).

[31] K.N. Barker and E.L. Allan, Research on drug-use-system errors, American Journal of the Health-System Pharmacy 52 (1995) 400–403.

[32] Institute for Safe Medication Practices, Over-reliance on computer systems may place patients at great risk, ISMP Medication Safety Alert, 1999. Huntingdon Valley, PA, ISMP, 1999.

[33] J.G. Anderson, Evaluation in health informatics: Computer simulation, Computers in Biology and Medicine 32 (2002) 151–164.

[34] J.G. Anderson, S.J. Jay, S.J. Clevenger et al., Physician utilization of a hospital information system: A computer simulation model, in: *Proceedings of the 12th Annual Symposium on Computer Applications in Medical Care*, Washington DC, Computer Society of the IEEE (1988), pp. 858–861.

[35] D.B. Fridsma, Error analysis using organizational simulation, in: *Procedures AMIA Annual Fall Symposium* (2000), pp. 260–264.

[36] D.B. Fridsma, Modeling medical protocols for organizational simulations: An information-processing approach, Computer in Mathematics Organizational Theory 4 (1998) 71–95.

[37] R.P. Betz and H.B. Levy, An interdisciplinary method of classifying and monitoring medication errors, American Journal of the Hospital Pharmacy 42 (1985) 1724–1732.

[38] K.V. Blum, S.R. Abel, C.J. Urbanski, and J.M. Pierce, Medication error prevention by pharmacists, American Journal of the Hospital Pharmacy 45 (1988) 1902–1903.

[39] N.M. Davis and M.R. Cohen, *Medication Errors: Causes and Prevention* (GF Stickley, Philadelphia, 1981).

[40] J.S. Lesar, L.L. Briceland, K. Delcoure et al., Medication prescribing errors in a teaching hospital, JAMA 263 (1990) 2329–2334.

[41] M.U. Vincer, Drug errors and incidents in a neonatal intensive [care unit, AJDS 143 (1989) 737–740.

[42] B. Hannon and M. Ruth, *Dynamic Modeling* (Springer-Verlag, New York, 1994).

[43] J.G. Anderson, Computer simulation in the health sciences: Modeling dynamic systems, in: *Proceedings of the Congress Nacional de Economia*, Las Palmas de Gran Canaria, Spain (1995), pp. 123–140.

[44] S.B. Soumerai and J. Avorn, Efficacy an cost-containment in hospital pharmacotherapy: State of the art and future directions, Milbank MEM Fund Q Health Soc 62 (1984) 447–474.

[45] D.F. Sittig and W.W. Stead, Computer-based physician order entry: The state of the art, Journal of the American Medical Informatics Association 1 (1994) 108–123.

[46] J.G. Anderson, S.J. Jay, J. Perry, and M.M. Anderson, Modifying physician use of a hospital information system: A quasi-experimental study, in: J.G. Anderson, C.E. Aydin, and S.J Jay, editors, *Evaluating Health Care Information Systems: Methods and Applications* (Sage Publications, Thousand Oaks, CA, 1994), pp. 276–287.

[47] D.W. Bates, Medication errors: How common are they and what can be done to prevent them? Drug Safe 5 (1996) 303–310.

[48] D.W. Simborg and H.J. Derewicz, A highly automated hospital medication system: Five years' experience and evaluation, Annals of Internal Medicine 83 (1975) 342–346.

[49] K. Brient, Bar-coding facilitates patient-focused care, Healthcare Informatics 12 (1995) 38–42.

[50] D.W. Bates, M. Cohen, L.L. Leape et al., Reducing the frequency of errors in medicine using information technology, Journal of the American Medical Informatics Association 8 (2001) 299–308.

[51] J.B. Sexton, E.J. Thomas, and R.L. Helmreich, Error, stress and teamwork in medicine and aviation: Cross-sectional surveys, BMJ 320 (2000) 745–749.

[52] H.L. Folli, R.L. Poole, W.E. Benitz, and J.C. Russo, Medication error prevention by clinical pharmacists in two children's hospitals, Pediatrics 79 (1987) 718–722.

[53] L.L. Leape, D.J. Cullen, M.D. Clapp et al., Pharmacist participation on physician rounds and adverse drug events in the intensive care unit, JAMA 282 (1999) 267–270.

[54] L.L. Leape, Error in medicine, JAMA 272 (1994) 1851–1868.

13
Implementing Computers in Ambulatory Care: Implications of Physician Practice Patterns for System Design

Carolyn E. Aydin and Diana E. Forsythe

Introduction

Research on computer use by physicians has begun to extend beyond informatics in hospitals and specialty medicine to include computing in outpatient settings [1,2,3]. Studies from the UK reveal concerns over depersonalization of the patient encounter and that additional time is required to gather more explicit data [1]. Most U.S. projects, however, have focused on identifying specific data needs and on workstation design. Little attention has been paid to how computers might be integrated into physicians' actual work patterns in the consulting room.

This chapter presents preimplementation data collected in the internal medicine division of a large physician group practice scheduled to implement an *electronic medical record (EMR)*. The EMR, developed in a collaboration between Hewlett Packard and the clinic, will integrate internal and external modular applications for clinical notes, order entry, test results, and so on, and provide a secure, single log-on, visually integrated environment for outpatient care customized to the needs of the clinic. The evaluation plan for the project included using qualitative methods to help system designers:

1. Understand the specific clinic setting and the ways in which the new system will fit into the everyday work patterns of those who will use it.
2. Understand users' perspectives on the system and how it might impact their daily work.
3. Make recommendations concerning system design, implementation, training, and support.

Note: This paper was first published in the Proceedings of the AMIA Annual Fall Symposium 1997, pp. 677–681.

Since many patients come from outside the clinic's immediate area, the practice has a particular need to ensure the timely flow of information to facilitate a diagnosis and treatment plan during the few days the patient is in town. While the clinic's paper record system is more efficient than most, recent projects include computerized lab results reporting, an order entry pilot, and telephone dictation in which clinical notes are transcribed into the computer by clerical staff. Direct physician entry of notes is also available, but only used by a limited number of physicians. The EMR will provide physicians with Episode and Problem Managers and will integrate all elements of the electronic medical record, including order entry, results reporting, clinical notes, and patient provided information.

Method

Participant observation is one of the ethnographic data gathering methods used by anthropologists and qualitative sociologists. In contrast to the use of observation to quantify the time spent in various tasks [2], we used participant observation to investigate individuals' perspectives on their own work through systematic observation and conversation with them as they engaged in their daily activities [3–7].

In the present study, 13 of the 19 physicians practicing in the first department scheduled for implementation were observed during consultations with patients. Observation of each physician ranged from 1 to 4 hours. In each case, the physician would enter the examining room, explain the study, and ask the patient's permission for an observer to be present. The researcher would then be introduced and remain in the exam room to observe and take notes, stepping out during the physical examination when asked to do so. The researcher also talked to physicians and other clinic staff about the EMR, including practice changes they anticipated or had already made with results reporting and clinical notes dictation. The study took place in February and May 1996, before scheduled implementation.

Findings

While study findings addressed a number of topics, this paper focuses on two of the most important: (1) the implications of physician movement and interrupted work sessions for design, and (2) parallels between the implementation of the clinical notes dictation system and the EMR.

Physician Movement and Interrupted Sessions

The "information work" of physicians and other healthcare professionals is distinct in that it is not restricted to one time or one place. Rather, they move from room to room, completing their notes and organizing information as they go, with frequent interruptions. For example, one physician first reviewed the chart very briefly outside of the room where the patient was waiting, then ushered the patient to his office/exam room where he interviewed the patient and made notes. Then, while the patient changed clothes, the physician took his paperwork and crossed the hall to another exam room to organize his thoughts and begin a working list of patient problems. The physician then returned to the first room to examine the patient and, after the patient left, organize the problem list, generate orders, and dictate his report.

Another physician went from one exam room to another rather than using her own office to see patients. She also spent considerable time in the corridor reviewing the chart before seeing each patient. She made notes throughout patient visits and then reread her notes, organized her orders, and summarized the visit after the patient left. She did not use the dictation system, but completed her notes using pen and paper.

In both examples, the physicians moved from room to room, each time taking up the information management and note taking process where they had left off in the previous location. In order to integrate the EMR into their current practice patterns, these physicians will probably need to log-on to several workstations in sequence. The Problem Manager, for example, is designed to help physicians organize their thoughts and work through the patient's problems while recording the information in the computerized patient record, generating orders linked to each problem at the same time. If a workstation is not readily available on which they can easily log in and out of unfinished sessions, however, they may be compelled to complete the problem list on paper during the course of their normal work, entering the information in the computer later (a largely clerical task). Since physicians and nurses tend to "know" their patients by their ailments and their medical history, most stated that they would want to review information about the patient at least briefly before entering the room. Thus, terminals need to be easily accessible and log-on/log-off functions need to be both simple and fast. Physicians should also be able to interrupt a work session and resume it easily from another workstation without each time having to go through an entire log-on/patient selection process.

Changing Practice Patterns: The Example of Clinical Notes Management

The most significant practice change at the time of observation was the implementation of Clinical Notes Management. Secretaries, nurses, and physicians all interact in some way with the Clinical Notes system. The system is designed to allow physicians or transcriptionists to enter a clinical note into the database. Physicians use the telephone to enter multiple codes and then follow one of several templates to dictate notes or letters. The dictation is then transcribed into the computer by transcription pools set up to relieve the added burden on secretaries created by the new system. While no one expressed strong negative feelings, the transition to dictation is having costs as well as benefits. Both secretaries and physicians commented that the dictation system has slowed some tasks.

The timing of the observation periods allowed us to observe physicians in different stages of learning the clinical notes system and to both observe and discuss with them how their practice patterns had been affected. By the second observation period, all but three of the department's physicians were dictating clinical notes, although some had just begun. These observations, detailed below, provide important clues to the ways in which physicians may adapt to the fully implemented EMR.

Learning to Use the Dictation System

Although all but three physicians were using the dictation system by May 1996, most did not log on to the computer to read or edit their notes. Physicians who were just beginning to dictate commented that the phone-based dictation system had slowed them down in some ways. Several physicians commented that while dictation reduced documentation time for long notes, it is slower for short notes than writing in the chart. One added that he kept forgetting to include the diagnosis and discharge instructions at the end, as prescribed by the protocol, and thus had to call back repeatedly. Others suggested that people create longer messages when dictating than when writing by hand, which may have also slowed them down. Physicians experienced with the system were observed dictating rapidly, however, saving time especially on long notes.

Time and Logistical Issues

Secretaries commented that with dictation, turnaround time could be slower. Physicians may do more elaborate short notes now (half a page instead of a scribbled 2–3 lines) and may feel less secure about what they're doing (since they are required to dictate according to a standard protocol). Slower turnaround time may also affect the work of secretaries and others who need the patient charts as well.

These staff comments were corroborated by observation of physicians. One said that she dictates notes between patients if she has time, but (as with handwritten notes) won't do so if it keeps other patients waiting. While observed, however, she was able to dictate on several patients between appointments; although at least three other patients were waiting, their charts were not yet back from the consultant visits, delaying the schedule. Full implementation of the Clinical Notes system throughout the practice should relieve this current bottleneck created by the paper-based system, ensuring that consultant notes are available to other clinicians electronically as soon as they are completed.

"Public" versus "Private" Clinical Notes

Handwritten clinical notes, while often illegible, also seem to feel much less "public," as though they "belong" to the individual physician and his or her patient. Dictated notes are not only more legible and easily accessible, they are also read by more people, both because they are easier to read and because transcription adds another person to the process. Thus a physician's practice becomes, in some sense, more exposed, or "public." While the physicians observed did not put the difference in these terms, several made relevant comments. One physician confided that she really didn't know how other physicians practice and envied the researcher her opportunity to observe. Several others seemed insecure about their own dictation, remarking that they "probably wrote too much." Some commented on the rigid conventions of the dictation system. When discussing the idea of dictating in the presence of patients, one physician noted that her colleague had recommended the practice. Although very comfortable with the dictation system, however, she herself had not tried dictating with patients in the room and was unsure how it would work. These observations reflect a shift from the "private" practice of medicine to something more public, in which not only the clinical note, but also the problem list that reflects the physician's thought process, may become more visible or legible to others in the patient record. It may also be dictated for the patient to hear.

Changing Practice Patterns

We observed physicians in various stages of adapting their practice to Clinical Notes dictation. Handwritten notes had always been the norm in this clinic. Physicians who had spent their entire careers there and had never had the experience of dictating seemed to find the change more difficult than those who had dictated elsewhere. Furthermore, physicians who used to complete all of their notes during the patient visit initially felt that the dictation system took extra time. This seemed particularly true of those who had been in the habit of remaining in the exam room to finalize the chart after the departure of the patient. While it seems quite possible to follow the same routine using the dictation system, at least one physician new at dictating took the chart back to his own office to dictate. He confided, however, that he found this interruption in his routine a problem because it disrupted his customary train of thought and he was afraid he would forget things. He now takes scratch notes when with the patient, then goes directly to the desk to complete his orders. Later, when he goes to dictate and do a problem list, however, he finds he may have forgotten an order because his thought processes and problem list were not complete at the end of the patient encounter. He commented: "Maybe I need to take more organized notes when with a patient. . . ."

Another physician new to dictation appeared quite competent and comfortable with the system, but confided that she disliked it. She said another physician had demonstrated how to dictate, using parts of the chart as reference materials, but she still feels as though she fumbles around when she dictates. She also indicated that it works well when she can keep up between patients, but if she is running late and cannot dictate between patients, she hand writes her information so she can remember it later when she dictates. Since physicians spend much of their time examining and sifting information to arrive at a diagnosis and treatment plan, ensuring that all functions of the EMR contribute to, rather than interrupt, this process is essential if the system is to enhance, rather than interfere with, practice.

Patient Presence

Physicians who hand write their notes frequently do so during the clinical encounter with the patient present. They simply stop the conversation at the end of a particular set of questions regarding a specific patient complaint or problem, making their notes while the patient waits. Others, however, do not stop the flow of the encounter. Instead they make short notes on scratch paper to cue themselves and depend on remembering the rest of what they will need later to write the long note. Some physicians (possibly those who make a point of not stopping the flow of the conversation) worry about turning away from the patient to use the computer: "You noticed I sat across from her? I'm wondering if patients will feel they're buying airline tickets. You know, you're clicking away like this . . ." (pantomiming typing while demonstratively turning his head away from the observer to indicate loss of eye contact).

Some physicians were observed using the dictation system while the patient was present. They saw this as enhancing patient education and reducing patient anxiety that the physician might be keeping something from them. Rather than stopping periodically during the exam (and then completing a long note at the end of the exam—usually after the patient leaves), these physicians dictated a long note while the patient was still present. They made specific efforts to involve the patients in the dictation process by explaining what they were going to do, maintaining eye contact with the patient and occasionally stopping the dictation to verify a point in the patient history with the patient. They emphasized what the patient had agreed to do (e.g., instead of indicating doubt that a patient would comply with an order, the physician would dictate: "Mrs. X has agreed to . . ."). One physician involved the patient by saying, "You can tell me if I'm saying anything wrong." While dictating with the patient present seemed to work well during our observations, it would not always be appropriate. As with computer use in the exam room, dictation in the presence of patients requires that the physician be secure with the system.

Entering or Editing Notes Online

Several physicians addressed trade-offs between dictation and entering or editing notes online. According to one experienced user, she only enters notes on-line when it is faster to type them than to dictate them. Another physician said, "I can talk a lot faster than I type. . . . I edit my own notes sometimes, but I don't type them." He felt that learning to type was a poor use of his time. None of the physicians could envision entering long notes online. One, however, pointed out that with a repeat patient, one could edit a previous long note to create a new one. It seems reasonable to infer that, even with maximum use of the clinical notes application by physicians, some dictation will continue to be the best option for long notes on patients new to the practice.

Changes in Clinical Notes

In summary, observation and interviews indicated that the new dictated electronic clinical notes are longer and more structured than handwritten notes. Physicians also noted that they seldom take time to edit their notes, either on line or by indicating changes to their secretaries. One physician noted that when he had been trained, it had seemed hard to edit notes online, but it may be easier now—he hadn't tried again, indicating the importance of having applications be easy to use. He also wondered when he would find time in his day to do the extra work of going back to edit notes. However, physicians no longer need to dictate final letters sent to patients and referring physicians; these are generated automatically from computerized notes and lab reports.

Discussion

Implementation of the EMR will result in change processes similar to those described for the dictation of clinical notes. One of the most significant EMR functions for clinical practice is the development of a problem list. While not required to do so, most physicians at the clinic already use problem lists. The structure and "rules" they use vary according to their experience and education. Development of the problem list appears to be an integral part of practice at this clinic, as physicians organize materials they have gathered on the patient, most of which will eventually be available online.

The problem list is logically generated before physician orders are entered. In this practice, however, it is essential that physician orders be completed *immediately* following the visit, since the patient is immediately sent to other areas for tests and consultations. Physicians complete their orders in the exam room and take them directly to the desk. *Thus, if the EMR is to be of maximum use to the physician, he or she must be comfortable enough with the system to use it in the patient's presence or immediately after the patient leaves (i.e., before orders are generated.)* This sequence of events implies a major change in physician practice. If the physician actually uses the EMR to organize information and generate the problem list, he or she will not be able to delay or batch the task to complete at the end of the day, as many do with their dictation of clinical notes, especially when they are behind. Based on observed practice, however, the temptation will be to wait and deal with the new and perhaps challenging system later. The result will be that physicians use the system merely to record a problem list developed earlier in order to generate the necessary orders.

If physicians are entering their orders online, and if the system *requires* them to link each order with a problem in the problem list, they will be forced to use the EMR as intended. This change in practice will require extensive support as physicians become familiar with the system and begin to use it. As with the dictation of long notes, however, once a "critical mass" is reached (perhaps after about 1 year), most continuing patients will already have problem lists that simply need to be updated and the biggest issue will be developing problem lists for new patients. Because of the major change in practice patterns required to get maximum use of the system, however, a substantial institutional commitment to training and support will be essential.

Summary and Recommendations

Physicians' information-related practice patterns vary, even within the same clinical setting. EMR implementation is likely to exert constraints upon at least some individuals' practice patterns. Including ethnography in the evaluation plan can help us understand how normal practice patterns may be affected, allowing informed inferences on how best to support implementation. Results for this clinic indicate that:

- Most physicians anticipate enough benefits from the EMR to be willing to use it; others said "When they make me do it, I will."
- To accommodate physician movement, computers must be accessible, easy to log into, and have provisions for interrupted sessions.
- Many were concerned about losing eye contact with patients, although research has shown this issue resolves as users become proficient [1].
- It is unrealistic to expect even good typists to enter their own long notes.
- Staged implementation introducing order entry before the Episode and Problem Managers may help physicians adapt gradually.
- Comprehensive training should include (1) provisions for physicians to see fewer patients during the learning period, allowing protected time for instruction, (2) simulated patient encounters to help physicians adapt their own practice patterns, and (3) tutors available on-site to answer questions in the clinical setting.

Note: Physician gender was changed randomly to provide anonymity to informants. The study was supported by Hewlett Packard.

References

[1] C.E. Aydin, P.N. Rosen, and V.J. Felitti, Transforming information use in preventive medicine: Learning to balance technology with the art of caring, in: *Proceedings of the 18th Annual Symposium on Computer Applications in Medical Care*, Washington, DC (1994), pp. 563–567.

[2] P.C. Tang, M.A. Jaworski, C.A. Felencer, N. Kreider, M.P. LaRosa, and W.C. Marquardt, Clinical information activities in diverse ambulatory care practices, in: *Proceedings of 1996 AMIA Annual Fall Symposium*, Washington, DC (1996), pp. 12–16.

[3] D. Fafchamps, C.Y. Young, and P.C. Tang, Modeling work practices: Imput to the design of a physician's workstation, in: *Proceedings of the 15th Annual Symposium on Computer Applications in Medical Care*, Washington, DC (1991), pp. 788–792.

[4] D.E. Forsythe, B.G. Buchanan, J.A. Osheroff, and R.A. Miller, Expanding the concept of medical information: An observational study of physicians' information needs, Computers and Biomedical Research 25 (1992) 181–200.

[5] B. Kaplan and H.P. Lundsgaarde, Toward an evaluation of an integrated clinical imaging system: Identifying clinical benefits, Methods of Information in Medicine 35 (1996) 221–229.

[6] D.E. Forsythe, Using ethnography in the design of an explanation system, Expert Systems with Applications 8(4) (1995) 403–417.

[7] B. Nardi, A. Kuchinsky, S. Whittaker, R. Leichner, and H. Schwarz, Video-as-data: Technical and social aspects of a collaborative multimedia application, Computer Supported Cooperative Work (CSCW) 4(1) (1996) 73–100.

14
Nursing Documentation Time During Implementation of an Electronic Medical Record

Lisa M. Korst, Alea C. Eusebio-Angeja, Terry Chamorro, Carolyn E. Aydin, and Kimberly D. Gregory

Introduction

Increased documentation needs during EMR implementation may necessitate increased staffing requirements in an already labor-intensive and demanding environment.

A work-sampling study was conducted over a 14-day study period, and 18 of 84 (21%) potential 4-hour observation periods were selected. During each period, a single observer made 120 observations and, on locating a specific nurse, immediately recorded that nurse's activity on a standardized and validated instrument. Categories of nursing activities included documentation, bedside care, bedside supportive care, nonbedside care, and nonpatient care.

A total of 2160 observations were made. The total percentage of nursing time spent for documentation was 15.8%, 10.6% on paper and 5.2% on the computer. The percentage of time spent on documentation was independently associated with day versus night shifts (19.2% vs. 12.4%, respectively).

Despite charting concurrently on both paper and computer, the amount of time spent on documentation was not excessive, and was consistent with previous studies in which neither electronic nor "double charting" occurred.

Despite the numerous and diverse endeavors to establish electronic medical records (EMR), limited success stories are noted [1] and few of these provide direct assistance to others who are trying to achieve the vision promulgated a decade ago by the Institute of Medicine [2]. Complex technical explanations for this general lack of progress predominate [3–5]; however, the ability of an organization to assist its staff through the behavioral and procedural changes required to rework such a fundamental aspect of normal operations is rarely addressed. Incorporating an EMR into an institutional environment inevitably generates a period of implementation that must be accommodated by staff and budgetary processes of the organization [6,7]. The clinical and financial ramifications of these implementation periods can discourage the "infusion" of EMR systems into American healthcare organizations [8]. Anderson et al. note the "unforeseen costs and organizational consequences, and even failure" of these systems [9] and, although experience with failure of EMR systems is not widely published, unsuccessful implementation efforts do occur [10–12].

A specific organizational concern related to the EMR is that nurses are frequently required to "double chart" during system implementation. Double charting is a vernacular term for the required entry of the same data elements in both computer and paperbased systems. Education and certification of hundreds of users on a new system and the completion of technical tasks to "go live" (e.g., achieving appropriate application configuration for the medical center environment, establishing server setup and networking, testing troubleshooting protocols, and meeting security and archival requirements) can generate an extensive period in which users must chart simultaneously on both paper and computer systems. Increased documentation needs can increase staffing requirements and costs in an already labor-intensive and demanding environment [13–18].

This study was done to determine, within the context of all nursing duties, the amount of time spent by nurses for documentation in the patient record during such an EMR implementation period on an intrapartum unit.

Methods

The study was undertaken at Cedars-Sinai Medical Center, a tertiary care, university-affiliated community hospital in Los Angeles, performing approximately 6700 births per year. The unit has 20 rooms: 12 labordelivery-recovery rooms and 8 labor rooms. An EMR system to document most of the labor and delivery process was installed in December 1998, and nurses were trained on the system during the first quarter of 1999. Nurses were instructed to chart on the computer in addition to maintaining their routine documentation on paper. Elements of computer documentation were a subset of the elements of normal paper documentation. Specifically, computer documentation included a summary of patient history; a flow sheet of nursing annotations about the labor, delivery, and recovery process; vital signs; and delivery summary. Additional paperbased documentation included comprehensive patient history; current problems, medications, and orders; and details of any operative process. The study took place from June 18 through July 1, 1999, and was approved by the Cedars-Sinai Medical Center Institutional Review Board.

A work-sampling study design was chosen for its ability to describe the proportion of nursing time spent on documentation activities relative to other duties. The rationale and details of such an approach have been well described by Sittig [19], and the work-sampling methodology has been contrasted with time and motion studies by Finkler et al. [20]. The potential categories of nursing activities were detailed before the study began and an observer, using a sampling mechanism to minimize bias, encountered the nurses in sequence to identify and chronicle their activities. From the percentage of all observations in a specific activity category, the percentage of all nursing time spent in that activity can be inferred.

A list of potential nursing activities in the intrapartum unit was modified from previously published studies [21,22], and tested over five 4-hour sessions before the study period. Activities were divided into five major categories: documentation, bedside care, bedside supportive care, nonbedside care, and nonpatient care activities (Table 14.1). Documentation activities included both paper and computer documentation, and providing assistance to other nurses learning to chart on the computer. Bedside care included both direct and indirect patient care; however, bedside supportive care was categorized separately (defined as those activities related to providing physical comfort, emotional support, instruction or information, and advocacy). Nonbedside care activities included intraunit transit, indirect care, reporting, advocacy, and assistance with operative deliveries. Non-

TABLE 14.1. Categories of nursing activity.

Category	Subcategory	Examples
Documentation*	Paper charting	Both bedside and nonbedside documentation of patient care
	Computer charting	Both bedside and nonbedside documentation of patient care
	Superuser	Assisting others with computer charting
Bedside care	Direct care	Positioning fetal heart rate monitor
	Indirect care	Preparing an IV at the bedside
Bedside supportive care	Advocacy support	Speaking to physician regarding a patient's needs
	Emotional support	Assisting the patient with pain management
	Instructional support	Educating the patient regarding breathing techniques
	Physical support	Assisting patient with pushing
Nonbedside care	Transit	Delivering blood specimens to nursing station
	Indirect care	Preparing medication
	Reports	Giving reports during shift change
	Cesarean room	Circulating in the operating room
	Advocacy	Communicating to the family in the waiting room
Nonpatient care	Meal break	Eating or drinking in the nursing lounge
	Social	Time spent in conversation unrelated to patient care
	Personal	Time spent for personal needs unrelated to meal breaks or socializing
	Not found	Unknown location
	Other	Administrative work
	Off unit	Obtaining meals or on a break off the unit

* Documentation (both computer and paper-based charting) could occur at the bedside or at a centralized nursing station.

patient care activities consisted of personal time (including restroom breaks), meal breaks, off-unit activities, and social interaction or conversations about non–patient-related activities. Only one of these five categories of activity was assigned per observation. Validation of the correct categorization of nursing activity was assured during the pilot period.

At the onset of the study period, the nurse manager informed staff that a study related to implementing the computer program would occur, and that they would be observed over the next 2 weeks. A single observer, a third-year medical student who had previously completed a month of obstetric training within the intrapartum unit, collected the data. The prior clinical rotation familiarized the observer with the unit, the nurses, and the types of nursing activities. Additionally, the observer, now comfortable with the personnel, could move throughout the unit without necessarily interrupting nursing activities. A 4-hour observation period was chosen to minimize observer fatigue. Over a 14-day study period, we randomly selected 9 of 42 (21%) 4-hour potential observation episodes during the day (7 A.M. to 7 P.M.) and 9 additional 4-hour episodes during the night (7 P.M. to 7 A.M.). For each of the 4-hour episodes (N = 18), 120 observations were collected, totaling 2160 total observations. Sample size requirements were determined using the following relationship: $n = P(1 - p)/\sigma^2$, where n = the total number of observations, P = expected percent of time required by the most important category of the study, and σ = standard deviation of the percentage (19). Thus, to establish that the percentage of time that nurses spend charting (conservatively) is 30% ± 2% with a 95% confidence interval (CI), $p = 0.3$, $2\sigma = 2\%$ ($\sigma = 0.01$), so that $n = 0.3(1 - 0.3)/(0.01)^2 = 2100$.

Recognizing that nursing activities are likely to be influenced by the daily census, for each observation period, the observer would note the number of patients and nurses on the unit at the start of the interval and the number of deliveries performed during the interval. The nurses on duty were observed in random order, and the activity category of each nurse recorded at the moment when she or he was found. If a nurse was not found within 5 minutes, her or his activity was labeled "Not Found." Patient activity was not observed or recorded.

Data were tabulated and analyzed using SAS statistical software, version 6.12 (Cary, NC). Analytical comparisons were made using the Student t test, or nonparametric tests, as appropriate. Probabilities are expressed ± the standard error. Statistical significance was defined as $P < .05$. Odds ratios comparing stratified data include 95% confidence interval (CI).

Results

For the 4-hour sampling periods (N = 18), the median number of nurses assigned to patients was 8 (range 7–12). The median patient census was 8 (range 3–14), and the median number of deliveries occurring during each of these periods was 2 (range 1–5). Of the 2160 data points collected, 1080 were collected on each shift. The estimated percentage of time spent by nurses on each activity is described in Table 14.2, with 15.79% (95% CI 14.25, 17.33) spent on all documentation: paper charting used 10.55% of nursing time, compared with 5.24% for computer charting. Nurses spent 11.39% of their time charting at the bedside, compared with 4.40% at other unit work areas.

The total estimated percentage of time spent in patient-care documentation differed between day and night shifts: 19.17% (95% CI 16.70%, 21.57%) and 12.41% (95% CI 10.44, 14.38) for days and nights, respectively. Because of this difference between day and night shifts, all five categories of nursing activities were compared between the two groups (Table 14.2). In addition to medical record documentation, the day shift spent a greater proportion of time providing direct and indirect bedside care and nonbedside care compared with the night shift.

The median total number of deliveries and the total number of nurses varied only slightly per shift: 9 nurses (range 7–12) for days versus 8 nurses (range 8–9) for nights; and 3 deliveries (range 2–5) during a day shift observational period versus 1 delivery (range 1–2) during a night shift. However, the median patient census varied noticeably per shift: 10 (range 6–14) for the day shift versus 4 (range 3–11) for the night shift ($P < .01$). For this reason, the observations were stratified by shift and each activity category was examined by how "busy" the unit was during the observation period (Table 14.3). A period with a census of 9 or more patients was defined as a

TABLE 14.2. Estimated percent of time used in nursing activities on an obstetrical unit by shift.

Activity	Shift	Percent estimate ± standard error	95% Confidence Interval (percent time)
Documentation*	Day	19.17 ± 1.20	16.70, 21.57
	Night	12.41 ± 1.00	10.44, 14.38
	Total	15.79 ± 0.78	14.25, 17.33
Bedside direct and indirect care†	Day	21.02 ± 1.24	18.59, 23.45
	Night	15.83 ± 1.11	13.66, 18.01
	Total	18.43 ± 0.83	16.79, 20.07
Bedside support	Day	11.48 ± 0.97	9.58, 13.38
	Night	8.98 ± 0.87	7.28, 10.69
	Total	10.23 ± 0.65	8.95, 11.51
Nonbedside care†	Day	29.44 ± 1.39	26.73, 32.16
	Night	14.07 ± 1.05	12.00, 16.15
	Total	21.76 ± 0.89	20.02, 23.50
Noncare†	Day	18.98 ± 1.19	16.64, 21.32
	Night	48.98 ± 1.52	46.00, 51.96
	Total	33.98 ± 1.02	31.98, 35.98

* Summary of percent estimates may vary slightly due to rounding; documentation includes computer and paper-based charting.
† Statistically significant difference.

TABLE 14.3. Odds ratios for nursing activities by unit census or "busyness" of the unit, stratified by shift.

Days

Activity	Percent when busy†	Percent when not busy†	Odds ratio	95% CI	P value
Charting	18.9% (136/720)	19.7% (71/360)	0.95	0.68–1.32	.806
Bedside care	22.6% (163/720)	17.8% (64/360)	1.35	0.97–1.89	.077
Support	10.3% (74/720)	13.9% (50/360)	0.71	0.48–1.06	.098
Nonbedside care*	31.7% (228/720)	25.0% (90/360)	1.39	1.03–1.87	.028
Nonpatient care*	16.7% (120/720)	23.6% (85/360)	0.65	0.47–0.90	.008
(reversed)			1.55	1.12–2.14	.008
Total	100% (720)	100% (360)			

Nights

Activity	Percent when busy	Percent when not busy	Odds ratio	95% CI	P value
Charting	15.0% (36/240)	11.7% (98/840)	1.34	0.87–2.06	.204
Bedside care*	22.1% (53/240)	14.1% (118/840)	1.73	1.19–2.53	.004
Support*	14.6% (35/240)	7.4% (62/840)	2.14	1.34–3.41	.001
Nonbedside care*	20.0% (48/240)	12.4% (104/840)	1.77	1.19–2.62	.004
Nonpatient care*	28.3% (68/240)	54.9% (461/840)	0.33	0.23–0.45	.000
(reversed)			3.08	2.23–4.26	.000
Total	100% (240)	100% (840)			

CI = confidence interval, $P < .01$.

* Statistically significant difference.

† A "busy" unit was defined as a census of 9 or more laboring patients.

"busy" period in an effort to split the observations into groups falling above or below the approximate median number of nurses available (i.e., the point at which nurses would be assigned the care of more than 1 patient in labor). The amount of time spent on documentation did not appear to be associated with the unit census; however, the proportion of time spent on most other nursing activities was related to the unit census, especially at night. A busy period was associated with an increased proportion of time spent on bedside care, supportive care, and nonbedside care activities.

Limitations

Although multiple limitations are inherent in the work-sampling method, few tools provide administrators with such a feasible and comprehensive view of their staff activities. Such methods are most comparable to time and motion studies, which can be much more precise because they make fewer assumptions, use contiguous observations, and can detail the duration of any specific task. However, because of the intensity of the observation needed in such studies, the activities of fewer individuals (and their idiosyncrasies) are examined, and the results may not necessarily be generalizable to the remaining staff. Further methodologic concerns are that work-sampling observations will inherently be biased by the sampling periods and that it is difficult to select sampling periods and the order of nurse observation completely "randomly." For example, whether a 4-hour sampling period was at the beginning, middle, or end of a shift can very well have been associated with the amount of time spent in documentation. Thus, although a large number of observations were made per shift, the distribution of those sampling periods adds another level of variance to the estimated percentage time spent in that activity.

As with any observational methodology, workers can change their work patterns on seeing the observer [19]. We feel this was not likely given (1) the instantaneous nature of the observations and (2) the high comfort level of the nurses with the observer. We used only one observer in this study to maintain the comfort level of the nurses with the observer and, therefore, interobserver variation was not estimated. This is a potential limitation to generalizing our findings; however, they do appear credible when evaluated in the context of similar published work. For example, our estimate of percent of nursing time spent in bedside supportive activities (10.23%) is comparable to estimates by Gagnon et al. (6%) and McNiven et al. (9%) [21,22].

Finally, work-sampling methods do not address the complexity of the nurse patient care relationship, but only measure the amount of time spent in performing observable activities [23]. For example, critical thinking and evaluation processes are often not observable, and multiple tasks can be occurring during any observation. Although we used a validated instrument for coding activities, the quality and complexity of that activity was never assessed.

Discussion

To improve efficiency and quality of patient care, hospitals are increasingly relying on computer technology to improve efficiency and accuracy in documentation [24–27]. To benefit from technologic advances in patient care, the study hospital implemented an EMR to document the progress of a woman in labor. The system continuously monitors uterine contractions and fetal heart rate and allows the user to chart the progress of labor, including interventions, at the bedside computer or at any computer on the unit that is part of the system. Many of the users initially expressed concerns that the new computerized method of charting would be more time-consuming and would detract from patient care. Our study was done during the transition from paper to computer charting, when the nurses were still charting both by paper and by computer. We found that less time was spent charting by computer than by paper (5.1% vs. 10.5%, respectively) and we estimated that the total amount of time (15.79%) spent documenting on both paper and the computer was comparable to reports based on paper charting alone [21,28].

This study should allay some administrative and user concerns regarding the magnitude of increased nursing resources during the implementation of an EMR. To our knowledge, this is the first study that specifically addresses the "double charting" situation. The additional time required does not appear to be excessive when compared with estimates of documentation time for systems based on paper alone. A work-sampling study in an obstetric unit estimated 10.2% of nursing time spent in medical record documentation outside of the patient's room [21]. In our study, less than 5% of all nursing documentation took place outside the patient's room. Computer workstations had been deliberately placed at the bedside to encourage nurses to stay with the patients in labor. Another study in a medical–surgical unit estimated 11% of total time was spent on nursing documentation on the day shift and 18% on the night shift [28]. We also noted important shift differences, with 19% of time spent on documentation during the day shift and 12% during the night shift. Additionally, the time spent during the night shift performing other nursing activities appeared to be highly associated with the unit census.

Concern about the potential for increased staffing requirements can paralyze EMR system implementation. Such operating costs can be difficult to budget. Although administrators may expect that an EMR will eventually save nurses time, evidence suggests that such systems will never allow any actual decrease in labor costs, but only enable nurses to decrease time spent on documentation and shift their time to direct patient care activities [29].

Pabst et al. [30] analyzed the effect of computerized documentation on nursing time. They found that switching to a computerized documentation system enabled nurses to spend less time on documentation and more time in direct patient care. Nurses could also update care plans more easily. They were not able, however, to increase patient loads with the saved time, and nurse managers were challenged to find ways to maximize the time saved as a result of the new technology. Given data regarding the importance of supportive personnel on labor outcome [31–36], opportunities to improve quality of care by increasing bedside supportive care could be realized if documentation time is minimized by implementing EMR.

The work-sampling methodology used in this study provided time estimates for documenting patient care and also multiple other nursing activities. Although these activities are tangential to the present investigation, they can offer some insight regarding efficiencies that can be gained in activities other than documentation. For example, the high proportion of nursing time used in non–patientcare activities (34%) suggests the possibility of using nonprofessional staff members instead of nurses for some activities, or redesigning the roles of existing personnel to include new responsibilities [23,37]. Alternatively, differences in the proportion of time spent in the various nursing activities between day and night shifts may encourage hospital administrators and nurse managers to consider innovative ideas for restructuring nursing time. For example, if less direct patient bedside care is needed at night, yet census status mandates a certain staffing ratio, some administrative duties or enhanced patient or nursing educational opportunities may be redirected to the night shift.

Summary

In summary, our data suggest that the implementation of an EMR in an intrapartum unit was not associated with excessive time spent on documentation. However, the data also suggest that other opportunities for improving nursing efficiency do exist. Work-sampling methods appear useful for estimating the allocation of nursing time and for suggesting areas in which staff activities can be optimized.

References

[1] R.A. Garibaldi, Computers and the quality of care—A clinician's perspective, N Engl J Med 338(4) (1998) 259–260.

[2] R. Dick and E. Steen, editors, Committee on Improving the Patient Record, Division of Health Care Services, Institute of Medicine, *The Computer-Based Patient Record, An Essential Technology for Health Care* (National Academy Press, Washington, DC, 1991).

[3] R.A. Miller and R.M. Gardner, Recommendations for responsible monitoring and regulation of clinical software systems, J Am Med Inform Assoc 4 (1997) 442–457.

[4] E.H. Shortliffe, The evolution of electronic medical records, Acad Med 74(4) (1999) 414–419.

[5] C.J. McDonald, The barriers to electronic medical record systems and how to overcome them, J Am Med Inform Assoc 4 (1997) 213–221.

[6] T.R. Prince and J.A. Sullivan, Financial viability, medical technology, and hospital closures, J Health Care Finance 26(4) (2000) 1–18.

[7] E. Miller and E. Arquiza, Improving computer skills to support hospital restructuring, J Nurs Care Quality 13(5) (1999) 44–56.

[8] J. Ash, Organizational factors that influence information technology diffusion in academic health sciences centers, J Am Med Inform Assoc 4 (1997) 102–111.

[9] J.G. Anderson, C.E. Aydin, and S.J. Jay, *Evaluating Health Care Information Systems: Methods and Applications* (Sage Publications, Thousand Oaks, CA, 1994) p. 289.

[10] B.L. Goddard, Termination of a contract to implement an enterprise electronic medical record, J Am Med Inform Assoc 7(6) (2000) 564–568.

[11] M.E. Frisse, Computers and productivity: Is it time for a reality check? Acad Med 73 (1998) 59–64.

[12] T. Chamorro, Computer-based patient record systems, Semin Oncol Nurs 17(1) (2001) 24–33.

[13] M.D. Sovie, Nursing staff in hospitals and nursing homes: Is it adequate? A review and commentary, Nurs Outlook 44(2) (1996) 100–101.

[14] P.M. Watson, M.S. Lower, S.M. Wells, S.J. Farrah, and C. Jarrell, Discovering what nurses do and what it costs, Nursing Management 22(5) (1991) 38–45.

[15] M.J. Fitzpatrick, M.J. McElroy, and S. DeWoody, Building a strong nursing organization in a merged, service line structure, J Nurs Admin 31(1) (2001) 24–32.

[16] E. Ammenwerth and R. Haux, A compendium of information processing functions in nursing: Development and pilot study, *Computers in Nursing* 18(4) (2000) 189–196.

[17] G.P. Lenehan, ED short staffing: It is time to take a hard look at a growing problem and strategies such as standard nursepatient ratios, J Emerg Nurs 25(2) (1999) 77–78.

[18] A.M. McDaniel, C. Matlin, P.R. Elmer, K. Paul, and G. Monastiere, Computer use in staff development: A national survey, Journal of Nursing Staff Development 14(3) (1998) 117–126.

[19] D.F. Sittig, Work-sampling: A statistical approach to evaluation of the effect of computers on work patterns in healthcare industry, Methods Inf Med 32 (1993) 167–174.

[20] S.A. Finkler, J.R. Knickman, G. Hendrickson, M. Lipkin Jr., and W.G. Thoompson, A comparison of work-sampling and time-and-motion studies in health services research, Health Serv Res 28(5) (1993) 577–597.

[21] A.J. Gagnon and K. Waghorn, Supportive care by maternity nurses: A work sampling study in an intrapartum unit, Birth 23 (1996) 1–6.

[22] P. McNiven, E. Hodnett, and L.L. O'Brien-Pallas, Supporting women in labor: A work sampling study of the activities of labor and delivery nurses, Birth 19(1) (1992) 3–8.

[23] L.D. Urden and J.I. Roode, Work sampling: A decision-making tool for determining resources and work redesign, J Nurs Admin 27 (1997) 34–41.

[24] T. Burkle, R. Kuch, A. Passian, U. Prokosch, and J. Dudeck, The impact of computer implementation on nursing work patterns: Study design and preliminary results, Medinfo 8 (1995), Pt. 2, 1321–1325.

[25] M. Berg, Medical work and the computer-based patient record: A sociological perspective, Methods Inform Med 37 (1998) 294–301.

[26] K.E. Dennis, P.M. Sweeney, L.P. Macdonald, and N.A. Morse, Point of care technology: Impact on people and paperwork, Nurs Econom 11 (1993) 229–237, 248.

[27] E. Evans, Using computers as clinical tools to improve patient care, Nephrology News Issues 9 (1995) 30–31, 35.

[28] V.V. Upenieks, Work sampling: Assessing nursing efficiency, Nurse Manager 29 (1998) 27–29.

[29] D. Adderly, C. Hyde, and P. Mauseth, The computer age impacts nurses, Computers in Nursing 15(1) (1997) 43–46.

[30] M.K. Pabst, J.C. Scherubel, and A.F. Minnick, The impact of computerized documentation on nurses' use of time, Computers in Nursing 14(1) (1996) 25–30.

[31] J. Kennell, M. Klaus, S. McGrath, S. Robertson, and C. Hinkley, Continuous emotional support during labor in a U.S. hospital, JAMA 265 (1991) 2197–2201.

[32] M. Sleutel and M. Guinn, As good as it gets?: Going online with a clinical information system, Computers in Nursing 17(4) (1999) 181–185.

[33] K.D. Scott, G. Berkowitz, and M. Klaus, A comparison of intermittent and continuous support during labor: A meta-analysis, Am J Obstet Gynecol 180(5) (1999) 1054–1059.

[34] R. Sosa, J. Kennell, S. Robertson, and J. Urrutia, The effect of a supportive companion on perinatal problems, length of labor, and mother-infant interaction, N Engl J Med 303 (1980) 597–600.

[35] J. Zhang, J.W. Bernasko, E. Leybovich, M. Fahs, and M.C. Hatch, Continuous labor support from lab or attendant for primiparous women: A meta-analysis, Obstet Gynecol 88(4) (1996) Pt. 2, 739–744.

[36] E. Hodnett, Caregiver support for women during childbirth (Cochrane review), in: *The Cochrane Library* (Update Software (Meta-analysis) 3, Oxford, 1999).

[37] L. Linden and K. English, Adjusting the cost-quality equation: Utilizing work sampling and time study data to redesign clinical practice, J Nurs Care Qual 8(3) (1994) 34–42.

15
Computer Charting: An Evaluation of a Respiratory Care Computer System

Robert D. Andrews, Reed M. Gardner, Sandy M. Metcalf, and Deon Simmons

Introduction

In efforts to increase the efficiency of medical care delivery, institutions are turning to computers as useful tools for processing and storing medical, financial, and administrative information. It has been reported that 25% to 35% of a health professional's time is spent doing paperwork [1–3], and although many hospital departments have computerized information systems, the clinical information in the patient's chart remains essentially unchanged [4–6]. This clinical information includes patient history, observations, medications, and progress notes used in diagnosis and treatment. The documentation of most procedures in respiratory care (RC) is similar in content. We report the usefulness of a computer-charting system in documenting and processing clinical information.

An Optimal System

The efficiency of any system is measured by the "useful" work completed compared to the energy required. The most efficient RC computer system would have the following characteristics:

- No repetition of work or reporting
- Easy access for entry and review
- Accurate and descriptive documentation
- Automatic performance of many functions from a single input (i.e., billing, reporting, checking for errors, alerting, and gathering of management statistics)
- Exact correlation between charting and billing
- Integration of RC information with that of other hospital departments
- Availability of information for diagnostic and research purposes

- Easy implementation
- Reliability (no downtime)
- Inexpensive equipment that pays for itself

Perhaps the best proof of a computer's usefulness is the degree to which people want to use it because it helps them do their jobs, not simply because its use is mandatory.

Institutional Background

LDS Hospital

LDS Hospital, a major referral center with 520 beds and 5 (4 adult, 1 newborn) intensive care units (ICUs), has been a leader in the development of computer applications in medicine. A highly developed hospital information system (HIS), known as HELP, integrates all patient information [7,8]. A Tandem "nonstop" computer system (Tandem, Cupertino CA) is connected to more than 300 terminals and 95 printers. It is highly reliable and has little downtime (0.2%) [9] because of its redundant processing and storage of data [10]. The computer has an integrated central billing system. The functions of order entry, reporting, data entry, and alerting are well developed for most departments. At least four terminals are available on every nursing division (each of which handles 48 patients), as is a printer. The ICUs have a terminal at each bedside.

Respiratory Care Department

Respiratory care presented several unique problems for computer implementation. By 1982 only about a dozen RC departments in the country had reached a level of substantial computerization; an equal number of departments had tried, but failed [11]. At LDS Hospital we introduced computer charting as an improvement on the written patient chart and to meet the clinical, financial, and management needs of RC.

The RC service is highly mobile. Therapists do not have a permanent workstation, as work is performed at the bedside and throughout the hospital. Therefore, entering computer information required having access to terminals in many locations or recording information on paper for later computer entry in the RC department. Thus, the logistics problems of where the data could be reviewed and how it could be entered in the patient's chart had to be solved.

Patient records vary in quality and detail because from one-third to one-half of them are in narrative which makes information difficult to collect and process [5,12–14]. Unlike computerized systems in clinical laboratories that process large amounts of numeric data, computerized RC information systems require a reporting "vocabulary" with a wide range of descriptions.

To be automated, patient records had to be converted from a narrative format to the computer's predefined vocabulary [6].

The RC computer system was developed from a very simple concept: "Chart accurately and let the computer do the rest of the paperwork." The system was designed to maximize the efficiency of documenting procedures and thereby improve the evaluation of medical care. In addition, documentation was required for hospital accreditation [15] and for verification that a procedure had been performed. The charting of clinical procedures was also used in nonmedical functions, such as management statistics and billing. Because the functions were integrated into the HIS, they became byproducts of the documentation process [16]. As paperwork was reduced, a higher percentage of the therapist's time could be spent doing the most useful work, patient care.

Respiratory care documentation has traditionally been written into the patient's chart using specific forms—those for notes, assessments, and ventilator monitoring—with each section organized chronologically. Documentation has allowed later review so that patient care can be assessed and changed if necessary. These processes of data entry, organization, storage, and review are very similar to the operation of a computer. To permit the computer to be used for patient charting, three programming functions of the HIS were instrumental: (1) One program allowed creation of questionnaires, to be used for data entry. This program also permitted the capture of billing information. (2) Another program allowed the creation of vocabulary used in charting by assigning the medical terminology to codes that were more easily stored in the computer's files. (3) A general reporting language was used to program the reports and statistics.

Description of the RC System

The RC computer system is a subsystem of the HIS; it depends on the central computer and uses nursing division terminals for data entry and review. It avoids duplication by using existing hardware and by using information from other hospital departments, such as admission, discharge, and transfer (ADT) information. The HIS controls and processes the flow of all patient information (Figure 15.1). RC charting is entered at the nursing divisions, is stored in patient data files and can be reviewed at any nursing division terminal. A 24-hour management report provides individual and departmental productivity records, and an alert report is used for both management and patient care monitoring. Permanent copies of all RC charting are automatically processed for delivery to Medical Records after a patient has been discharged. The HIS is integrated with a billing computer system that processes financial transactions and provides the hospital with productivity reports. Thus, all reporting and billing are extracted directly from the computerized clinical charting.

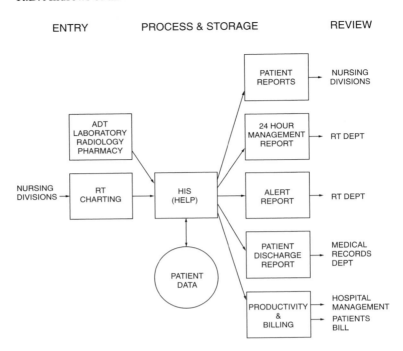

FIGURE 15.1. The RC computer system uses the hospital information system (HIS) for the processing of medical information.

Currently the RC department is not fully computerized—order entry, workload allocation, and newborn nursery charting are still done manually. The charting of ventilator data was recently implemented, because bedside terminals are now available in the ICUs where ventilators are used. Approximately 90% of RC charting and charge capture is now computerized.

Charting

The charting process is initiated by selecting the "Respiratory Therapy Charting" option on the computer terminal at the nursing station. Entries are made by selecting multiple-choice items from the menu, by number entry, or by typing in free text (Figure 15.2). The questionnaire-entry format follows a logical sequence that corresponds with the department's charting requirements. Entries can include the charting of more than one procedure at a time, which allows procedures that are frequently done together to be charted without redundant questions and multiple data entries. To speed the process, only questions pertinent to the specific procedure are asked.

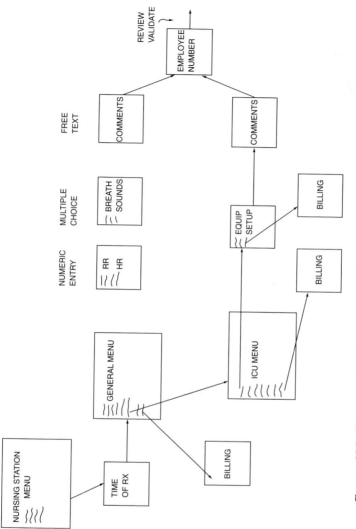

Figure 15.2. Computer charting uses menu selection for entering results of RC procedures.

Follow-up questions are also specific to certain entries; this results in a highly variable pathway that allows flexibility yet decreases the time required for data entry. The only questions to which answers are mandatory are those pertaining to medical-legal or billing issues; most questions can be left unanswered, allowing the therapist to chart only that which is necessary. The therapist is responsible for complete and accurate charting. A procedure attempted but not completed is also documented in order to verify that an attempt was made and to explain why it was not done. All entries require an employee identification number, which serves as an electronic "signature."

Review of Charting

The review of charting is available by using a review option on any hospital terminal. This option is on the same menu for review of laboratory, blood gas, and radiology results. Because results can be reviewed from any terminal, it is not necessary to be on a particular ward to obtain a patient's chart. The report is a text report (Figure 15.3) that resembles written entries (Figure 15.4).

Automatic Routine Reporting

Every morning at 03:00 a program automatically generates three routine reports for the RC department: (1) a complete printout of RC charting on patients discharged the previous day, (2) a 24-hour management report, and (3) an alert report. These three reports are the only hard-copy printouts that are automatically generated routinely by the RC system. This early morning use of the computer is efficient and provides information that can be assessed by supervisors at the beginning of the day.

The 24-hour management report lists the work that has been charted for that period by each therapist (Figure 15.5). The report identifies the patient, work units, and duration of each procedure. It is a record of each therapist's

```
08/18/84.17:00      -02-
02 INTERFACE:CANNULA;  FLOW RATE:  5.0 L/MIN;  8 HRS ON 02;
                                                      THPST#/DUR/ENTRY: 32000/ 10/19:18
08/19/84.15.45      -MEDICATION NEBULIZER- -CPT-
PATIENT INTERFACE: MOUTHPIECE;  POSITION: DANGLE;  MEDICATION: ALUPENT, 10 MG, DILUENT: NORMAL SALINE; PRE BREATH SOUNDS: RHONCHI,
THROUGHOUT INSPIRATION; MECHANICAL PERCUSSION: FOR 20 MIN, LEFT/FLAT, RIGHT/FLAT, BOTH LUNGS; COUGH: WHEN ENCOURAGED,
MODERATE, PRODUCTIVE;  PATIENT CONDITION: ALERT, COOPERATIVE;  POST BREATH SOUNDS: IMPROVED;
                    HEART RATE:  78/   / 80   RESP RATE:  8/   /10          THPST#/DUR/ENTRY: 46547/ 30/16:44

08/18/84.11.40      -PULMONARY EXERCISE- -MEDICATION NEBULIZER- -CPT-
PATIENT INTERFACE: MOUTHPIECE;  POSITION: SITTING; MEDICATION: ALUPENT, 16 MG; DILUENT: NORMAL SALINE; PRE BREATH SOUNDS:
WHEEZING, THROUGHOUT INSPIRATION, BOTH LUNGS; IC: 1000 CC; 10 BREATHS DURING PULMONARY EXERCISE; MECHANICAL PERCUSSION:
FOR 20 MIN, TRENDELENBURG/RIGHT, TRENDELENBURG/LEFT, BLL; COUGH: FREQUENT, STRONG, PRODUCTIVE;  SPUTUM: SPONTANEOUS,
QUANTITY:  3 CC, YELLOW, THICK;  PATIENT CONDITION: ALERT, COOPERATIVE;  POST BREATH SOUNDS: IMPROVED;  COMMENT: RX TOL WELL;
          HEART RATE:  84/84/ 84   RESP RATE:  24/   /24               THPST#/DUR/ENTRY: 46637/ 60/13:17

08/18/84.11:30      -MEDICATION NEBULIZER-
PATIENT INTERFACE: MOUTHPIECE;  POSITION: DANGLE;  MEDICATION: ALUPENT, 15 MG. DILUENT: NORMAL SALINE; PRE BREATH SOUNDS: WHEEZING,
THROUGHOUT ENSPIRATION, BOTH LUNGS; COUGH: SPONTANEOUS, STRONG, NON-PRODUCTIVE;  PATIENT CONDITION: ALERT, COOPERATIVE;
POST BREATH SOUNDS: UNCHANGED;  COMMENT: RX TOL WELL;
                    HEART RATE:  76/   / 80                             THPST#/DUR/ENTRY: 46637/ 20/11:34
```

FIGURE 15.3. An example of computer charting.

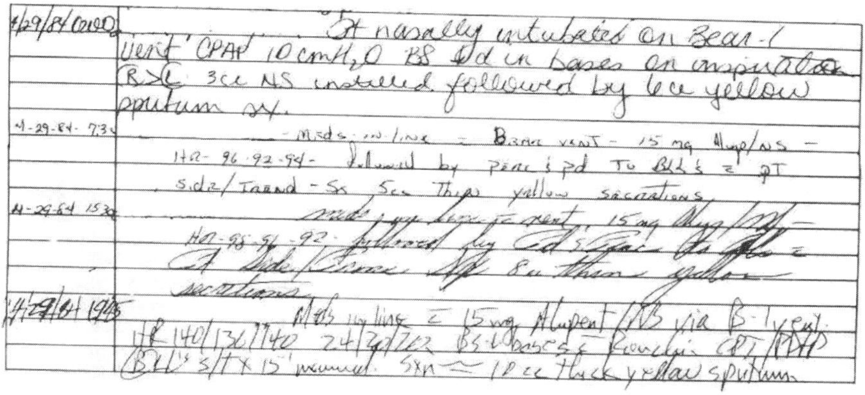

FIGURE 15.4. An example of manual charting.

productivity. Supervisors review the report to confirm that assigned procedures were completed, so that missed procedures or missed charting can be
identified and corrected. The management report also provides a department summary, listing a breakdown of total procedures performed and the
reasons when treatments were not completed (Figure 15.6). The 24-hour

RESPIRATORY CARE THERAPIST REPORT   17 AUG 1984

24 HOUR MANAGEMENT REPORT

THERAPIST # 46482   LINDA STANCHFIELD   AUG 17, 1984   00:00 - AUG 17, 1984   23:59

DATE	TIME	ROOM	PATIENT	TREATMENTS	RVU'S	UNITS	DUR	PC	TA	CT	ENTRY
08-17	12:00	E609	PATIENT, A	MEDICATION NEBULIZER	23.24	1	30		164	4.6	16:00
08-17	12:00	E609	PATIENT, A	NEBULIZER MONITORING	2.39	1	10		128	1.6	14:17
				HPN EQUIPMENT SET UP	20.61						
				ON O2	67						
08-17	08:00	E609	PATIENT, A	MEDICATION NEBULIZER	23.24	1	20		209	3.6	11:46
08-17	07:30	E609	PATIENT, A	NEBULIZER MONITORING	16.73	7	10		402	1.6	14:21
08-17	07:30	E609	PATIENT, A	O2	4.69	7	10		398	1.6	14:15
08-17	07:00	E610	PATIENT, B	NEBULIZER MONITORING	19.12	8	10		419	1.6	14:08
				ON O2	5.36						
08-17	13:45	W623	PATIENT, C	PULMONARY EXERCISE	16.04	1	20		33	3.6	14:33
				MEDICATION NEBULIZER	23.24						
08-17	09:30	W623	PATIENT, C	PULMONARY EXERCISE	16.04	1	20		284	2.6	14:32
				MEDICATION NEBULIZER	23.24						
08-17	13:30	DSCH	PATIENT, D	MEDICATION NEBULIZER ** NOT DONE **	0	0	6		83	1.6	14:67
					0						
08-17	12:00	DSCH	PATIENT, D	MEDICATION NEBULIZER ** NOT DONE ** NOT ON UNIT	0	0	6		191	1.6	14:66
					0						
08-17	07:40	DSCH	PATIENT, D	MEDICATION NEBULIZER	23.24	1	20		226	1.6	11:44
08-17	07:00	E614	PATIENT, E	O2	6.36	8	10		423	1.6	14:12
08-17	12:30	E612	PATIENT, F	IPPB	27.34	1	35		108	4.6	14:49
				CPT	24.61						
08-17	10:30	E612	PATIENT, F	IPPB	27.34	1	35		224	4.6	14:46
				CPT	24.61						
08-17	08:30	E612	PATIENT, F	IPPB	27.34	1	20		366	4.6	14:41
08-17	07:30	W629	PATIENT, G	NEBULIZER MONITORING	19.12	8	10		406	2.6	14:23
				ON O2	5.36						
08-17	07:30	E516	PATIENT, H	NEBULIZER MONITORING	19.12	8	10		408	1.6	14:27
08-17	07:15	W538	PATIENT, I	MEDICATION NEBULIZER	23.24	1	20		416	2.6	14:28

POINTS: 14.0   TOTALS: 419.19   300   0   46.0
                     AVERAGES: 270.2   2.6

FIGURE 15.5. The 24-hour management report provides a record of all procedures
documented by each therapist.

RESPIRATORY CARE DEPARTMENT REPORT   17 AUG 1984
24 HOUR MANAGEMENT REPORT

RUN AT 03 31   18 AUG 84
RUN TIME   24 MIN
                                        TOTALS

AVE POINTS	11.8	POINTS	318.3	ENTRIES	446	AVE ENTRIES 16.6
AVE RVU'S	354.79	RVU'S:	9579.43	ENTRY TIME:	796	AVE TIME: 1.8
RVU / DUR	1.36	THERAPISTS DUR:	7021	AVE TURNAROUND TIME	100.7	
THERAPISTS	.27	CHARGES	8014.76	%RVU'S COMPLETED	97.6	% CHARGES COMPLETED 98.4

TREATMENT TOTALS

TREATMENTS COMPLETED	TOTAL (INITIAL)		RVU'S	CHARGES
PULMONARY EXERCISE:	87	(14)	1538.08	814.70
MEDICATION NEBULIZER:	85	(12)	2008.20	941.80
IPPB:	16	(1)	508.52	204.60
CPT:	53	(3)	1353.53	1066.00
INTERMITTENT NEBULIZER:	1	(1)	35.54	14.00
ASSESSMENT:	38	(17)	935.18	176.70
02:	1600 HRS		1206.00	3600.00
NEBULIZER MONITORING:	313 HRS		748.07	287.96
SUCTION:	2		27.34	13.00
HYPERBARIC CHAMBER:	150 MIN		266.50	201.00
INTERHOSPITAL TRANSPORT:	60 MIN		60.00	66.00
MED NEBULIZER – IN LINE:	30		246.00	120.00
INTRAHOSPITAL TRANSPORT:	240 MIN		240.00	264.00
THORACIC DEMO:	1		61.52	35.00
USN EQUIPMENT SET UP:	3		41.01	30.00
HPN EQUIPMENT SET UP:	7		143.57	70.00
02 EQUIPMENT SET UP:	11		160.37	110.00
STANDBY:	20 MIN		20.00	0
			9579.43	8014.76

REASONS TREATMENTS NOT DONE

NOT ON UNIT:	1	23.24	10.90
ASLEEP:	1	15.04	7.90
RECEIVING OTHER CARE:	1	15.04	7.90
NAUSEATED:	1	24.61	20.00
DUE TO WORKLOAD:	3	45.12	23.70
REFUSED CARE:	2	30.08	15.80
ADVISED NOT TO GIVE:	1	24.61	20.00
UNABLE TO COMPLETE:	1	15.04	7.90
OTHER:	2	38.28	18.80
	13	231.06	132.90

FIGURE 15.6. The 24-hour management report also provides a departmental summary of procedures performed and the reasons when procedures were not completed.

report provides management data extracted directly from patient charting and forms the basis for long-term individual and departmental reports.

The alert report (Figure 15.7) is used to monitor for both management and medical errors. The listing for Patient B is an example of a management alert to an overcharge resulting from double charting. If hourly therapy, such as oxygen, is documented for more than 24 hours in a single day, an alert is printed so that the charting and billing can be corrected. A medical alert might indicate a need for closer patient assessment. If a patient is on continuous oxygen therapy for a prolonged period of time and has never had a blood gas test, an alert is printed. Alert capability will be expanded to include the monitoring of medical necessity protocols [17,18].

Billing

Billing is an automatic byproduct of the computer charting of a completed procedure. An example of a therapist's chart is shown in Figure 15.3. This

```
4N84    PATIENT, A
        *** NO BLOOD GAS IN LAST 4 DAYS ***

4N89    PATIENT, B
        $$$ 2 DAYS AGO > 24 HRS 02 CHARGES / DAY $$$
        *** CONTINUOUS 02 DISCONTINUED OR INTERRUPTED YESTERDAY ***

4N89    PATIENT, C
        *** NO BLOOD GASES ***
```

FIGURE 15.7. Alert report identifies possible errors and oversights in computer charting and patient care.

documentation of oxygen therapy results in a bill for 8 hours of oxygen. The next treatment shows medications-nebulizer therapy and chest physical therapy (CPT), which are billed. Everything is charted for clinical reasons, and the program automatically bills when appropriate. Treatments ordered but not done are reported in the chart but are not billed. Thus, billing accuracy depends on the therapist's charting accuracy. Mistakes can still occur, such as charting the wrong patient or charting the same procedure twice.

These errors can be found easily by therapists as they review the charting or by supervisors as they review the 24-hour management report, and the errors can be easily corrected by supervisory personnel. Billing accuracy is not merely of concern to the hospital and patient, but also determines RC productivity, which is used to justify the staffing requirements of the RC department. The 24-hour management report determines the individual therapist's productivity as well as that of the RC department as a whole.

Evaluation Methods

The RC computer system was evaluated in four ways: (1) therapists' appraisal, (2) observation of work patterns, (3) audit of the quality and content of charting, and (4) productivity analysis. The evaluation was made before computer charting (PRE) and after computer charting (POST).

Therapists' Appraisal

Questionnaires were distributed to the therapists (63 PRE and 55 POST) to be filled out anonymously 2 months before and 2 months after the establishment of computer charting (March 1984). The questionnaires were used to determine therapists' expectations, problems, suggestions, and preferences.

Work Patterns

PRE and POST individual work patterns were compared. After 2 months of computer charting, an inquiry of head nurses and ward clerks was made to obtain feedback on possible interference or congestion at nursing station terminals. The department managers of both Billing and Medical Records were also interviewed.

Quality and Content of Charting

We compared the quality and content of computer charting against manual documentation by auditing medications-nebulizer therapy, one of the most common RC procedures. Guided by departmental standards for this treatment, we checked documentation for inclusion of (1) therapist signature, (2) medications delivered, (3) comments (patient's condition, effects of therapy, and adverse reactions), (4) changes in breath sounds, (5) heart rate before and after treatment, (6) sputum production, (7) cough effort, and (8) patient position. Chart legibility was also evaluated. For this study, patients' charts were selected at random before and after implementation of computer charting. Five hundred manually charted procedures (performed on 22 patients by 49 therapists) were evaluated for content and quality and compared to 500 computer-charted procedures (performed on 29 patients by 51 therapists). The only item that was a mandatory entry on the computer was "therapist signature."

Productivity

PRE and POST statistics of work volume and productivity were compared for all procedures preformed by the RC department during a 6-month period (February through July 1984). Four PRE pay periods (the 8 weeks preceding computer implementation) were compared to the first 8 pay periods (167 weeks) of POST data. Hospital data on productivity and work volume were generated from procedures billed; RC department data were generated from the supervisors' accounts of completed work assignments. These two sources were evaluated with regard to changes in productivity and work volume. An unpaired t test was used for comparison of PRE and POST data.

Results of Evaluation

Therapists' Appraisal

Questionnaires returned by the therapists (49 PRE and 50 POST) indicated job position, location, and shift worked. Virtually all therapists were familiar with the use of computer terminals for reviewing information (96% had used a hospital terminal before), and it took only about 3 days for most of them to feel comfortable doing computer charting. Results of the questionnaires are presented in Table 15.1. Of the 50 therapists who returned the POST survey, 32 (64%) favored computer charting, compared to 10 (20%) who preferred manual charting.

Work Patterns

Computer charting reduced a four-step process (charting the procedure, filling out a charge slip, processing the charge slip and transferring it to billing, and posting the charges into the computer) to only one step—computer charting the procedure. The secretary's job was changed from that of processing charges to auditing billing mistakes and making sure that all printouts of discharged patients were delivered to Medical. Records. Shift supervisors generally had about 30 minutes added to their workload as a result of reviewing the 24-hour management report. Entering billing charges in the Kardex system was eliminated, which, according to estimates from the Industrial Engineering Department, saved each therapist 10 minutes a day. Many therapists felt that charting was faster using the computer.

Other departments affected by the computer were Nursing, Billing, and Medical Records. Access to nursing station terminals was not found to be a major problem. Occasionally problems resulted if a therapist entered several procedures at once and deprived others of access to the terminal. Because computer charting completely bypassed the Billing Department, posting RC charges was eliminated; this saved the Billing Department about 30 minutes per day. The Medical Records Department agreed to put the patient reports onto the patient's chart; this added about 30 minutes of work per day in this department. The net result of RC computer charting on other departments was one of redistribution of effort, with no major overall change.

Quality and Content of Charting

Computer charting was found to be more complete than manual charting in every case except the documentation of medication, which remained the same (Figure 15.8). Both the manual and computer charts had four instances (0.8%) in which the medication was not specified. Legibility and signature were both 100% on the computer. Figures 15.3 and 15.4 illustrate the difference in legibility between computer and manual charting. It was noted that not only was there an improvement in meeting the department's requirements for charting, but often the requirements were exceeded. Computer charting was found to be more informative, concise, and compact.

TABLE 15.1. Results of survey completed anonymously by therapists two months before and two months after computer charting was established.

1. Approximately how many minutes do you spend in charting a treatment?

	<2 min	2–5 min	6–10 min	>10 min	No response
PRE	2 (4%)	27 (55%)	19 (39%)	1 (2%)	
POST	11 (22%)	30 (60%)	7 (14%)	1 (2%)	1 (2%)

2. (POST) How does computer charting time compare to charting manually?

Faster	About the same	Longer	No response
18 (36%)	21 (42%)	9 (18%)	2 (4%)

3. (POST) To do the same amount of work for your job, how much time has the computer saved or added?

	# Responses	Total minutes
Min/shift the computer has saved	16	414
Min/shift the computer has added	9	345

4. How many times during a shift do you use a hospital terminal?

	<2 min	2–5 min	6–10 min	>10 min	No response
PRE	3 (6%)	10 (20%)	19 (39%)	14 (29%)	3 (6%)
POST	2 (4%)	6 (12%)	13 (26%)	28 (56%)	1 (2%)

5. (POST) For the following aspects, how do you feel computer charting compares to manual charting?

	Much better	Better	About the same	Worse	Much worse	No response
Quality of time spent:	7 (14%)	21 (42%)	16 (32%)	2 (4%)	2 (4%)	2 (4%)
Ease of entering:	12 (24%)	19 (38%)	12 (24%)	5 (10%)		2 (4%)
Ease of review:	8 (16%)	17 (34%)	8 (16%)	14 (28%)	1 (2%)	2 (4%)
Accuracy:	12 (24%)	14 (28%)	13 (26%)	8 (16%)	1 (2%)	2 (4%)
Productivity:	13 (26%)	24 (48%)	9 (18%)	2 (4%)		2 (4%)

6. How often do you have trouble getting access to a terminal on the ward?

	Very rarely	Occasionally	Often	Almost always	No response
PRE	17 (35%)	27 (55%)	2 (4%)		3 (6%)
POST	23 (46%)	22 (44%)	2 (4%)	1 (2%)	2 (4%)

7. (PRE) How often do you have trouble getting access to a patient's chart?

Very rarely	Occasionally	Often	Almost always
9 (19%)	31 (63%)	7 (14%)	2 (4%)

8. Do you feel computer charting will make your job any easier?

	Yes	No	No response
PRE	17 (35%)	20 (41%)	12 (24%)
POST	29 (58%)	9 (18%)	12 (24%)

9. (POST) Which do you prefer, computer charting or manual charting?

Computer charting	Manual charting	No response
32 (64%)	10 (20%)	8 (16%)

10. (POST) What difference, if any, do you feel computer charting has made in the quality of patient care?

Better	No change	Worse	No response
16 (32%)	30 (60%)	2 (4%)	2 (4%)

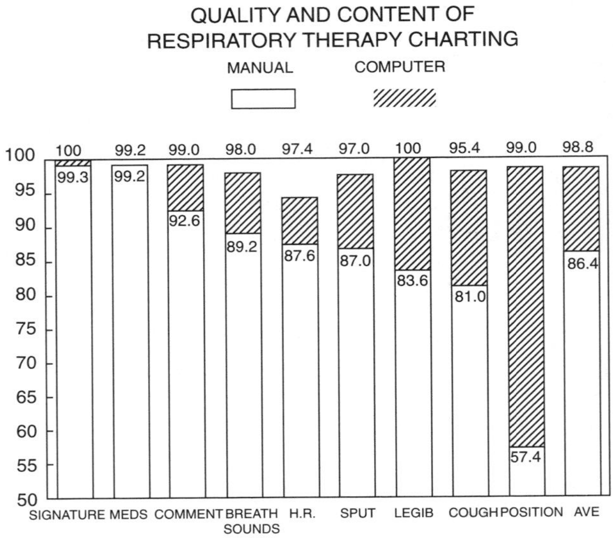

QUALITY AND CONTENT OF
RESPIRATORY THERAPY CHARTING

MANUAL   COMPUTER

FIGURE 15.8. Percentages of acceptable charting from an audit of 500 procedures of manual charting and 500 procedures of computer charting. Numbers atop bars are percentages of acceptable computer charts; numbers in bars are percentages of acceptable manual charts.

Productivity

Productivity data are presented in Table 15.2. Significant (p ≤ 0.03) increases after computer charting was instituted are shown for both productivity and work volume. Hospital data calculated from billed procedures showed that productivity increased 18.2%; RC records showed that productivity (average workload completed per therapist) increased an average of 13.7%. Hospital data showed that work volume increased 20.9%, while RC department records showed that it increased 16.4%. The number of employees who worked during both periods was not significantly different (51.23 PRE vs. 52.40 POST).

Discussion

Implementation of the computer-charting system was trouble free, and therapists learned the system quickly. Therapists' response was very positive. The preference for using the system was not only very high, but higher than anticipated. Whereas only 35% (17/49) of those who returned the PRE questionnaire felt computer charting would make their job easier, 64% (32/50) of those who returned the POST questionnaire expressed a preference for computer charting. About one third of the responding therapists reported that computer charting was faster (Table 15.1, items 2 and 3); however, 56% of therapists returning the POST survey felt that their charting time was better spent and 74% felt productivity was better (Table 15.1, item 5), indicating that the computer may have been helpful in ways other than speed of charting.

The computerized clinical records were more descriptive, legible, and complete than were the manual reports (Figure 15.8). Overall, computer charting was found to be 12.4% more complete than manual charting. The only item in the study that did not show a significant improvement was medication documentation, which has now been made a mandatory entry on the computer. This will ensure 100% compliance and is justified because the delivery of medication is the primary objective of medications-nebulizer therapy.

Because computer charting can be programmed so that a therapist must reply to a question in order to proceed through the entry process, an

TABLE 15.2. Productivity and work-unit data for the 8 weeks preceding and the 16 weeks following the implementation of computer charting.

Pay period (2 weeks)		Hospital data (procedures billed)		RC department data (supervisors' accounts)	
PRE	FTE	Productivity	Work Units	Productivity	Work Units
1	49.96	93	221,869	87	206,834
2	50.40	95	229,005	88	211,680
3	49.88	91	217,955	91	215,482
4	54.68	86	226,560	98	255,902
Average	51.23	91.3	223,847	91.0	222,475
POST					
5	48.82	118	275,346	92	213,832
6	51.05	109	267,750	98	237,383
7	54.44	103	268,834	103	267,845
8	50.62	107	260,645	107	258,162
9	50.55	112	271,524	112	271,524
10	50.91	103	250,040	106	258,114
11	54.88	105	277,183	104	273,302
12	57.92	106	294,009	106	291,916
Average	52.40	107.9	270,666	103.5	259,010
P	NS	0.0002	0.00004	0.0054	0.0300
% Increase	2.3	18.2	20.9	13.7	16.4

FTE = full-time equivalent therapists paid during pay period.
Productivity = the % of work completed compared to the amount of work expected to be completed for the number of FTEs.
Work units = the number of minutes spent doing productive work (determined by hospital Industrial Engineering). One work unit = one productive minute of work.
P = P value from unpaired t test of PRE and POST results.
NS = not significant.

argument can be made that the answering of all questions should be mandatory, assuring 100% compliance. Although mandatory entry seems to be the ideal solution, it has the disadvantage of not allowing the therapist to exercise discretion over what is charted. Mandatory entry may force the reporting of irrelevant or incorrect information. Certainly information is better left unreported than reported incorrectly. The ultimate responsibility for complete charting is the therapist's. Computer documentation significantly improved charting without forcing the outcome.

Every procedure allows the entry of comments in a free-text format; therefore, a procedure can be documented entirely on comments and still be complete. However, free-text entries are not so useful as structured data (selections that are stored in the computer in coded format). As an example, if patients receiving a certain bronchodilator were to be monitored for changes in breath sounds, the computer could be programmed easily to find the data if the information was structured. If the information was free text, accurate retrieval and monitoring would not be possible. Currently, structured data accounts for more than 95% of RC charting.

An argument can be made that too much information is charted, resulting in "information overload," whereby irrelevant information reduces the impact of relevant information on decision making [8,9–22]. Just what information is the most useful is a question that will require further study.

Evaluation of productivity was hampered by the fact that all accounting methods and charges had been changed 8 weeks prior to computer implementation. Unfortunately, this limited the amount of useful PRE data to only four pay periods.

Because the RC department maintains a nearly constant work force, fluctuations in work volume affect the productivity of the department. The results in Table 15.2 show that there were increases in productivity, according to both hospital and departmental calculation, after computer implementation (18.2% and 13.7%, respectively). Work volume also increased (20.9% and 16.4%, respectively), while the number of therapists did not increase significantly.

There were three possible reasons for the apparent improvement in productivity: (1) The work volume increased, requiring the therapists to work more efficiently. (2) The computer assured that work charted was charged for, and this accuracy increased the work volume. This explanation assumes that in the PRE period, some work was done but not accounted for. We were unable from the data available to make a quantitative assessment of this factor. Nevertheless, the computer assures concordance of clinical and financial record keeping and minimizes lost charges. (3) Computer charting helped the therapists do their job more efficiently and thus allowed them to handle heavier workloads. The manual Kardex system was replaced, saving 10 minutes per therapist per shift. The therapist survey showed that 74% of the therapists thought computer charting allowed them to be

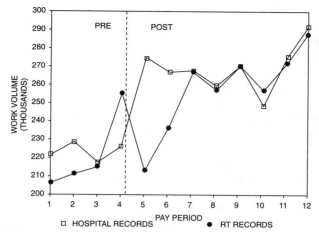

Figure 15.9. Comparison of work volume from hospital records and work volume from departmental records. Computer charting started at point marked by dotted line (March 1984).

more productive, but they also indicated that the timesavings was not very substantial.

We conclude that all three factors mentioned above, or a combination of them, could have been responsible for the increase in productivity, although it remains unclear to what extent each factor may have been responsible. One fact was clear: during the period when therapists were busier and 18% more productive, they were using the computer. Computer charting did not decrease productivity.

Figure 15.9 shows that after Pay Period 6, about 6 weeks after implementation of computer charting, procedures billed and procedures assigned became highly correlated ($r = 0.96$ for Pay Periods 7 though 12). These results confirmed that computer charting provided a high degree of confidence that every item billed was documented as being performed. The poor correlation for Pay Periods 5 and 6 can be partially explained. Computer charting processes billing information immediately, whereas manual charting processes billing at least a day later. Pay Period 5, the first after conversion to computer charting, reflected the billing of all procedures during that pay period, plus the carryover billing of some procedures completed in the previous pay period hence, hospital billing records and RC records differed in the work volume reported. Also, the 24-hour management report was not implemented until Pay Period 6, so errors may have gone unnoticed before that date.

Information that is stored in the computer is used in ways that are impractical with manual methods. The alert program provides automatic quality assurance by routinely searching all current patients' records for possible needs for corrective. The facet of computerized charting with the greatest potential for development is in the expansion of the automatic monitoring of patient care. Information could be incorporated into assessment protocols that automatically monitor the efficacy of treatments. Patients' assessments could be reviewed so that care could be optimized. The medical staff could be provided computer-generated reminders for use in treatment assessment [22], The information charted could also be useful for other departments. For example, a program monitoring infectious disease could take into consideration a change in breath sounds in a patient suspected of having a pulmonary infection. RC charting is now incorporated into computerized ICU-rounds reports and patient-summary reports. These reports extract the most recent and useful data and display them in a concise format for optimal use [6,9,21].

The RC computer system is efficient because it has streamlined the process of documentation while extracting the most "useful" information. Without having to provide costly cumulative paper reports, the RC system provides better access for entry and review. Overall, computer charting is preferred by therapists over manual charting, making their job easier while improving the quality of information charted. Computer charting has added a high degree of confidence that there will be good correlation of clinical, administrative, and financial records. The computerization of charting RC procedures demonstrates the advantages of using clinical information for the benefit of the therapist, the department, the hospital, and the patient.

References

[1] R.A. Jydstrup and M.J. Gross, Cost of information handling in hospitals, Health Serv Res 1 (1966) 253–271.

[2] K. Jacobwitzk, L. Strodtman, T. Lomas, and T. Turax, Microcomputer-based data management system for nursing assessment of the diabetic patient, in: *Proceedings of the 5th Annual Symposium on Computers in Medical Care* (1981), pp. 755–759.

[3] M.F. Collen, L.S. Davis, E.E. Van Brunt, and J.F. Terdiman, Functional goals and problems in large-scale patient record management and automated screening, Fed Proc 33 (1974) 2376–2379.

[4] J.D. Bronzino, *Computer Applications for Patient Care* (Addison-Wesley, Menlo Park CA, 1983).

[5] S.L. Mertz, S.R. Ash, and J. Farrell, The CNS in the ICU: A bedside notation system for nurses, in: *Proceedings of the 6th Annual Symposium on Computers in Medical Care* (1982), pp. 577–581.

[6] G.O. Barnett, The application of computer-based medical-record systems in ambulatory practice, New England Journal of Medicine 310 (1984) 1643–1650.

[7] T.A. Pryor, R.M. Gardner, P.D. Clayton, and H.R. Warner, The HELP system, Journal Medical Systemic 7 (1983) 87–102.

[8] B.R. Warner, *Computer Assisted Medical Decision Making* (Academic Press, New York, 1979).

[9] R.M. Gardner, B.J. West, T.A. Pryor, et al., Computer-based ICU data acquisition as an aid to clinical decision making, Crit Care Med 10 (1982) 823–830.

[10] O. Serlin, Fault tolerant systems in commercial applications, Computer 17 (1984) 19–30.

[11] G. Jeromin, Computerization: Are we ready? Respiratory Care 27 (1982) 797–798.

[12] L.E. Garrett, W.W. Stead, W.E. Hammond, C.J. McDonald, and M. Buecher, A method of handling subjective and physical data; experience with two systems, in: *Proceedings of the 6th Annual Symposium on Computers in Medical Care* (1982), pp. 232–235.

[13] R.D. Zielstorff, J.L. Roglieri, K. Marble, et al., Experience with a computer-based medical record for nurse practitioners in ambulatory care, Comput Biomed Res 10 (1977) 61–73.

[14] M.F. Collen, Patient data acquisition, Med Instrum 12 (1978) 222–225.

[15] Joint Commission on Accreditation of Hospitals, Accreditation manual for hospitals, 1982 edition (American Hospital Association, Chicago).

[16] D.J. Mishelevich, A.L. Robinson, C. Rogers, M.E. DuPriest, and E.I. Mize, Respiratory therapy as a component of an integrated hospital information system: The Parkland On-line Information System (POIS), Respiratory Care 27 (1982) 846–854.

[17] Blue Cross and Blue Shield Association, Medical necessity guidelines: Respiratory care (inpatient) (Chicago, September 1982).

[18] ACCP-NHLBI, National conference on oxygen therapy, Chest 86 (1984) 234–247.

[19] M.R. Grier, The need for data in making nursing decisions, in: H.H. Werley and M.R. Grier, editors, *Nursing Information Systems* (Springer, New York, 1981), pp. 15–31.

[20] W.R. Ayers, The potentials and limitations of computers in medical practice: Update—Computers in Medicine 1 (1983) 35–39.

[21] K.E. Bradshaw, R.M. Gardner, T.P. Clemmer, J.F. Orme, F. Thomas, and B.J. West, Physician decision-making: Evaluation of data used in a computerized ICU, Int J Clin Monitor and Comput 1 (1984) 81–41.

[22] C.J. McDonald, Protocol-based computer reminders, the quality of care and the non-perfectibility of man, New England Journal of Medicine 295 (1976) 1351–1355.

[23] G.O. Barnett, R. Winickoff, J.L. Dorsey, M.M. Morgan, and R.S. Lurie, Quality assurance through automated monitoring and concurrent feedback using a computer-based medical information system, Medical Care 16 (1978) 962–970.

16
Research and Evaluation: Future Directions

JAMES G. ANDERSON and CAROLYN E. AYDIN

During the 1970s, efforts to develop and introduce computers into health-care settings focused primarily on components of inpatient and outpatient systems. Inpatient systems included hospital information systems, clinical laboratory systems, and support systems for radiology and emergency medicine. There was also a parallel development of systems to support outpatient care such as ambulatory medical records, physician office systems, and telecommunications for medical consultation [1–3].

Advances in computer technology and artificial intelligence during the 1980s led to the development of expert systems and other clinical decision support systems [4]. In addition, the use of inpatient and outpatient systems became widespread as more healthcare organizations began to adopt applications such as order entry and support systems for ancillary departments [5]. In the 1990s, the need for cost-effective delivery of health services led to integrated databases and computer-based systems supporting outcomes research, identification of physician practice patterns, utilization review, and total quality management programs [6,7]. Concerns about patient safety also accelerated planning and implementation of computerized physician order entry (CPOE) and more comprehensive electronic health records [8].

Since the publication of the first edition of this book in 1994, important advances have also been made in the *evaluation* of healthcare information systems. In 1994 we noted the lack of comprehensive and unifying models to aid in understanding the success and failures of new systems. Such models would take into account the relative importance of the environment, both external and internal, the organization and its policies, characteristics of potential users of the system, and the attributes of the technology itself. Much work has been done in this area in the last decade. In the introduction to Chapter 1 of the present volume, we directed the reader to new theoretical frameworks and related perspectives that complement and extend the "social interaction" perspective described in that chapter. On the methodological front, the chapters in this book describe recent developments in system evaluation that give informaticians valuable new tools for conducting system evaluations. The increased recognition of the importance of organizational issues in the evaluation of new technologies has also resulted in the creation of active working groups in both the International Medical Informatics Association (IMIA) in 1993 and the American Medical Informatics Association (AMIA) in 1996.

Despite these advances, however, expensive system failures persist. Many groups and institutions implementing new systems remain unaware of the importance of system evaluation or reluctant to allocate the resources required for an adequate evaluation. In addition, acceptance by primary care physicians of new electronic medical records, electronic prescribing systems, and point-of-care decision support systems has been limited. A recent survey of primary care physicians in the United States [9] found that only 20% to 25% of primary care physicians reported using these information technology applications in their practice. In contrast, studies have shown that 52% of primary care physicians in New Zealand and 59% in the UK were using electronic medical records, while 44% of physicians in Australia, 52% in New Zealand, and 87% in the UK were using electronic prescribing [10].

As this book goes to press, the President's Information Technology Advisory Committee's Draft Report calls for accelerated adoption of information technology in the healthcare sector [11]. They recommend the adoption of (1) electronic health records to maximize the information available to healthcare providers at the point of care; (2) computer-assisted decision support to increase compliance with evidence-based medicine; (3) electronic order entry in both outpatient and inpatient practice settings; and (4) interoperable electronic information interchange. In order to facilitate the implementation of these recommendations, President Bush has proposed $100 million to be spent on promoting health information technology.

In light of past experience, however, the implementation of many of these newer systems, as well as new adoptions of more established systems, will result in unforeseen costs and organizational consequences, or even fail, because developers and administrators neglect their social impacts [12–16]. The methods and applications included in this book provide an overview of current knowledge and emphasize the importance of a multimethod approach to system evaluation based on an understanding of the complex social and behavioral processes occurring within healthcare organizations. The dissemination of this knowledge to those involved in system design and implementation, however, remains a challenge.

The purpose of this book has been to provide a practical guide for determining (1) appropriate evaluation questions based on specific underlying models of change, and (2) the most effective methods available to evaluate anticipated impacts and answer the questions posed. Too many informaticians remain unaware or unconvinced of the importance of system evaluation, or are unable to make the case for the required funds to the organization's administration. Too often evaluation experts continue to "preach to the choir," without reaching out to convince decision makers of the importance of an adequate evaluation. The challenge for researchers in system evaluation today is to identify appropriate venues and strategies that will ensure that healthcare administrators are both (1) aware of the importance of system evaluation to a successful implementation, and (2) willing to make the necessary organizational commitment to conducting and using appropriate evaluation methods throughout the implementation process.

References

[1] J.G. Anderson, Clinical information systems, in: A. Kent, editor, *Encyclopedia of Library and Information Science*, Vol. 69, Supplement 32 (Marcel Dekker, New York, 2000), pp. 33–53.

[2] J.G. Anderson, Computer-based ambulatory information systems: Recent developments, Journal of Ambulatory Care Management 23(2) (2000) 53–63.

[3] National Center for Health Services Research, Computer applications in health care, DHHS Publication No. (PHS)80-3251 (1980).

[4] W.J. Clancey and T. Shortliffe, editors, *Readings in Medical Artificial Intelligence: The First Decade* (Addison-Wesley, Reading, MA, 1984).

[5] C.L. Packer, Historical changes in hospital computer use, Hospitals 59 (1985) 115–118.

[6] S.J. Jay and J.G. Anderson, Computers in medicine: Dreams and realities, Hospital Physician 25 (1989) 3–13.

[7] A.W. DeTore, Medical informatics: An introduction to computer technology in medicine, American Journal of Medicine 85 (1988) 399–403.

[8] L.T. Kohn, J.M. Corrigan, and M.S. Donaldson, editors, *To Err Is Human: Building a Safer Health System* (National Academy Press, Washington, DC, 2000).

[9] J.G. Anderson and E.A. Balas, Computerization of primary care in the United States (unpublished manuscript, 2004).

[10] U.S. trails other English-speaking countries in use of electronic medical records and electronic prescribing, HarrisInteractive Health Care News 1(28) (2001).

[11] President's Information Technology Advisory Committee, Health care delivery and information technology (HIT) subcommittee: Draft recommendations. Available: www.nitrd.gov.pitac.

[12] J.G. Anderson and S.J. Jay, editors, *Use and Impact of Computers in Clinical Medicine* (Springer-Verlag, New York, 1987).

[13] A.F. Dowling, Do hospital staff interfere with computer system implementation? Health Care Management Review 5 (1980) 23–32.

[14] E. Gardner, Information systems: Computers full capabilities often go untapped, Modern Healthcare May 28 (1990) 38–40.

[15] K. Lyytinen, Expectation failure concept and systems analysts' view of information systems failure: Results of an exploratory study, Information and Management 14 (1988) 45–56.

[16] K. Lyytinen and R. Hirschheim, Information systems failures: A survey and classification of the empirical literature, Oxford Surveys in Information Technology 4 (1987) 257–309.

Index

Health Informatics Series
(formerly Computers in Health Care)

(continued from page ii)

Consumer Informatics
Applications and Strategies in Cyber Health Care
R. Nelson and M.J. Ball

Public Health Informatics and Information Systems
P.W. O'Carroll, W.A. Yasnoff, M.E. Ward, L.H. Ripp,
and E.L. Martin

Advancing Federal Sector Health Care
A Model for Technology Transfer
P. Ramsaroop, M.J. Ball, D. Beaulieu, and J.V. Douglas

Medical Informatics
Computer Applications in Health Care and Biomedicine, Second Edition
E.H. Shortliffe and L.E. Perreault

Filmless Radiology
E.L. Siegel and R.M. Kolodner

Cancer Informatics
Essential Technologies for Clinical Trials
J.S. Silva, M.J. Ball, C.G. Chute, J.V. Douglas, C.P. Langlotz, J.C. Niland,
and W.L. Scherlis

Clinical Information Systems
A Component-Based Approach
R. Van de Velde and P. Degoulet

Knowledge Coupling
New Premises and New Tools for Medical Care and Education
L.L. Weed

Healthcare Information Management Systems
Cases, Strategies, and Solutions, Third Edition
M.J. Ball, C.A. Weaver, and J.M. Kiel

Organizational Aspects of Health Informatics, Second Edition
Managing Technological Change
N.M. Lorenzi and R.T. Riley

Information Technology Solutions for Healthcare
K. Zieliński, M. Duplaga, and D. Ingram